THE NEUROLOGY OF GASTROINTESTINAL DISEASE

Volume 3 in the Series

Major Problems in Neurology

JOHN N. WALTON, TD, MD, DSc, FRCP

Consulting Editor

OTHER MONOGRAPHS IN THE SERIES

PUBLISHED

Barnett, Foster and Hudgson: **Syringomyelia,** *1973*

Dubowitz and Brooke: **Muscle Biopsy: A Modern Approach,** *1973*

FORTHCOMING

Hutchinson and Acheson: **The Natural History of Cerebral Vascular Disease**

Currie: **Immunological Aspects of Neurology**

Cartlidge and Shaw: **Medical Aspects of Head Injury**

Lewis and Pallis: **The Neurology of Renal Disease**

The Neurology of Gastrointestinal Disease

CHRISTOPHER A. PALLIS, MA, DM, FRCP

Reader in Neurology, Royal Postgraduate Medical School, Consultant Neurologist, Hammersmith Hospital, London.

PAUL D. LEWIS, BSc, MD, MRCP

Lecturer in Pathology (Neuropathology), Royal Postgraduate Medical School, Consultant Pathologist and Neurologist, Hammersmith Hospital, London.

1974

W. B. Saunders Company Ltd

London · Philadelphia · Toronto

W. B. Saunders Company Ltd: 12 Dyott Street
London WC1A 1DB

West Washington Square
Philadelphia, Pa. 19105

833 Oxford Street
Toronto, Ontario M8Z 5T9

The Neurology of Gastrointestinal Disease ISBN 0-7216-7046-6

 Library of Congress Catalog Card Number 73-89191.

Printed by The Whitefriars Press Ltd, London and Tonbridge

Print Number: 9 8 7 6 5 4 3 2 1

Foreword

At first sight the reader may be surprised to find a volume on 'The Neurology of Gastrointestinal Disease' appearing in a series devoted to Major Problems in Neurology. But all physicians engaged in neurological practice have been alerted increasingly in recent years to the importance of the neurological complications of internal medical disorders, complications which seem to be increasing in prominence as well as in complexity. This fact underlines the well-established principle that all neurologists should have a thorough grounding in internal medicine and that general physicians or internists must be aware of those manifestations of disordered nervous function which may well arise in their patients. To such specialist physicians and to gastroenterologists this volume will have a major attraction, as it will to all who accept and acknowledge the complex interrelationships of disease processes involving several bodily systems.

As series editor, therefore, I make no apology for inviting Drs Pallis and Lewis to write this book, the first of several on the neurological manifestations of general medical disease which will be interwoven eventually into this series. The recognition of such syndromes and symptom-complexes can indeed be regarded as a major problem in neurology, not only in the diagnostic sense but also in view of the light which such manifestations cast upon the aetiology and pathogenesis of diseases which are essentially confined to the nervous system on the one hand and the gastrointestinal tract on the other.

The partnership of Dr Christopher Pallis, a clinical neurologist, and Dr Paul Lewis, a neuropathologist, is especially appropriate for the task in hand as they work in a major postgraduate medical centre which houses a great many specialist medical departments and an outstanding department of gastroenterology, a hospital where multidisciplinary conferences are regularly held and where cross-consultations between specialties are very frequent. I believe that their coverage of the subject is comprehensive yet succinct, clearly-written and logically arranged. The fruits of their combined clinical and investigative experience are embodied in this important commentary, which will be an invaluable source of reference and an indispensable vade mecum for the physician in neurology or gastroenterology who is called into consultation to advise upon the management of a patient with a gastroenterological disorder who develops neurological symptoms or vice versa. I believe that this exciting monograph will be warmly welcomed.

Newcastle upon Tyne, 1973 John N. Walton

Preface

Specialisation is a necessary evil: it narrows our outlook but concentrates our energy. In the pre-specialist era Jan van Heurne, a Leyden physician who was one of the founders of our tradition of bedside teaching, wrote a book on *Diseases of the Head* (van Heurne, 1594). Most of the book is neurological. The author deals at length with headache, fits, strokes, paralysis, tremor, dementia, rabies and insanity, not to mention sneezing, incubi and succubi. However, his approach—inevitably, at the time—is regional rather than systematic, and the need to be comprehensive leads him to include chapters on alopecia, acne, lice and greying of the hair. His treatise is thus something of a rag-bag. We fear that our monograph, overlapping as it does two well-defined areas, but belonging strictly to neither, may possibly suffer from the same defect. Writing as neurologists—rather than gastroenterologists—we will be reviewing information on a mass of unrelated diseases which have as sole common denominator the fact that they may have neurological complications. At the same time, we hope that our clearing of the ground may be of help to others working in our specialty.

Seeing the title of this book, a prospective reader might think only of intestinal malabsorption. Malabsorption is certainly central to our concern but we can assure those prepared to travel with us that our study will take us wider afield, into subjects such as the prevailing nutritional habits in certain parts of the world, the bacteriology of the small bowel, South American trypanosomiasis, the classification of amyloidosis, the relation between the brain and the pancreas, and a number of other esoteric areas. We have even ventured into controversial fields such as the definition of sprue and of coeliac disease which others, with more experience, would doubtless have side-stepped.

In the course of writing we have had to learn—after first unlearning—a good deal of gastroenterology. It has been exciting for us to discover what has been happening in that subject since we began our specialist training as neurologists a decade or two ago, and became effectively cut off from developments in other compartments of medicine. It is a sad commentary on the structure of modern medicine that a need is now widely felt to synthesise areas of knowledge not so long ago enthusiastically being separated. But this is also a commentary on present-day science—and at a deeper level on present-day society—where groups of people are having increasing difficulty not only in conveying detailed information to one another but even in understanding the basic concepts to which others are committed.

Our monograph does not aspire to the status of a textbook of gastroenterology and we have felt it to be beyond our brief to discuss the primary treatment of the various disorders referred to. Our aim is to cover a field of neurology which may be unfamiliar to some working in specialised institutes or departments of nervous diseases. We hope to teach some gastroenterology to neurologists, and perhaps even a little neurology to gastroenterologists. We are in the awkward position of knowing that at any given moment half of our readers will be inadequately equipped critically to assess what we say, but that *everything* in these pages will at some time come under the expert scrutiny of someone or another. One of the hazards of straying into no man's land is, of course, the hazard of being sniped at from both sides. Another danger is that, as we venture into their territory, we may appear to gastroenterologists to be carrying coals to Newcastle. Writing primarily for neurologists this is, in a sense, unavoidable. We do not share the pessimism of La Bruyère observing (in 1688) that we all come too late to say anything which has not been said already. It is a question of how we convey our message, why we convey it, and to whom it is conveyed. We have sought to present some of the older observations in a new light, and not just to move old bones from one graveyard to another.

This is probably the first detailed survey of a new medical territory, and it is impossible for us to say if we have charted it adequately. We suspect that our coverage will seem increasingly patchy as advances are made and the scope of 'gastroenterological neurology' becomes better defined. One of our problems has been the assessment of old, and often incomplete, observations (both clinical and pathological) which have been generally accepted, widely quoted in subsequent writings and integrated into a whole structure of neuromythology. We hope to convince the reader who disagrees with our interpretations of these early reports that the original data at least allowed room for doubt: in our assessments we have frequently found ourselves buffeted between the Scylla of nihilism and the Charybdis of credulity, and if we have erred, it has in some cases been towards charity, in others towards cynicism. We have nevertheless felt the need critically to look at many of these old reports. In 1974 we should be able to take a dispassionate and historical view of topics which have been in a state of continuous development or were, in the past, a source of controversy.

Many have helped us in our work and we would like here to acknowledge the debt we owe them. It is immense. Without their help it is doubtful whether this volume would have seen the light of day. Working in an institution like the Royal Postgraduate Medical School creates particular problems, however. One such is that helpful experts want to share with you, to the full, the subtleties and intricacies of their expertise. In the contemporary era, when the life of any new fact is only a few years, such enthusiasm may be a mixed blessing. It may even result in a certain loss of focus. As we are not aiming primarily at a gastroenterological readership, we have deliberately sought to remain this side of the gastroenterological growing points. Our first and foremost thanks are nevertheless due to our colleagues in the Gastroenterology Department at Hammersmith Hospital, whose stimulating discussions (and even disagreements on some basic issues) convinced us that their discipline was in full and vigorous evolution. We wish in particular to thank Dr G. Neale, who read the whole text and made many useful suggestions.

Our thanks are also due to Dr A. V. Hoffbrand for helpful comments concerning the absorption and malabsorption of folic acid and vitamin B_{12}, to Professor M. D. Milne for critically reviewing the chapter on Hartnup disease, to Professor G. M. Taori, of the Christian Medical College, Vellore, for sharing with us, before they were published, his experiences of the neurological complications of tropical sprue, to Professor W. T. Smith, for drawing our attention to relevant data concerning nutritional B_{12} deficiency myelopathy in monkeys, to Dr D. Gompertz for helping us formulate some biochemical propositions in a language even remotely comprehensible to biochemists, to Professor W. B. Matthews of Oxford, for his comments about a much-reported patient of his, with diverticulosis and myelopathy (see p. 74), 'published by everyone who had had anything to do with her' except himself, and to Sir Charles Symonds for moral support in the argument concerning the relative significance of peripheral neuropathy and of disease of the posterior columns in producing the neurological semeiology of vitamin B_{12} deficiency.

Our thanks are finally due to the Library staff at the Royal Postgraduate Medical School for cheerful and unremitting help in unearthing old references, to J. P. and Mrs Catherine Chmaj for numerous typings of the manuscript, and to all those who by their encouragement kept us at it, when at times we felt the task to be beyond our competence or to require more energy than our conjoined reserves could possibly muster.

References

Heurne, J. van (1594). *De morbis qui in singulis partibus humani capitis insidere consueverunt*. Leyden: Raphelengius.

La Bruyère, J. de (1688). *Les Charactères: Des Ouvrages de l'Esprit*. Paris: Michallet.

Contents

CHAPTER ONE

Malabsorption and the Nervous System

The nervous system, like any other part of the body, is critically dependent on an adequate intake of nutrients, properly absorbed and delivered in appropriate form to the sites at which they will be used. Many books, reviews and articles describe the neurological sequelae, in various animals, of *experimental* deprivation of protein, carbohydrate, fat, minerals and vitamins. An equally impressive literature documents the neurological effects on man of '*naturally*' occurring dietary deficiency (Denny-Brown, 1947; Spillane, 1947; Follis, 1948; Cruickshank, 1952; Brozek and Grande, 1960). There are no studies, however, specifically relating nutritional disorders of the human nervous system to disordered function of the alimentary tract. This is one of the lacunae we are seeking to fill.

Most nutritional disorders of the nervous system are not primarily due to gastrointestinal disease. They are the result of reduced dietary intake, and will only be referred to briefly, as they are mainly beyond the scope of this monograph. An important exception is the vitamin B_{12} deficiency state, which is far more often due to malabsorption than to reduced ingestion (see Chapter 5).

Several factors are usually involved in producing the clinical manifestations of a nutritional deficiency. To long-standing dietary deficits may be added the effects of a more abruptly reduced intake. Painful conditions of the mouth or throat may cause dysphagia. Anorexia, nausea and vomiting may further reduce ingestion. These latter symptoms may themselves, however, be the effect—as well as the cause—of a vitamin-deficient diet. They may result, for instance, from a diet containing insufficient thiamine. Similar considerations apply to nicotinic acid deficiency, where glossitis and stomatitis may be both cause and effect of reduced intake, and may further reduce ingestion. Diarrhoea, whether due to a primary gastrointestinal disorder or to the effects of vitamin deficiency (as in pellagra) may impair absorption of what little is ingested. Other dietary deficiencies, for instance of protein, may certainly cause changes in intestinal villous structure and may possibly cause malabsorption (Stanfield, Hutt and Tunnicliffe, 1965; Tandon et al, 1968; Mayoral et al, 1967; Viteri et al, 1973). Increased metabolic demands due to fever, thyrotoxicosis, surgery or pregnancy may also contribute to creating a nutritional deficiency.

It is useful to distinguish between disorders of digestion and disorders of absorption, particularly in relation to the metabolism of protein, fat and carbohydrate. Digestive disorders are a common cause of malabsorption (they are a more frequent cause of steatorrhoea, for instance, than disease of the intestinal mucosa). The distinction is perhaps less relevant in relation to those substances of greatest neurological import, namely the vitamins. Vitamin deficiencies, when not due to reduced intake, are far more likely to be due to malabsorption than to faulty digestion. Problems of storage, in the liver or elsewhere, are particularly relevant in relation to the vitamins. Thiamine is hardly stored at all and the vomiting of pyloric stenosis may result in Wernicke's encephalopathy in a matter of weeks. There are, on the other hand, vast stores of vitamin B_{12} in the liver. This explains why it may take years to produce subacute combined degeneration of the spinal cord following partial gastrectomy.

In discussing how malabsorption affects the nervous system, we will try to focus attention on two narrow fields. The first deals with the effect of the intestinal defect on the availability of the relevant substance, the second with the effect of reduced availability on the nervous system. We will confine ourselves to describing the occurrence and pathogenesis *in man* of such neurological disorders as are directly or indirectly attributable to malabsorption. We admit to having experienced a certain temptation to stray from these narrow terms of reference. However interesting to the neurologist the ataxia of valine-deprived rats (Rose and Eppstein, 1939) may be, we have fortified ourselves with the thought that isolated valine deficiency is not known to occur in man. Nevertheless, despite the irrelevance of certain animal models, we have had occasionally to refer to experimental work in the nutritional field, if only to throw some light on otherwise obscure areas of human neuropathology.

We will first review the neurological complications of malabsorption as they relate to protein (including specific amino-acids). Although rare, some of these disorders—for instance Hartnup disease—are of considerable theoretical importance. They epitomise a 'prototype' of disordered absorption, due to genetic causes. We will say a few words about malabsorption of fat (which may have some neurological significance) but not of carbohydrate (which has none). We will then discuss the malabsorption of vitamins, again emphasising the neurological repercussions. The question of vitamin B_{12} deficiency will be gone into at some length. The subject merits detailed treatment, for B_{12} deficiency contributes substantially to the neurology of gastrointestinal disease. But before embarking on this survey we must briefly summarise modern concepts of absorption and of the various influences likely to disturb it.

References

Brozek, J. & Grande, F. (1960). Abnormalities of neural function in the presence of inadequate nutrition. In *Handbook of Physiology. Section 1: Neurophysiology*, ed. Magoun, H. W., Vol. III, Ch. 79. Washington: American Physiological Society.

Cruickshank, E. K. (1952). Dietary neuropathies. *Vitamins and Hormones*, **10**, 1–45.

Denny-Brown, D. (1947). Neurological conditions resulting from prolonged and severe dietary restriction. *Medicine (Baltimore)*, **26,** 41–113.
Follis, R. H. (1948). *The Pathology of Nutritional Diseases*. Springfield: Thomas.
Mayoral, L. B., Tripathy, K., Garcia, F. T., Klahr, S., Bolanos, D. & Ghitis, J. (1967). Malabsorption in the tropics: a second look. I. The role of protein malnutrition. *American Journal of Clinical Nutrition*, **20,** 866–883.
Rose, W. C. & Eppstein, S. H. (1939). Dietary indispensability of valine. *Journal of Biological Chemistry*, **127,** 677–684.
Spillane, J. D. (1947). *Nutritional Disorders of the Nervous System*. Edinburgh: Livingstone.
Stanfield, J. P., Hutt, M. S. R. & Tunnicliffe, R. (1965). Intestinal biopsy in kwashiorkor. *Lancet*, **2,** 519–523.
Tandon, B. N., Magotra, M. L., Saraya, A. K. & Ramalingaswami, V. (1968). Small intestine in protein malnutrition. *American Journal of Clinical Nutrition*, **21,** 813–819.
Viteri, F. E., Flores, J. M., Alvarado, J. & Behar, M. (1973). Intestinal malabsorption in malnourished children before and during recovery. Relation between severity of protein deficiency and the malabsorption process. *American Journal of Digestive Diseases*, **18,** 201–212.

CHAPTER TWO

Absorption and Malabsorption

In an adult human being the surface area available for intestinal absorption may attain 200 m^2. It consists of a continuous sheet of epithelium, one cell thick, thrown into folds and ridges from which arise millions of finger-like villi. The absorptive surface is increased still further as a result of the hundreds of microvilli present on the luminal surface of each columnar epithelial cell (or enterocyte). Important enzymes are located along this 'brush border'.

The enterocytes are produced in the crypts between the villi and migrate to sites on the villous surface, where they become functionally active. The life span of the enterocyte rarely exceeds 72 hours, degenerated cells being shed into the intestinal lumen. Creamer (1964) has suggested that the appearance of the intestinal mucosa under the dissecting microscope, at any given point in time, depends on the balance between the rate at which these cells are produced and the rate at which they are shed.

MECHANISMS OF ABSORPTION

Absorption takes place through this sheet of columnar cells. Nearly four decades ago a well-known monograph claimed that the problem of intestinal absorption seemed 'to contain no facts which require the supposition of special vital forces'. Everything could be explained by 'diffusion, osmosis, and filtration of dissolved substances' (Verzár and McDougall, 1936). Although inaccurate even at the time (the active transport of glucose had been described several decades earlier), the situation today is vastly more complex and a number of mechanisms have to be considered. In discussing these we will lay emphasis on the absorption of substances of special relevance to the nervous system.

Passive diffusion

Many water-soluble substances are absorbed by passive diffusion. This is thought to take place through 'water-pores' in the lipid (or lipoprotein) membrane of the columnar cells. These pores are said to have a radius of about 3 to 4 Å which would prevent the diffusion of substances of molecular weight above 200 (Hogben, 1960). The undoubted absorption by this process of rather larger water-soluble molecules suggests that the pores may be considerably bigger. It should be stressed that no one has ever seen such 'pores', their alleged dimensions being beyond the limits of resolution of conventional electron microscopy. Whether they in fact 'exist' or whether their postulation merely provides a more or less satisfactory hypothesis to explain certain physiological observations must, for the time being, be left undecided.

Of the water-soluble substances of neurological interest absorbed in this way we may mention such vitamins as pyridoxine (Brain, Stewart and Booth, 1963), riboflavine, nicotinic acid and pantothenic acid (Turner and Hughes, 1962). There is controversy concerning the absorption of thiamine. Monoglycerides, fat-soluble vitamins (with the possible exception of vitamin A) and many fat-soluble drugs are also absorbed by passive diffusion—this time through the lipid outer layer of the enterocyte. As far as drugs are concerned, their absorption is in fact closely related to their lipid solubility. Many are either weak acids or weak bases (and therefore largely un-ionised) and can be absorbed directly through the lipid membrane. Salicylates and phenytoin are absorbed in this way.

The intestinal handling of triglycerides constitutes a special example of passive diffusion and deserves special mention. Digestion consists of a preliminary emulsification in the stomach followed by a 'chemical' phase in which pancreatic lipase breaks down each triglyceride molecule into a molecule of 2-monoglyceride and two molecules of fatty acid. The reaction is buffered by bicarbonate. During the 'physical' phase of digestion these lipolytic products, which are insoluble in water, are dispersed by conjugated bile acids (bile salts) in a process known as micellar solubilisation.* As a result of this process the surface area of a given amount of dietary fat is vastly increased, permitting it to come into apposition with the enormous surface provided by the microvilli. It has been estimated that 1 gram of dietary fat, present as a spherical globule in water, will have a volume of just over 1 cm^3, a diameter of 1·25 cm and an oil–water interfacial area of about 5 cm^2—about the area of a postage stamp. Emulsification followed by micellar solubilisation will result in a very considerable reduction in particle diameter and in a commensurately enormous increase in oil–water interfacial area. For 1 gram of dietary fat this area may now reach over 1300 m^2, equivalent to the size of six tennis courts!

---

* Bile acids are sterol acids, synthesised by the liver from cholesterol. Cholesterol is insoluble in water, while the bile acids are polar and soluble in water. Molecules of bile acid have a peculiar configuration and are said to be 'amphipathic'. This means that they are asymmetrically structured, their polar (hydrophilic) and non-polar (hydrophobic) regions being disposed on opposite faces of the molecule. In watery solutions, and at a certain concentration, such molecules behave in a characteristic manner, resolving their contradictory affinities for water by forming small aggregates known as micelles. In these molecular aggregates the polar groups of the molecules are outwardly directed, while the centre of the micelle is formed by the inwardly-directed, non-polar hydrocarbon chains. Other fatty substances may dissolve in these chains, resulting in the formation of 'mixed micellar aggregates' of conjugated bile salts and, for instance, the products of fat digestion.

Micellar solubilisation seems to lead to optimum conditions for a fat-soluble substance to penetrate the enterocyte, although it is not known how exactly this takes place at the molecular level. Whether one considers the small intestine as a whole—or the ultrastructure of an individual microvillus—there is no evidence to date of any specific absorption-site for lipids. There is no evidence that energy is expended in the process whereby monoglyceride enters the mucosal cell.

Active transport

If we take two sugars of equal molecular weight (such as glucose and mannose) it can easily be shown that the first readily enters the enterocyte whereas the latter hardly enters at all. Similarly, particular amino-acids are differentially absorbed, according to whether they are presented to the enterocyte as their dextro- or laevo-isomers. Observations such as these imply the operation of some mechanism other than the size of the 'pores' in regulating the entry into the cell of certain water-soluble substances. This mechanism is known as *active transport.*

Active transport is responsible for the absorption of many substances essential to nutrition. Most sugars (Wilson and Landau, 1960), nearly all L-amino-acids (Wiseman, 1968) and some D-amino-acids (Daniels, Newey and Smyth, 1969), some peptides (Matthews, 1972), bile salts, iron, calcium and other electrolytes (Wilson, 1962), and probably even fatty acids (Bloch, Haberich and Lorenz-Meyer, 1973) are absorbed by this mechanism. Of special significance to the theme of this monograph is the fact that vitamin B_{12} is also absorbed by active transport.

Active transport requires energy supplied by cellular metabolism, is inhibited by low temperatures and by certain poisons, demonstrates the phenomenon of competitive inhibition by similar compounds, and becomes saturated by excess of the particular substance transported. The process takes place against an electrochemical concentration gradient and probably arose initially as a result of special membrane adaptations to augment the absorption of certain molecules beyond that allowed by passive diffusion. Active transport usually involves specific processes for various molecules or types of molecule. The active transport of glucose, for instance, involves the recognition of the molecule by certain membrane structures, presumably proteins, followed by the translocation of the particular substance from the outside to the inside of the membrane. The process of 'identifying' particular molecular shapes, usually distinguishing them even from their own stereo-isomers, seems to be extremely specific. As will be discussed in a later section (see p. 17) groups of amino-acids seem to share common transport systems.

The modern concept of 'active transport' is that it takes place through the operation of 'carriers'. A carrier is a hypothetical molecule in the cell membrane, soluble in the membrane itself and capable of diffusing through it. The substance to be transported attaches itself to an 'active site' on the carrier. The carrier with the attached substance forms a complex, itself lipid-soluble. The carrier then passes through the membrane, releasing the substance on the other side. The 'empty' carrier then returns for more, operating a sort of molecular shuttle service. Carriers resemble enzymes in that both have active sites, permitting attachment of substances of particular chemical configuration. They differ from enzymes in that when an 'absorbate' leaves a carrier it does so in the same form as that in which it originally became attached, whereas in the case of enzymes the substrate leaves as a different substance or substances. No carrier molecules have as yet been identified with certainty, perhaps because they are fundamental parts of the cell structure, and that disrupting the cell alters the chemical structure of the carrier (Smyth, 1971).

Some active transport mechanisms, for instance those involving glucose and galactose, have been shown to be Na^+-dependent, at least in certain experimental animals (Crane, 1968). Both the substrate and sodium ions are reversibly attached to a 'carrier' which brings about translocation of the particular carbohydrate through the membrane. The monosaccharide can be transported against its concentration gradient, the energy for this process being provided at least in part by a concentration gradient of Na^+ across the membrane, itself maintained by the Na^+ pump effectively removing Na^+ from the enterocyte (Holmes, 1971). The significance, if any, of sodium-dependent active transport in man is not known.

Another interesting feature of 'active transport' to which much attention has recently been directed is the existence of allosteric effects. By this is meant the effect which a substrate, attaching itself to a binding site, has on the affinity of an adjacent binding site for a quite different substrate.

Facilitated diffusion

Facilitated diffusion (Wilson, 1962) is the term used to describe absorption occurring more rapidly than can be accounted for by passive diffusion and which can also be reduced by competitive inhibition. Such absorption need not take place against a concentration gradient. Xylose may be absorbed by this mechanism.

Pinocytosis

Amoebae feed by engulfing particles in their immediate vicinity. Phagocytic cells also function in this way and it was once suggested that intestinal microvilli might 'capture' lipid particles in this manner (Palay and Karlin, 1959). Quantitatively speaking, pinocytosis probably plays no significant role in normal fat absorption. In certain species protein molecules (such as maternal antibodies) may be absorbed by pinocytosis during the first few weeks of life (Saunders and Isselbacher, 1966). There is some evidence suggesting that the vitamin B_{12}–intrinsic factor complex (Wilson, 1963) and dietary folate (Hoffbrand and Peters, 1969) may be absorbed by this mechanism.

These various mechanisms have been described individually for the benefit of those who have not followed developments in this field over the past decade. Some of the concepts just mentioned have doubtless already been superseded in this rapidly advancing field. In relation to vitamin A for instance (see p. 112), although entry into the enterocyte may be by passive diffusion, the esterification of retinol to retinyl esters, the formation of other lipids (triglycerides, cholesteryl esters and phospholipids) in the mucosal cell, their packaging into chylomicrons, and perhaps chylomicron secretion into lymph channels all require energy, making it more appropriate to discuss the overall absorption of vitamin A in terms of its component processes, rather than in blanket terms such as 'active transport' or 'passive diffusion'.

SITES OF ABSORPTION

It is the exception rather than the rule for specific substances to be absorbed at specific intestinal sites. Bile salts are reabsorbed in the terminal ileum (Lack and Weiner, 1961); so is vitamin B_{12}. Localised bowel disease can certainly result in vitamin B_{12} deficiency and in profound disturbances in the enterohepatic circulation of bile salts. Most other substances are, however, absorbed throughout the length of the small intestine. This is true whatever the exact mechanism whereby they gain entry to the mucosal cell. It is a valid generalisation that absorptive defects from localised gastrointestinal lesions are rare.

In practice, the site at which the bulk of an oral dose of a given substance is absorbed will depend on several factors. These are clearly discussed by Booth, Kanaghinis and Stewart (1963), and by Booth (1965) and comprise:

(a) the mechanism of absorption (i.e. whether by active transport or by passive diffusion);

(b) the distribution of the appropriate mechanism in different portions of the intestinal tract;

(c) the relation between the rate of absorption of a given substance and its transit rate in the small intestine.

Let us consider a substance which is absorbed by passive diffusion, or by an active transport mechanism distributed throughout the intestine. When fed by mouth the absorption of such a substance will be predominantly proximal. Where exactly absorption takes place will, however, vary with the dietary load. A large load of a substance absorbed by active transport may well result in proximal absorption sites rapidly becoming saturated. Absorption will then also take place more distally. The rate of absorption is also relevant. Rapidly absorbed substances (most vitamins of the B group, folic acid, glucose, iron) enter mucosal cells situated in the jejunum, more slowly absorbed substances (such as monoglycerides and amino-acids) will be absorbed distally (i.e. in the ileum) as well. Transit times through the ileum are more prolonged than through the jejunum, an arrangement which ensures distal absorption of substances which for one reason or another have not been fully absorbed more proximally.

Dual mechanisms of absorption exist for certain substances such as tryptophan (Booth and Kanaghinis, 1963), iron (Conrad and Crosby, 1963) and vitamin B_{12} (Ross et al, 1954). Bile acids conjugated to glycine may be passively absorbed from the jejunum, whereas other conjugated bile acids are actively absorbed from the ileum.

One further factor is of relevance in determining whether localised intestinal disease will cause significant malabsorption or not, namely the reserve capacity of the bowel for the substance concerned. One reason why neurological disease due to vitamin deficiency is uncommon in patients with gastrointestinal disorders is the existence of this vast reserve capacity of the small intestine, in relation to vitamins absorbed by passive diffusion. For instance, in 24 hours an adult can probably absorb 500 times his daily requirement of pyridoxine (Booth, 1965). This clearly shows how severe an intestinal disorder will have to be for it to cause pyridoxine deficiency. A similar vast reserve capacity exists in relation to fat. Under ordinary circumstances, appetite alone limits the intestinal absorption of this substance and despite the large number of causes of steatorrhoea (discussed later) total malabsorption of fat is quite exceptional. Such reserve capacity does not exist, however, for substances such as vitamin B_{12}, only 2 to 4 μg of which may be absorbed daily, an amount approximately equal to daily requirements.

Digestion takes place both within the intestinal lumen and—particularly in relation to carbohydrates—at the brush border of the intestinal cell, which is rich in disaccharidases. The products of digestion then enter the cell by one of the mechanisms we have just discussed. The process of absorption is not complete once entry into the enterocyte has been achieved. The relevant substances still have to be delivered to where they will be required, either directly via the portal blood stream or via the intestinal lymphatics. Water-soluble substances and short- or medium-chain fatty acids, being moderately water-soluble, may enter the portal blood directly. Long chain fatty acids are reesterified to triglycerides, probably within the endoplasmic reticular tubules of the enterocytes. This is an energy-dependent process. Chylomicrons (consisting of triglyceride, free fatty acids, cholesterol, cholesterol esters, phospholipid and protein) are synthesised in the endoplasmic reticulum of the enterocytes, stored in the Golgi-storage network and discharged from the cell by a process of reversed pinocytosis. They enter the lymph through spaces between cells and fenestrations in the lacteal walls.

MALABSORPTION

Modern concepts of malabsorption stress biological processes taking place at the surface or within the substance of the enterocyte, or at its interface with lymphatic channels and the portal capillaries. Less emphasis than formerly is placed on disorders of intestinal motility or on maldigestion as causes of malabsorption. In the case of fat, it is true, conditions such as pancreatic insufficiency or defective release or reabsorption of bile are clearly of fundamental importance in the aetiology of steatorrhoea. Such disturbances are beyond the scope of this chapter and interested neurologists are referred to standard textbooks of gastroenterology.

We will here seek to focus attention on certain general principles pertaining to the absorption of substances of significance to the nervous system. Our discussion will not seek to be exhaustive, our purpose being merely to stress the wide range of relevant pathogenetic mechanisms (see Figure 2.1 and Table 2.1) rather than to discuss any of them in depth.

An increasing number of disorders characterised by *genetically determined malabsorption* of certain substances have recently been described. Such conditions as Hartnup disease, the 'blue diaper syndrome', and 'oast-house urine disease' (or at least one of its variants) are of this type and are discussed

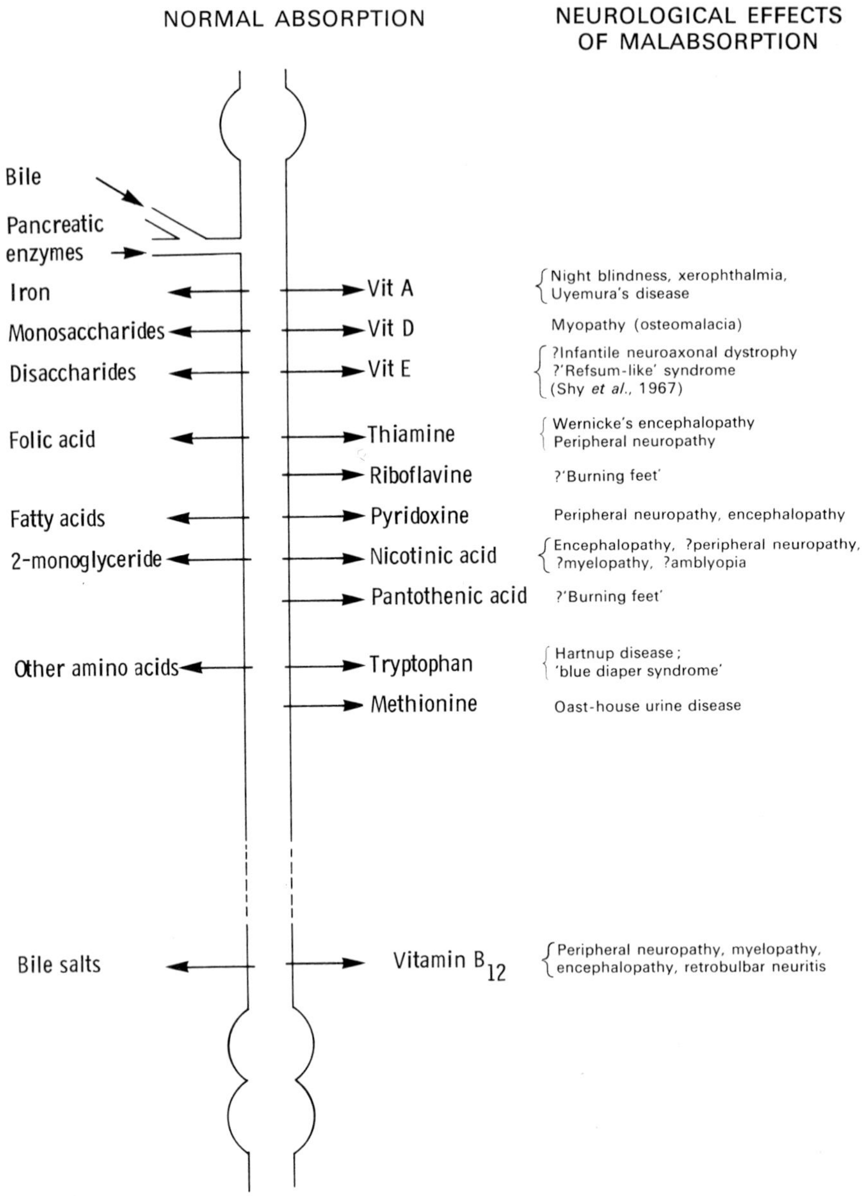

Figure 2.1. Normal absorption and some neurological effects of malabsorption (after Booth, 1968). On the right are listed those nutrients malabsorption of which may have neurological repercussions. The sequence is arbitrary, the purpose of the diagram being merely to show that most neurologically significant substances are absorbed from the proximal or middle thirds of the small intestine—with the exception of vitamin B_{12}.

Table 2.1

Mechanisms Whereby Malabsorption may be Related to Neurological Disease

Gastrointestinal defect	Substance malabsorbed	Associated* neurological disorder
1. Localised gastric lesions		
(a) pernicious anaemia	Vitamin B_{12}	Neuropathy, myelopathy, etc.
(b) congenital IF deficiency	Vitamin B_{12}	Neuropathy, myelopathy, etc.
(c) partial gastrectomy	Vitamin B_{12}	Neuropathy, myelopathy, etc.
	Vitamin D	Osteomalacic myopathy
2. Localised lesions of small intestine		
(a) predominantly proximal	? Water-soluble vitamins	? Hypovitaminosis B (q.v.)
	Vitamin D	? Osteomalacic myopathy
	Folic acid	Probably none
(b) predominantly distal	Vitamin B_{12}	Neuropathy, myelopathy, etc.
3. Bacterial contamination of small bowel (jejunal diverticulosis, blind-loops, strictures)	Vitamin B_{12}	Neuropathy, myelopathy, etc.
4. Congenital absorptive defect	'Neutral' amino-acids	Hartnup disease
	Tryptophan	'Blue diaper syndrome'
	Methionine	'Oast-house urine disease'
	Folic acid	Mental retardation, seizures, ataxia, choreoathetosis*
	Vitamin B_{12}	Neuropathy, myelopathy
5. Transmucosal transport disorders associated with steatorrhoea	Fat-soluble vitamins	Xerophthalmia
		Keratomalacia
		? Osteomalacic myopathy
(a) endocrine causes		
(b) post-irradiation		
(c) drug-induced		
6. Defective synthesis of chylomicrons	? Vitamin E (carrier lipoprotein not synthesised in liver)	Bassen–Kornzweig disease*
7. Infiltration of villous cores	Fats (defective chylomicron release)	Encephalopathy of Whipple's disease*
8. Competition for essential nutrients (e.g. fish tapeworm)	Vitamin B_{12}	Neuropathy, myelopathy, etc.

* By association we do not necessarily imply a causal relationship (particularly in respect of the items marked with an asterisk).

on pages 17 to 21. Congenital intrinsic factor deficiency and congenital malabsorption of vitamin B_{12} (of which several variants have now been recognised) are further genetically determined conditions of both paediatric and neurological interest, and are briefly discussed on pages 68 and 81. Congenital folate malabsorption (see p. 126) is of interest in that it is associated with a severe neurological disturbance whereas acquired folate malabsorption probably never has any neurological repercussions (see Chapter 7).

Many patients with malabsorption have obvious structural changes of the intestinal mucosa due to coeliac disease, tropical sprue or regional enteritis. Or they can be shown to have various types of blind loop or stricture, or various types of inflammation or infiltration of the bowel wall. Resection of variable lengths of bowel for Crohn's disease, or following volvulus or superior mesenteric artery occlusion have provided opportunities for interesting physiological studies, which have taught gastroenterologists a great deal about absorption but are of limited neurological interest. The subject is well reviewed by Booth (1965). Malabsorption of vitamin B_{12} in conditions other than Addisonian pernicious anaemia will be discussed at length under the appropriate headings. The role of bacterial contamination of the small bowel in relation to vitamin B_{12} absorption is reviewed in the chapter dealing with lesions such as jejunal diverticulosis, strictures and blind loops. Malabsorption of vitamin B_{12} is also referred to in the sections on coeliac disease and on tropical sprue, and in the discussion on infestation with the fish tapeworm *Diphyllobothrium latum*.

Neurologists are sometimes confronted with a patient presenting with steatorrhoea and an obvious or less obvious generalised endocrine disorder (such as Addison's disease, hypothyroidism, hypoparathyroidism, thyrotoxicosis or diabetes mellitus) which may itself be a cause of neurological symptoms. The question of steatorrhoea is an extremely complex one, but apart from its frequent association with hypovitaminosis A (and occasionally hypovitaminosis D) it seldom has any neurological sequelae per se. It is therefore important to avoid overenthusiastic attribution of the neurological signs and symptoms to the gastrointestinal defect. That endocrine disorders may at times interfere with intestinal fat transport, by mechanisms as yet poorly understood, is now well established. McBrien, Jones and Creamer (1963) recorded steatorrhoea in four patients with adrenal insufficiency and similar findings have been reported in hypoparathyroidism (Jackson, 1957), hypothyroidism (Kelley and Stewart, 1964) and thyrotoxicosis (Crane and Evans, 1966). Steatorrhoea in diabetics (see also p. 253) may be due to associated pancreatitis, to unrelated coeliac disease, to autonomic neuropathy, which may allow bacterial colonisation of the small bowel to take place, or to causes as yet poorly understood (Vinnik, Kern and Struthers, 1962). Endocrine disorders like the Zollinger–Ellison syndrome, the carcinoid syndrome and medullary carcinoma of the thyroid, although established causes of diarrhoea and, occasionally, steatorrhoea, have in themselves no significant neurological repercussions liable to lead to diagnostic error.

The effects of radiation on the bowel (Reeves et al, 1959) may also cause malabsorption, possibly by altering the rate of intestinal cell turnover. The spinal cord may also be involved in such cases and we have seen at least one patient in whom a chronic paraplegia due to radiation myelopathy was complicated by chronic malabsorption (and eventually by perforation) from radiation enteritis. The administration of certain drugs such as folic acid antagonists, and colchicine (Hawkins, 1961) may cause malabsorption by a similar mechanism, i.e. by slowing down cell replacement. Phenindione (Juel-Jensen, 1959), triparanol (McPherson and Summerskill, 1963) and neomycin (Jacobson, Chodos and Faloon, 1960; Thompson, Heath and

MacMahon, 1969) may all cause malabsorption, the latter possibly by precipitating micellar components through ionic binding of fatty acids. Of these various drugs neomycin alone may cause neurological side-effects (such as neuromuscular block) in its own right and this might conceivably lead to diagnostic problems.

Infiltration of the bowel wall, as in certain types of amyloidosis or in Whipple's disease, leads to steatorrhoea but seldom to malabsorption severe enough to cause neurological signs; the relevant facts are discussed in greater detail under the appropriate headings. Protein-losing enteropathy such as may occur in intestinal lymphangiectasia, Ménétrier's disease (giant rugal hypertrophy of the stomach), ulcerative colitis, severe coeliac disease or any severe inflammatory disorder of the bowel may be associated with hypoproteinaemia, but this of itself does not seem to entail any neurological sequelae.

Turning finally to the release into the circulation of substances adequately absorbed into the mucosal cell, we must mention the rare condition of abetalipoproteinaemia (or Bassen–Kornzweig disease). In this condition there is impaired synthesis of chylomicrons (and in particular of the protein 'net' surrounding the lipid core of the globule) (see p. 239). When the villus is obstructed, as in Whipple's disease (see p. 207) formed chylomicrons may fail to enter the core of the villus, and hence the lymph. Both conditions are associated with steatorrhoea, present characteristic appearances on intestinal biopsy, and may have striking neurological associations.

References

Bloch, R., Haberich, F. J. & Lorenz-Meyer, H. (1972). Untersuchungen zur Transport-Kinetik mittelkettiger Fettsäuren am Dünndarm. *Pflügers Archiv für die gesamte Physiologie des Menschen und der Tiere*, **335**, 198–212.

Booth, C. C. (1965). Physiopathology of intestinal absorption. In *Recent Advances in Gastro-enterology*, ed. Badenoch, J. & Brooke, B. N., Ch. 10. London: Churchill.

Booth, C. C. (1968). Effect of location along the small intestine on absorption of nutrients. In *Handbook of Physiology*, ed. Code, C. F., Section 6, Vol. III, pp. 1513–1527. Washington D.C.: American Physiological Society.

Booth, C. C. & Kanaghinis, T. (1963). A dual mechanism of absorption of L-tryptophan. *Journal of Physiology*, **167**, 18P.

Booth, C. C., Kanaghinis, T. & Stewart, J. S. (1963). Sites of absorption in the small intestine. In *Surgical Physiology of the Gastrointestinal Tract*, ed. Bruce, J. & Smith, A. N. pp. 152–160. Edinburgh: Royal College of Surgeons.

Brain, M. C., Stewart, J. S. & Booth, C. C. (1963). The absorption of tritiated pyridoxine in the rat and in man. *Radioaktive Isotope in Klinik und Forschung*, ed. Fellinger, K. & Hofer, R., Band V, pp. 475–483. Munich: Urban & Schwarzenberg.

Conrad, M. E. & Crosby, W. H. (1963). Intestinal mucosal mechanisms controlling iron absorption. *Blood*, **22**, 406–415.

Crane, R. K. (1968). Absorption of sugars. In *Handbook of Physiology*, ed. Code, C. F., Section 6, Vol. III, pp. 1323–1351. Washington D.C.: American Physiological Society.

Crane, C. W. & Evans, D. W. (1966). Thyrotoxic steatorrhoea. *British Medical Journal*, **2**, 1575.

Creamer, B. (1964). Variations in small intestinal villous shape and mucosal dynamics. *British Medical Journal*, **2**, 1371–1373.

Daniels, V. G., Newey, H. & Smyth, D. H. (1969). Stereochemical specificity of neutral aminoacid transfer systems in rat small intestine. *Biochimica et biophysica acta*, **183**, 637–639.

Hawkins, C. F. (1961). Haematological abnormalities. *Proceedings of the Royal Society of Medicine*, **54**, 495–497.

Hoffbrand, A. V. & Peters, T. J. (1969). The subcellular localisation of pteroyl polyglutamate hydrolase and folate in guinea pig intestinal mucosa. *Biochimica et biophysica acta*, **192**, 479–485.

Hogben, C. A. M. (1960). The alimentary tract. *Annual Review of Physiology*, **22**, 381–406.

Holmes, R. (1971). Carbohydrate digestion and absorption. *Journal of Clinical Pathology*, **24**, Supplement (Royal College of Pathologists) **5**, 10–13.

Jackson, W. P. U. (1957). Steatorrhoea and hypoparathyroidism. *Lancet*, **1**, 1086–1087.

Jacobson, E. D., Chodos, R. B. & Faloon, W. W. (1960). An experimental malabsorption syndrome induced by neomycin. *American Journal of Medicine*, **28**, 524–533.

Juel-Jensen, B. E. (1959). Sensitivity to phenindione; report of a case of severe diarrhoea. *British Medical Journal*, **2**, 173–174.

Kelley, M. L. Jr. & Stewart, J. M. (1964). Myxedema and intestinal malabsorption (non-tropical sprue?) with severe hypomotility of the gastrointestinal tract. Report of a case. *American Journal of Digestive Diseases*, **9**, 79–86.

Lack, L. & Weiner, I. M. (1961). In vitro absorption of bile salts by small intestine of rats and guinea pigs. *American Journal of Physiology*, **200**, 313–317.

McBrien, D. J., Jones, D. V., & Creamer, B. (1963). Steatorrhoea in Addison's disease. *Lancet*, **1**, 25–26.

McPherson, J. R. & Summerskill, W. H. J. (1963). An acute malabsorption syndrome with reversible mucosal atrophy. *Gastroenterology*, **44**, 900–904.

Matthews, D. M. (1972). Rates of peptide uptake by small intestine. In *Peptide Transport in Bacteria and Mammalian Gut*. Ciba Foundation Symposium. Amsterdam: Elsevier.

Palay, S. L. & Karlin, L. J. (1959). Electron microscopic studies of the intestinal villus. *Journal of Biophysical and Biochemical Cytology*, **5**, 373–383.

Reeves, R. J., Sanders, A. P., Islay, J. K., Sharpe, K. W. & Bayliss, G. J. (1959). Fat absorption from the human gastro-intestinal tract in patients undergoing radiation therapy. *Radiology*, **73**, 398–401.

Ross, G. I. M., Mollin, D. L., Cox, E. V. & Ungley, C. C. (1954). Hematologic responses and concentration of vitamin B_{12} in serum and urine following oral administration of vitamin B_{12} without intrinsic factor. *Blood*, **9**, 473–488.

Saunders, S. J. & Isselbacher, M. D. (1966). Intestinal absorption of amino acids. *Gastroenterology*, **50**, 586–595.

Shy, G. M., Silberberg, D. H., Appel, S. H., Mishkin, M. M. & Godfrey, E. H. (1967). A generalised disorder of nervous system, skeletal muscle and heart resembling Refsum's disease and Hurler's syndrome. *American Journal of Medicine*, **42**, 163–178.

Smyth, D. H. (1971). Intestinal transfer mechanisms, measurements and analogies. *Journal of Clinical Pathology*, **24**, Supplement (Royal College of Pathologists), **5**, 1–9.

Thompson, G. R., Heath, J. & MacMahon, M. T. (1969). Interaction of neomycin with micellar fatty acids and cholesterol. *Clinical Science*, **37**, 569.

Turner, J. B. & Hughes, D. E. (1962). The absorption of some B-group vitamins by surviving rat intestine preparations. *Quarterly Journal of Experimental Physiology and Cognate Medical Sciences*, **47**, 107–133.

Verzár, F. & McDougall, E. J. (1936). *Absorption from the Intestine*. London: Longmans Green.

Vinnik, I. E., Kern, F. Jr. & Struthers, J. E. Jr. (1962). Malabsorption and the diarrhea of diabetes mellitus. *Gastroenterology*, **43**, 507–520.

Wilson, T. H. (1962). *Intestinal Absorption*. Philadelphia & London: Saunders.

Wilson, T. H. (1963). Intestinal absorption of vitamin B_{12}. *Physiologist*, **6**, 11–26.

Wilson, T. H. & Landau, B. R. (1960). Specificity of sugar transport by the intestine of the hamster. *American Journal of Physiology*, **198**, 99–102.

Wiseman, G. (1964). *Absorption from the Intestine*. London: Academic Press.

Wiseman, G. (1968). Absorption of amino-acids. In *Handbook of Physiology*, ed. Code, C. F., Section 6, Vol. III, pp. 1277–1308. Washington D.C.: American Physiological Society.

CHAPTER THREE

Protein and Amino-Acids

PROTEIN MALNUTRITION AND CEREBRAL FUNCTION

It is not known for how long the human brain continues to produce neurones after birth. The process, most active in the second and third trimesters of fetal life, draws to a close at term. The periventricular matrix layer, the source in the fetus of cerebral neurones and later of neuroglia, persists in the human neonate, and it is possible that in primates—as in rodents—limited, regional formation of neurones continues during the first postnatal month. It is probable that in the cerebellum granule cells may also be produced for a while after birth.

Even if neuronal *formation* is limited after birth, neuronal *enlargement* certainly occurs and is of vital importance. Dendritic arborisation becomes more extensive and complex. Moreover, the formation of neuroglia is a continuing process: new glial cells are produced in the primate brain for several years after birth (Lewis, 1968). Further the process of myelination involves a vast increase in the cytoplasmic mass of the oligodendroglia.

It is thus clear that events of vital importance are taking place in the infant's brain, and it would be surprising if it were not at risk from nutritional deprivation during the early months of life. It has been suspected for some years that protein–calorie malnutrition at this time might impair normal cerebral development (Carothers, 1953; Trowell, Davies and Dean, 1954). In recent years it has been confirmed that such deprivation delays both the functional and biochemical development of the brain (Smart and Dobbing, 1971; Adlard and Dobbing, 1971), and appears to produce a permanent deficit both in cell number and in brain weight (Winick, 1969; Dobbing, Hopewell and Lynch, 1971). Decreased head size and intelligence have also been documented in protein-deprived infants (Cravioto, de Licardie and Birch, 1966; Stoch and Smythe, 1967). Studies of total DNA content and rate of DNA formation in nutritionally-deprived animals have thrown some light on the possible mechanism of these changes (Patel, Balázs and Johnson, 1973), though how protein lack causes diminished cell production or function in the brain remains obscure.

The whole subject of protein malnutrition and its effect on intelligence is an explosive one with enormous social and political implications. The subject must be mentioned here, however, for there are fragments of evidence, both from children with kwashiorkor and others with a grossly inadequate diet, that protein deprivation may itself lead to structural changes and to changes in the absorptive capacity of the bowel (Stanfield, Hutt and Tunnicliffe, 1965; Mayoral et al, 1967; Tandon et al, 1968), changes which will of course aggravate the nutritional deficit. We must add, however, that there is little evidence that protein malnutrition in early life is ever due *predominantly* to a disorder of the gastrointestinal tract. Moreover, there are no specific neurological complications of the protein-losing enteropathies of later life.

PROTEIN ABSORPTION

It was once thought that proteins within the intestinal lumen were completely hydrolysed to their component amino-acids prior to absorption. It is now known that the situation is far more complex. During the first two weeks of life entire protein molecules, such as antibodies, may, in some species, be absorbed relatively unchanged. A few peptides, which are hydrolysed with difficulty, may be absorbed as such (Prockop and Sjoerdsma, 1961). Although dietary protein appears in the portal blood almost entirely in the form of amino-acids, the hydrolysis of dietary protein to free amino-acids proceeds far more rapidly than could be accounted for by the action of pancreatic proteases alone. Mucosal polypeptidases, situated at the brush border of the enterocytes are now known to hydrolyse some oligopeptides with uptake of the resultant amino-acids. There is also probably a substantial uptake by the enterocyte of di- and tri-peptides, followed by hydrolysis to amino-acids within the mucosal cell itself. Some free amino-acids may also be liberated from oligopeptides by desquamated cells within the intestinal lumen.

Free amino-acids are absorbed by active transport, although facilitated diffusion may sometimes play a role (Booth, 1963). Correct stereoisomerism is necessary, the L-forms being much more readily absorbed than the D-forms. The active transport of amino-acids is probably both pyridoxine-dependent (Akedo et al, 1960; Huang, 1961) and sodium-dependent (Saunders and Isselbacher, 1966). Useful recent reviews of amino-acid absorption have been published by Fisher (1967), Wiseman (1968) and Matthews (1969).

Although disorders due to deficiencies of intestinal disaccharidases are well recognised, no disorders due to deficiencies of mucosal peptidases have yet been described (Matthews, 1971). It is doubtful whether general malabsorption of protein, such as may occur with gastric, pancreatic, or intestinal disease has per se any specific effect on the nervous system.

SOME DISORDERS OF AMINO-ACID TRANSPORT

The absorption of free amino-acids and the uptake and subsequent hydrolysis of oligopeptides are separate processes. In hereditary disorders of amino-acid transport it is only the absorption of certain free amino-acids that is impaired.

Several hereditary disorders of amino-acid transport have been described. In some the disorder is confined to the alimentary tract, in others to the renal tubule, whereas in some both sites are involved. Some of these disorders have neurological complications, with which they may in fact present.

If amino-acids are considered in relation to transport across the intestinal mucosa (or across the cells lining the renal tubule) they seem to fall into four main groups:

(a) *Monoamino-monocarboxylic (neutral) amino-acids:* alanine, serine, threonine, valine, leucine, isoleucine, phenylalanine, tyrosine, tryptophan, asparagine, histidine, cysteine, methionine and citrulline.

(b) *Dibasic amino-acids:* lysine, arginine, ornithine, and the neutral amino-acid cystine.

(c) *Dicarboxylic acids:* glutamic acid and aspartic acid which are extensively converted to alanine by transaminases during the absorptive process.

(d) *The imino acid and glycine group:* proline, hydroxyproline and glycine.

Three disorders with neurological complications will be discussed: Hartnup disease; tryptophan malabsorption syndrome (the 'blue diaper syndrome'); and methionine malabsorption. All are predominantly disorders of mono-amino-monocarboxylic amino-acid transport.

Hartnup disease

This is an autosomal recessive disorder characterised *clinically* by an intermittent cutaneous eruption resembling pellagra and by episodic neurological disturbances (usually of cerebellar type), and *biochemically* by diminished intestinal absorption (and increased faecal excretion) of most mono-amino-monocarboxylic acids (including tryptophan), by a constant renal aminoaciduria of characteristic pattern, and by the intermittent excessive excretion of indican and of indolic acids in the urine. The condition seems to be the homozygous manifestation of a rare non X-linked allele. In Hartnup disease absorptive disorders of a similar nature affect both intestinal mucosa and renal tubule. The former is of paramount importance in explaining the neurological and several of the biochemical features.

Despite the physiological defect there are usually no gastrointestinal symptoms in this condition. Persistent neonatal diarrhoea has however been described (Halvorsen and Halvorsen, 1963).

Biochemical abnormalities. The amino-acid tryptophan is a precursor of nicotinamide, and deficiency of nicotinamide causes pellagra. Following an oral dose of L-tryptophan, patients with Hartnup disease develop a smaller rise of serum tryptophan than do normal controls. They also show an increased faecal excretion of the amino-acid. Part of the tryptophan which escapes absorption in the small bowel is degraded to indole and indolic acids by colonic bacteria. These substances, themselves of no nutritional value, are absorbed and then excreted in the urine as indican and indolylacetic acid (Milne et al, 1960a; Asatoor et al, 1963; Milne, 1964). The administration of neomycin interferes with bacterial activity in the colon and markedly reduces the indicanuria. These characteristic biochemical disturbances have been reported in the absence of clinical manifestations of the condition (Seakins and Ersser, 1967; Pomeroy et al, 1968).

In patients with Hartnup disease a disproportionate amount of *absorbed* L-tryptophan seems to be diverted from the kynurenine–nicotinamide metabolic pathway and, instead, converted to indolylacetic acid and its glutamine conjugate which are excreted in excess in the urine (Milne et al, 1960b). Taken in conjunction with the constant loss of tryptophan in urine and faeces this might contribute to the pellagrous features of the disease. It is doubtful whether it will adequately explain the neurological episodes, however. Cerebellar ataxia is certainly not a prominent feature of pellagra.

A characteristic pattern of aminoaciduria is the most constant biochemical feature of Hartnup disease. It involves the 'neutral' (monoamino-monocarboxylic) amino-acids, with the exception of methionine. It also seems to involve the 'dibasic' amino-acid lysine. Despite massive aminoaciduria, patients with Hartnup disease show only minimal evidence of protein malnutrition. Recent work suggests that they may maintain protein nutrition by absorbing oligopeptides (Asatoor et al, 1970). Many of the patients are, however, of slightly reduced stature (Colliss, Levi and Milne, 1963).

Neurological aspects. The neurological episodes in the 43 hitherto reported cases of Hartnup disease (Jepson, 1972) are rather more pleomorphic than the original descriptions suggested. They may follow intercurrent infections and are usually—but not always—associated with the appearance of the typical rash. An inadequate or irregular diet seems to be a frequent precipitating factor.

An ataxic disorder of gait is the most common presentation. Intention tremor and nystagmus have been reported on several occasions. Muscle pains, inexplicable weakness, headache, attacks of 'collapsing', delirium and other psychiatric manifestations have all been described. The neurological symptoms may fluctuate but usually recover completely, most often after a period of a few weeks. Although the administration of nicotinamide seems to hasten improvement, particularly of the cutaneous lesion, spontaneous improvement of the neurological disability has been recorded several times. About a quarter of the patients are mentally retarded but the impression of steady mental deterioration, conveyed by the original reports, has not been substantiated. If anything, these patients tend to get better as the years go by.

Hartnup disease should be suspected in any case of pellagra without adequate dietary cause and in any child with intermittent cerebellar symptoms, particularly if there is a family history of similar disturbance.

Neuropathology. To date we have only found evidence of a single necropsy report mentioning examination of the brain in a case of Hartnup disease (Daute, Dietel and Ebert, 1966). In the last two years of her life, a 10-year-old girl had suffered from intermittent fever, headache and loss of appetite. No neurological signs had been noted a year before her death, but before she died—of cachexia—bilateral extensor plantars were recorded. Sections of her brain were said to show loss of occasional Purkinje cells in the cerebellum, and occasional foci of perivascular glial proliferation. Lesions of the bowel (an ulcerative enterocolitis), liver, kidney and skin were clearly described in this report. Unfortunately, little emphasis was placed on detailed examination of the central nervous system.

It is interesting to speculate whether the patient described in great detail by Greenfield and Holmes (1939)—and long considered a classic illustration of the neuropathology of pellagra (uncomplicated by other avitaminoses)—might not have been a case of Hartnup disease! The patient, a boy of five years, had been brought up on a diet containing 'plenty of fresh vegetables, milk and butter', his parents being farmers. At the age of four he had an attack suggestive of pellagra from which, after several weeks, he had made a spontaneous recovery. A year later he died of bronchopneumonia complicating measles, just as he was recovering from a recent, severe neurological disorder characterised by ataxia, dysarthria, nystagmus, bilateral pyramidal signs associated with a widespread recurrence of the pellagrous rash. At necropsy upper and lower motor neurones were involved, as were the spino-cerebellar pathways, the dentate nuclei, and the 'neurones which have their cell station in the dorsal root ganglia'.

Pathogenesis and management of neurological disturbances. The absorption from the colon of toxic substances (produced by the action of bacteria on unabsorbed amino-acids) might be at the root of these disturbances. The exact nature of the responsible agents is unknown. Milne (1964, 1967) has suggested that in addition to indolic acids derived from tryptophan, patients with Hartnup disease might have to cope with increased amounts of histamine derived from histidine, of phenylethylamine derived from phenylalanine, and, in addition, with tryptamine, tyramine, isoamylamine and other amines derived from the decarboxylation of amino-acids. Theoretically these neurological complications might respond to the sort of regime used in the management of hepatic pre-coma.

Hartnup disease is of considerable neurological interest in that it clearly establishes that a disorder characterised by constant aminoaciduria can produce *intermittent* neurological symptoms. This intermittency suggests the periodic operation of some additional factor. Some of the attacks of cerebellar ataxia in Hartnup disease seem to be related to intercurrent infection (Baron et al, 1956—Cases 1 and 3; Weyers and Bickel, 1958). Systemic infections tend to produce an acid urine (as a result of increased tissue breakdown and starvation ketosis). The excretion of indolylacetic acid is less in an acid urine than in an alkaline urine (Milne et al, 1960a). If the neurological symptoms of Hartnup disease are in any way related to the presence of indolic acids in the blood, the excretion of these acids could be increased by simple alkalinisation of the urine. We have no knowledge as to whether this form of therapy, first suggested by Milne et al (1960b) has ever been tried in a patient with Hartnup disease in relapse. Large doses of indolylacetic acid produce ataxia in experimental animals (Baruk et al, 1958) but the substance does not appear to be significantly toxic in man (Mirsky, 1957).

Tryptophan malabsorption syndrome ('blue diaper syndrome')

This is a very rare genetically-determined disorder affecting the intestinal absorption of tryptophan. The absorption of other monoamino-monocarboxylic acids is normal and the defect does not involve the renal tubule. There is consequently no aminoaciduria.

In this condition unabsorbed tryptophan is acted upon by colonic bacteria and the absorbed products are excreted in the urine as indican. On hydrolysis and oxidation the indican yields the dye indigotin (hence the name 'blue diaper syndrome').

In the original description by Drummond and his co-workers (1964) the condition was associated, in two brothers, with hypercalcaemia and nephrocalcinosis. Both infants had shown failure to thrive, recurrent unexplained fever, marked irritability and constipation. The facies was normal. There was no gross mental retardation, although the exact mental state of these children was difficult to assess as one developed renal insufficiency and the other died following operation for a subdural haematoma. The relation of the disorder of calcium homeostasis to the disorder of tryptophan absorption is obscure as the authors claim that oral tryptophan raised the serum calcium in one of the infants. The oral administration of certain amino-acids, including tryptophan, to rats can greatly enhance calcium absorption (Wasserman, Comar and Nold, 1956; Wasserman et al, 1957).

Methionine malabsorption syndrome

In 1964 Hooft and his colleagues described a mentally defective girl of two years who was liable to convulsions, attacks of hyperpnoea and periodic diarrhoea. She had white hair, blue eyes and a characteristic smell emanated from her. On a normal diet her urine and faeces contained α-hydroxybutyric acid. Methionine and branched-chain amino-acids were present in large amounts in the faeces.

Feeding methionine increased the amounts of α-hydroxybutyric acid and of methionine in the faeces and caused diarrhoea. The frequency of the convulsions lessened—and the electroencephalogram improved—when the patient was fed a diet low in methionine. Under these circumstances α-hydroxybutyric acid disappeared from the urine and faeces, and branched-chain amino-acids from the faeces.

The authors postulated a defect in the intestinal absorption of methionine, with conversion (by colonic bacteria) of unabsorbed methionine to α-hydroxybutyric acid.

The condition resembles that described by Smith and Strang (1958) as 'oast-house urine disease' (an oast-house is a kiln for drying hops). The two children described by these authors were also mentally defective, with white hair, and also suffered from convulsions and attacks of hyperpnoea. The urine contained not only α-hydroxybutyric acid, but also methionine and an excess of tyrosine, phenylalanine and branched-chain amino-acids. The condition seemed to be characterised by impaired intestinal and renal absorption of methionine and possibly of other amino-acids. These cases emphasise the importance of a keen sense of smell in paediatric neurology. Several short-chain (or branched-chain) fatty acids and their related keto-acids have characteristic odours.

It has recently been shown that there is a defective uptake of amino-acids in patients with Whipple's disease and in patients with coeliac disease (Brice,

Owen and Tyor, 1965). Although neurological symptoms may occur in both these conditions—and are discussed under the appropriate headings—there is no evidence that they are due to amino-acid malabsorption.

References

Adlard, B. P. F. & Dobbing, J. (1971). Vulnerability of developing brain. III. Development of four enzymes in the brains of normal and undernourished rats. *Brain Research*, **28**, 97–107.

Akedo, H., Sugawa, T., Yoshikawa, S. & Suda, M. (1960). Intestinal absorption of amino-acids. I. The effect of vitamin B_6 on the absorption of L-amino-acids through the intestine. *Journal of Biochemistry (Tokyo)*, **47**, 124–130.

Asatoor, A. M., Cheng, B., Edwards, K. D. G., Laut, A. F., Matthews, D. M., Milne, M. D., Navab, F. & Richards, A. J. (1970). Intestinal absorption of two dipeptides in Hartnup disease. *Gut*, **11**, 380–387.

Asatoor, A. M., Craske, J., London, D. R. & Milne, M. D. (1963). Indole production in Hartnup disease. *Lancet*, **1**, 126–128.

Baron, D. N., Dent, C. E., Harris, H., Hart, E. W. & Jepson, J. B. (1956). Hereditary pellagra-like skin rash with temporary cerebellar ataxia, constant renal aminoaciduria and other bizarre biochemical features. *Lancet*, **2**, 421–428.

Baruk, H., Launay, J., Berges, J., Perles, R. & Conte, C. (1958). Effets neuropsychiques chez l'animal de quelques dérivés indoliques: sérotonine, tryptamine, acide β-indol-acétique et indol. *Annales Médico-Psychologiques (Paris)*, **116**, 115–125.

Booth, C. C. (1963). Absorption from the small intestine. In *The Scientific Basis of Medicine Annual Reviews*. London: Athlone Press.

Brice, R. S., Owen, E. E. & Tyor, M. P. (1965). Aminoacid uptake and fatty acid esterification by intestinal mucosa from patients with Whipple's disease and nontropical sprue. *Gastroenterology*, **48**, 584–592.

Carothers, J. C. (1953). *The African Mind in Health and Disease: A Study of Ethnopsychiatry*. World Health Organisation Monograph Series, No. 17.

Colliss, J. E., Levi, A. J. & Milne, M. D. (1963). Stature and nutrition in cystinuria and Hartnup disease. *British Medical Journal*, **1**, 590–592.

Cravioto, J., de Licardie, E. R. & Birch, H. G. (1966). Nutrition, growth and neurointegrative development: An experimental and ecologic study. *Pediatrics*, **38**, 319–372.

Daute, K. H., Dietel, K. & Ebert, W. (1966). Das Hartnupsyndrom. Bericht über einen tödlichen Krankheitsverlauf. *Zeitschrift für Kinderheilkunde*, **95**, 103–113.

Dobbing, J., Hopewell, J. W. & Lynch, A. (1971). Vulnerability of developing brain. VII. Permanent deficit of neurons in cerebral and cerebellar cortex following early mild undernutrition. *Experimental Neurology*, **32**, 439–447.

Drummond, K. N., Michael, A. F., Ulstrom, R. A. & Good, R. A. (1964). The blue diaper syndrome: familial hypercalcaemia with nephrocalcinosis and indicanuria. *American Journal of Medicine*, **37**, 928–948.

Fisher, R. B. (1967). Absorption of proteins. *British Medical Bulletin*, **23**, 241–246.

Greenfield, J. G. & Holmes, J. MacD. (1939). A case of pellagra—the pathological changes in the spinal cord. *British Medical Journal*, **1**, 815–819.

Halvorsen, K. & Halvorsen, S. (1963). Hartnup disease. *Pediatrics*, **31**, 29–38.

Hooft, C., Timmermans, J., Snoek, J., Anterer, I., Ouaert, W. & van den Hends, C. H. (1964). Methionine malabsorption in a mentally defective child. *Lancet*, **2**, 20.

Huang, K. C. (1961). Intestinal absorption of L-tyrosine derivatives. *Federation Proceedings*, **20**, 246.

Jepson J. B. (1972). Hartnup disease. In *The Metabolic Basis of Inherited Disease*, ed. Stanbury, J. B., Wyngaarden, J. B. & Fredrickson, D. S. New York: McGraw-Hill.

Lewis, P. D. (1968). Mitotic activity in the primate subependymal layer and the genesis of gliomas. *Nature*, **217**, 974–975.

Matthews, D. M. (1969). Absorption und Malabsorption von Eiweissverdauungsprodukten. *Klinische Wochenschrift*, **47**, 397–414.

Matthews, D. M. (1971). Protein absorption. *Journal of Clinical Pathology*, **24**, Supplement (Royal College of Pathologists), **5**, 29–40.

Mayoral, L. B., Tripathy, K., Garcia, F. T., Klahr, S., Bolanos, D. & Ghitis, J. (1967). Malabsorption in the tropics: a second look. I. The role of protein malnutrition. *American Journal of Clinical Nutrition*, **20**, 866–883.

Milne, M. D. (1964). Disorders of aminoacid transport. *British Medical Journal*, **1**, 327–336.

Milne, M. D. (1967). Hereditary abnormalities of intestinal absorption. *British Medical Bulletin*, **23**, 279–284.

Milne, M. D., Crawford, M. A., Girao, C. B. & Loughridge, L. (1960a). The excretion of indolylactic acid and related indolic acids in man and the rat. *Clinical Science*, **19**, 165–179.

Milne, M. D., Crawford, M. A., Girao, C. B. & Loughridge, L. W. (1960b). The metabolic disorder in Hartnup disease. *Quarterly Journal of Medicine*, **29**, 407–421.

Mirsky, J. A. (1957). Insulinase, insulinase inhibitors and diabetes mellitus. *Recent Progress in Hormone Research*, **13**, 429–471.

Patel, A. J., Balázs, R. & Johnson, A. L. (1973). Effect of undernutrition on cell formation in the rat brain. *Journal of Neurochemistry*, **20**, 1151–1165.

Pomeroy, J., Efron, M. L., Dayman, J. & Hoefnagel, D. (1968). Hartnup disorder in a New England family. *New England Journal of Medicine*, **278**, 1214–1216.

Prockop, D. J. & Sjoerdsma, A. (1961). Significance of urinary hydroxyproline in man. *Journal of Clinical Investigation*, **40**, 843–849.

Saunders, S. J. & Isselbacher, M. D. (1966). Intestinal absorption of amino acids. *Gastroenterology*, **50**, 586–595

Seakins, J. W. T. & Ersser, R. S. (1967). Effects of aminoacid loads on a healthy infant with the biochemcial features of Hartnup disease. *Archives of Disease in Childhood*, **42**, 682–688.

Smart, J. L. & Dobbing, J. (1971). Vulnerability of developing brain. II. Effects of early nutritional deprivation on reflex ontogeny and development of behaviour in the rat. *Brain Research*, **28**, 85–95.

Smith, A. J. & Strang, L. B. (1958). Inborn error of metabolism with urinary excretion of α-hydroxy-butyric acid and phenylpyruvic acid. *Archives of Disease in Childhood*, **33**, 109–113.

Stanfield, J. P., Hutt, M. S. R. & Tunnicliffe, R. (1965). Intestinal biopsy in kwashiorkor. *Lancet*, **2**, 519–523.

Stoch, M. B. & Smythe, P. M. (1967). The effect of undernutrition during infancy on subsequent brain growth and intellectual development. *South African Medical Journal*, **41**, 1027–1030.

Tandon, B. N., Magotra, M. L., Saraya, A. K. & Ramalingaswami, V. (1968). Small intestine in protein malabsorption. *American Journal of Clinical Nutrition*, **21**, 813–819.

Trowell, H. C., Davies, J. N. P. & Dean, R. F. A. (1954). *Kwashiorkor*. London: Arnold.

Wasserman, R. H., Comar, C. L. & Nold, M. M. (1956). The influence of aminoacids and other organic compounds on the gastrointestinal absorption of calcium^{45} and strontium^{89} in the rat. *Journal of Nutrition*, **59**, 371–383.

Wasserman, R. H., Comar, C. L., Schooley, J. C. & Lengemann, F. W. (1957). Interrelated effects of L-lysine and other dietary factors on the gastrointestinal absorption of calcium^{45} in the rat and chick. *Journal of Nutrition*, **62**, 367–376.

Weyers, H. & Bickel, H. (1958). Photodermatose mit Aminoacidurie, Indolaceturie und cerebralen Manifestationen (Hartnup-syndrom). *Klinische Wochenschrift*, **36**, 893–897.

Winick, M. (1969). Malnutrition and brain development. *Journal of Pediatrics*, **74**, 667–679.

Wiseman, G. (1968). Absorption of amino-acids. In *Handbook of Physiology*, Section 6, Vol. III, ed. Code, C. F., pp. 1277–1308. Washington: American Physiological Society.

CHAPTER FOUR

Vitamin Deficiencies in Patients with Malabsorption

When neurological signs or symptoms are found in a patient with a gastro-intestinal disorder the almost reflex response of most physicians is to suspect malabsorption of vitamin B_{12}. Vitamin B_{12} deficiency may well turn out to be the cause of the patient's complaints but it is important to bear in mind that other vitamin deficiencies (and possibly deficiencies of other factors altogether) may sometimes be responsible. For instance, some of the neurological complications of partial gastrectomy (Williams et al, 1969), of jejunal diverticulosis (Cooke et al, 1963) and of adult coeliac disease (Cooke and Smith, 1966) seem to be unrelated to hypovitaminosis B_{12}. Whether deficiencies of other vitamins of the B complex are implicated, or even perhaps of fat-soluble vitamins, has seldom been systematically investigated, using modern techniques.

Vitamin deficiencies can often be detected before they produce physical signs. The rate at which tissue desaturation occurs (whether due to dietary lack, malabsorption or excessive demand) will depend on the size of the tissue stores. This will vary considerably from vitamin to vitamin. Thiamine is hardly stored at all, while tissue stores of vitamin B_{12} are such that they may delay the appearance of neurological symptoms for several years after gastrectomy or distal gut resection. Once tissue desaturation has reached a critical level changes occur in the specific enzyme activity catalysed by the vitamin. A 'metabolic lesion' has appeared. The vitamin B_{12}-deficient patient will start excreting methylmalonic acid in his urine. The pyridoxine-deficient patient will start excreting xanthurenic acid in response to a tryptophan load. To begin with, these biochemical disturbances, occurring at a cellular or humoral level, may leave no tell-tale signs that the clinician can detect. It is only when they reach a critical stage and provoke morphological repercussions that a clinically identifiable disorder emerges and that a clinical diagnosis of vitamin deficiency becomes possible.

It is surprising how seldom clinicians attempt to ascertain the possible presence of such deficiencies. Many seem unaware of how to set about establishing or documenting their existence. There is a tendency to dismiss the problem as 'nutritional', almost implying thereby that it is beyond the realm of rational investigation. To counteract this nihilistic attitude we will review some of the clinical and biochemical features of those vitamin deficiencies which are of neurological significance. We will stress what is known of the absorption and storage of those vitamins, deficiency of which may cause neurological signs and symptoms in man, and review some of the cases in which deficiency could reasonably be attributed to malabsorption. Although we will confine ourselves to vitamins of the B complex and to vitamin A, we recognise that certain other vitamin deficiencies may have repercussions on the nervous system. Vitamin C deficiency, for instance, may occasionally produce intracranial bleeding, but we have found no account of such an event arising on the basis of malabsorption. Vitamin D deficiency may be associated with diffuse bone pain but also with myopathy, in certain patients with osteomalacia (see Chapter 9). Vitamin E, which is certainly poorly absorbed in a number of conditions, is of uncertain importance in *human* neurological disease. It is referred to, in the context of Bassen–Kornzweig disease (abetalipoproteinaemia) on p. 239. Vitamin K deficiency in neonates—not of course due to malabsorption—is also a well-recognised cause of intracranial haemorrhage, but to our knowledge such an occurrence has not been described in the context of an obstructive jaundice (or of any other form of malabsorption).

In any patient with gastrointestinal disease and signs or symptoms of *peripheral neuropathy*, investigations should of course seek to establish whether there is vitamin B_{12} deficiency. Deficiencies of thiamine, riboflavine, nicotinic acid, pyridoxine and perhaps pantothenic acid should also be considered and if possible ruled out. The presence of thiamine deficiency will be easy to establish. If *burning feet* is the main complaint attention should centre on malabsorption of pyridoxine, riboflavine and pantothenic acid, although, as will be discussed, the definitive cause of this syndrome has not been established. Folate deficiency should be sought for (and, when present, treated on its merits) despite controversy as to whether it is ever responsible for neurological signs (see Chapter 7).

It should be remembered that weakness and sensory symptoms in patients with malabsorption may be due to causes other than polyneuropathy. These include hypokalaemia and tetany, and estimations of serum potassium, calcium, and if possible magnesium are important in any patient with gastrointestinal disease complaining of heaviness or of tingling in the limbs. Evidence of *myelopathy* should lead to a search for deficiency of vitamin B_{12} and possibly of nicotinic acid too. *Myopathy* should lead to a search for underlying osteomalacia, itself probably related to malabsorption of vitamin D. As will be described, such a myopathy has been reported following gastrectomy, in coeliac disease and in patients with tropical sprue. The presence of *ocular or visual symptoms* raises the possibility of vitamin A deficiency, but optic neuropathy may also complicate vitamin B_{12} deficiency and possibly deficiency of other water-soluble vitamins. An acute or subacute *encephalopathic state* may be due to thiamine deficiency (Wernicke's encephalopathy), but also to nicotinic acid deficiency (Jolliffe's syndrome). The occurrence of such an episode in the context of jejunal diverticulosis will be reported.

Table 4.1

Some Effects of Vitamin Deficiency (Water-soluble Vitamins)

Vitamin deficiency	CNS	Gut	Eye (anterior segment)	Mouth	Skin	Other
Thiamine	Peripheral neuropathy (beri-beri) Wernicke's encephalopathy Paroxysmal rigidity with aphonia (infants) Irritability-anorexia syndrome	Anorexia Vomiting Intestinal atony Epigastric distress	Nil	Nil	Nil	Heart failure Parotid enlargement Pancreatic oedema
Riboflavine	? 'Burning feet' syndrome	Nil	Corneal vascularisation Conjunctivitis, photophobia, lachrymation, blepharospasm ? Corneal epithelial dystrophy	Angular stomatitis Cheilosis Glossitis	Naso-labial seborrhoea Scrotal and vulval dermatitis	Occasional normocytic normochromic anaemia
Nicotinic acid	Pellagrous dementia Acute encephalopathy (Jolliffe's syndrome) ? Peripheral neuropathy ? Myelopathy ? Nutritional amblyopia	Diarrhoea	Nil	Gingivitis Stomatitis Glossitis	Pellagrous rash	
Pyridoxine	Peripheral neuropathy ? 'Burning feet' syndrome Infantile convulsions	Nil	Nil	Cheilosis Glossitis	Atrophy of epidermis and hair follicles Naso-labial seborrhoea	Hypochromic anaemia Lymphopenia
Pantothenic acid	? 'Burning feet' syndrome	Intestinal atony	Nil	Nil	? As above	

Table 4.1 *(continued)*

Vitamin deficiency	CNS	Gut	Eye (anterior segment	Mouth	Skin	Other
Vitamin B_{12}	Peripheral neuropathy Myelopathy Encephalopathy Optic neuropathy	? Impaired absorption of vitamin B_{12} itself	Nil	Glossitis	? Hyperpigmentation	Megaloblastic anaemia
Folic acid	Probably none	Nil	Nil	Nil	? Hyperpigmentation	Megaloblastic anaemia
Ascorbic acid	Cerebral and intraneural haemorrhage (rare)	? Haemorrhage	Nil	Gingivitis	Petechiae Ecchymoses	Microscopic haematuria

Table 4.2

Some Effects of Vitamin Deficiency (Fat-soluble Vitamins)

Vitamin deficiency	CNS	Gut	Eye (anterior) segment	Mouth	Skin	Other
Vitamin A	Impaired dark-adaptation Uyemura's syndrome	Nil	Xerophthalmia Keratomalacia	Nil	Follicular hyperkeratosis ? Phrynoderma	Haematuria 'Bronchitis'
Vitamin D	Osteomalacic myopathy	Nil	Nil	Nil	Nil	Rickets, osteomalacia
Vitamin E	?Myopathy	Nil	Nil	Nil	Nil	?Haemolytic anaemia Very low levels in Bassen–Kornzweig disease (no causal relationship)
Vitamin K	Cerebral haemorrhage Retinal haemorrhage	Nil	Nil	Nil	Petechiae Ecchymoses	Nil

Table 4.3
Normal Concentrations of Vitamins in Whole Blood, Serum and Erythrocytes

	Mean concentration (ng/ml) and 95% range		Reference
Thiamine (total)			
Whole blood	28	(20–75)	Baker et al, 1964
Serum	21	(18–62)	,, ,, ,,
Erythrocytes	100	–	Marks, 1968
Riboflavine (total)			
Whole blood	66·8	(49–104)	Kerppola, 1955
Erythrocytes	224	(180–262)	Burch et al, 1948
Nicotinic acid			
Whole blood	–	(3900–9600)	Baker and Sobotka, 1962
Whole blood	6550	(5320–7780)	Goldsmith, 1964
Serum	–	(16–50)	Baker and Sobotka, 1962
Pyridoxal phosphate			
Plasma (age: < 1)	16·3	(6·5–57·1)	Hamfelt, 1964
Plasma (age: 20–29)	11·3	(3·8–21·6)	,, ,,
Plasma (age: 30–59)	7·1	(2·4–12·4)	,, ,,
Plasma (age: > 60)	3·4	(0–13·5)	,, ,,
B_6 (total activity)			
Whole blood	37	(20–45)	Baker et al, 1966
Serum	44	(30–80)	,, ,, ,,
Erythrocytes	20	(13–31)	,, ,, ,,
Pantothenic acid			
Whole blood	560	(220–1900)	Baker and Sobotka, 1962
Whole blood	464	(382–546)	Hatano, 1962
Vitamin B_{12}			
Whole blood (pg/ml)	–	(120–450)	Baker et al, 1961
Serum (pg/ml)	611	(277–945)	Barakat and Ekins, 1963
Serum (pg/ml)	356	(100–900)	Mollin and Ross, 1957
Erythrocytes (pg/ml)	74	(59–88)	Baker et al, 1957
*Folate**			
Whole blood	89	(47–149)	Rachmilewitz, 1965
Serum	8·2	(3·5–15·0)	,, ,,
Erythrocytes	327	(184–655)	Mollin and Hoffbrand, 1965
Vitamin A			
Serum	324	(207–471)	Campbell and Tonks, 1962
Vitamin D			
Serum (children) (iu/l)	–	(860–2100)	Job et al, 1967
Serum (adults) (iu/l)	2000	(700–3100)	Thomas et al, 1959
Vitamin E			
Serum (men)	10·6	(5·6–15·6)	Bieri et al, 1964
Serum (women)	10·4	(5·0–15·8)	,, ,, ,,

* *L. casei* method.

Vitamin B_{12} deficiency may also be responsible. A search for a gastrectomy scar should certainly be carried out before any patient is certified insane. *Stupor* may occasionally be due to the rare condition of central pontine myelinolysis, which, although of unknown aetiology, occurs too often in a context of water and electrolyte imbalance and of nutritional deficiency for the association to be fortuitous.

General examination and clinical assessment of the patient may provide useful clues as to whether a vitamin deficiency is present. The effects of various vitamin deficiencies on the nervous system, eye, mouth, skin, gut, blood, and other tissues are summarised in Tables 4.1 and 4.2. Table 4.3 provides information not readily available in tabular form concerning 'normal' concentrations of various vitamins in whole blood, serum, or erythrocytes. How these vitamin deficiencies arise in the context of gastrointestinal disease, and how they affect the nervous system will be discussed under the heading of each particular vitamin. These sections will also include information concerning the biochemical diagnosis of the relevant vitamin deficiencies. Details relating to the microbiological assay of vitamins are beyond the scope of this study. The reader is referred to special articles relating to such neurologically significant vitamins as thiamine (Pearson, 1967a), riboflavine (Pearson, 1967b), nicotinic acid (Goldsmith and Miller, 1967), pyridoxine (Sauberlich, 1967), pantothenic acid (Bird and Thompson, 1967), and vitamin B_{12} (Skeggs, 1967).

Referring to the vitamins, Greengard (1970) wrote that 'no class of drugs has been the target of so much quackery, misunderstanding, misrepresentation and misuse'. One might add that there are few drugs in relation to which there is such a wide disparity between the extent of prescription and the paucity of clinical research relating to absorption and storage *in man.* Very little is known, for instance, about how certain components of the B complex (such as pantothenic acid) are absorbed under normal and pathological conditions, or about where certain other components, such as nicotinic acid, are stored. We have found no systematic study of the effects of diarrhoea on vitamin absorption. The detailed studies of absorption *in vitro*, using everted sacs of *rat* intestine—or the *in vivo* studies of *rabbits* with Thiry-Vella fistulae—are only marginally relevant to our clinical preoccupations.

References

Baker, H., Frank, O., Fennelly, J. J. & Leevy, C. M. (1964). A method for assaying thiamine status in man and animals. *American Journal of Clinical Nutrition*, **14**, 197–201.

Baker, H., Frank, O., Ning, M., Gellene, R. A., Hutner, S. H. & Leevy, C. M. (1966). A protozoological method for detecting clinical vitamin B_6 deficiency. *American Journal of Clinical Nutrition*, **18**, 123–133.

Baker, H., Frank, O., Pasher, I., Sobotka, H. & Hutner, S. H. (1961). Physiology—vitamin levels in blood and serum. *Nature*, **191**, 78.

Baker, H., Pasher, I., Sobotka, H., Hutner, S. H., Aaronson, S. & Ziffer, H. (1957). Vitamin B_{12} distribution between plasma and cells. *Nature*, **180**, 1043–1044.

Baker, H. & Sobotka, H. (1962). Microbiological assay methods for vitamins. *Advances in Clinical Chemistry*, **5**, 173–235

Barakat, R. M. & Ekins, R. P. (1963). An isotopic method for the determination of vitamin B_{12} levels in blood. *Blood*, **21**, 70–79.

Bieri, J. G., Teets, L., Belavady, B. & Andrews, E. L. (1964). Serum vitamin E levels in a normal adult population in the Washington D.C. area. *Proceedings of the Society for Experimental Biology and Medicine*, **117,** 131–132.

Bird, O. D. & Thompson, R. Q. (1967). Pantothenic acid. In *The Vitamins (Chemistry, Physiology, Pathology, Methods)*, ed. György, P. & Pearson, W. N., Vol. II, Ch. 7. New York: Academic Press.

Burch, H. B., Bessey, O. A. & Lowry, O. H. (1948). Fluorometric measurements of riboflavin and its natural derivatives in small quantities of blood serum and cells. *Journal of Biological Chemistry*, **175,** 457–470.

Campbell, D. A. & Tonks, E. L. (1962). Biochemical findings in retinitis pigmentosa. *British Journal of Ophthalmology*, **46,** 151–164.

Cooke, W. T. & Smith, W. T. (1966). Neurological disorders associated with adult coeliac disease, *Brain*, **89,** 683–722.

Cooke, W. T., Cox, E. V., Fone, D. J., Meynell, M. J. & Gaddie, R. (1963). The clinical and metabolic significance of jejunal diverticula. *Gut*, **4,** 115–131.

Goldsmith, G. A. (1964). *Nutrition* (Vitamins, Nutrient Requirements and Food Selections), ed. Beaton, G. H. & McHenry, E. W., Vol. 2, p. 109. New York: Academic Press.

Goldsmith, G. A. & Miller, O. N. (1967). Niacin. In *The Vitamins (Chemistry, Physiology, Pathology, Methods)*, ed. György, P. & Pearson, W. N., Vol. II, Ch. 5. New York: Academic Press.

Greengard, P. (1970). Water soluble vitamins. I. The vitamin B complex. In *The Pharmacological Basis of Therapeutics*, ed. Goodman, L. S. & Gilman, A. 4th edition. Ch. 73. New York: MacMillan.

Hamfelt, A. (1964). Age variation of vitamin B_6 metabolism in man. *Clinica chimica acta*, **10,** 48–54.

Hatano, M. (1962). Microbiological assay of pantothenic acid in blood and urine. *Journal of Vitamin (Kyoto)* **8,** 134–142.

Job, J. C., Milhaud, G., Autener, I. & Rossier, A. (1967). Les anomalies du métabolisme calcique chez les enfants hypothyroïdiens. *Semaine des Hôpitaux de Paris* (Annales de Pédiatrie), **43,** 2412–2417 (*P* 648–653).

Kerppola, W. (1955). The content of riboflavin and riboflavin-containing coenzymes in the blood in health and in various diseases in particular schizophrenia, neurocirculatory asthenia and tuberculosis. *Acta medica Scandinavica*, **153,** 33–48.

Marks, J. (1968). *The Vitamins in Health and Disease*. London: Churchill.

Mollin, D. L. & Hoffbrand, A. V. (1965). The diagnosis of folate deficiency. *Series haematologica*, **3,** 1–18.

Mollin, D. L. & Ross, G. I. M. (1957). Europäisches Symposium über Vitamin B_{12} und Intrinsic Factor (Hamburg, 1956). In *Vitamin B_{12} und Intrinsic Factor*, ed. Heinrich, H. C. p. 413. Stuttgart: Enke.

Pearson, W. N. (1967a). Thiamine. In *The Vitamins (Chemistry, Physiology, Pathology, Methods)* ed. György, P. & Pearson, W. N., Vol. II, Ch. 3. New York: Academic Press.

Pearson, W. N. (1967b). Riboflavin. In *The Vitamins (Chemistry, Physiology, Pathology, Methods)* ed. György, P. & Pearson, W. N., Vol. II, Ch. 4. New York: Academic Press.

Rachmilewitz, M. (1965). Folic acid deficiency: clinical studies. *Series haematologica*, **3,** 19–37.

Sauberlich, H. E. (1967). Pyridoxine. In *The Vitamins (Chemistry, Physiology, Pathology, Methods)*, ed. György, P. & Pearson, W. N., Vol. II, Ch. 6. New York: Academic Press.

Skeggs, H. R. (1967). Vitamin B_{12}. In *The Vitamins (Chemistry, Physiology, Pathology, Methods)*, ed. György, P. & Pearson, W. N., Vol. II, Ch. 9. New York: Academic Press.

Thomas, W. C., Morgan, H. G., Connor, T. B., Haddock, L., Bills, C. E. & Howard, J. E. (1959). Studies on antiricketic activity in sera from patients with disorders of calcium metabolism and preliminary observations on the mode of transport of vitamin D in human serum. *Journal of Clinical Investigation*, **38,** 1078–1085.

Williams, J. A., Hall, G. S., Thompson, A. G. & Cooke, W. T. (1969). Neurological disease after partial gastrectomy. *British Medical Journal*, **2,** 210–212.

CHAPTER FIVE

Vitamin B_{12} Deficiency in Gastrointestinal Disease

SOME BIOLOGICAL CONSIDERATIONS

Vitamin B_{12}-dependent reactions in man

Twenty-two years elapsed between the report by Minot and Murphy (1926) that orally administered liver had a beneficial effect in pernicious anaemia and the isolation of a red crystalline substance from such tissue by Smith and Parker (1948) in Britain and Rickes and his co-workers (1948) in the United States. Progress was slow because there was no naturally occurring animal disease resembling pernicious anaemia. Patients with pernicious anaemia in relapse had to be used for assays and they did not prove very satisfactory laboratory animals. The active substance, vitamin B_{12}, was moreover only present in liver in minute amounts. A further quarter of a century has now passed and our knowledge of the function of vitamin B_{12} in man remains fragmentary: an untidy miscellany of chemical, pathological and clinical data only marginally related to the vast vitaminological literature documenting its role in the lives of bacteria. Detailed reviews and monographs dealing with the biochemistry of vitamin B_{12} have been published (Smith, 1965; Moore and Folkers, 1968; Barker, 1968; Weissbach and Taylor, 1968; Hogenkamp, 1968).

Vitamin B_{12} is essential to human nutrition. Deficiency results in certain well-defined clinical manifestations, and the main brunt falls on haemopoietic tissue, epithelial surfaces, and the nervous system. The first two have been extensively studied but, for obvious reasons of accessibility, the biochemical effects of vitamin B_{12} deficiency on the nervous systems have scarcely been investigated at all.

Vitamin B_{12} belongs to a group of compounds known as cobalamins. Deoxyadenosylcobalamin (the main form of dietary vitamin B_{12}) and methylcobalamin (the major form of vitamin B_{12} found in human plasma) are known to be involved in a large number of enzyme systems in bacteria (Hoffbrand,

1971).* To date there are only two definite enzymic reactions, in man, in which vitamin B_{12} derivatives have been shown to participate as cofactors. The first is responsible for the conversion of L-methylmalonyl-CoA to succinyl-CoA. In this reaction 5′-deoxyadenosyl-B_{12} acts as coenzyme for the enzyme L-methylmalonyl-CoA mutase. The second is the methylation of homocysteine to methionine, a step in which methyl-B_{12} acts as a coenzyme in the methyltransferase reaction, a reaction also involving folate. Neither of these reactions, it must be stressed, can as yet be related to the neuropathology of human vitamin B_{12} deficiency.

Although the effects of vitamin B_{12} deficiency on peripheral nerves and spinal cord are profound, very little is known about how they arise, at the level of molecular biology. Many workers have produced hypotheses attempting to link the sparse biochemical data concerning known B_{12}-dependent enzymic reactions in man with the neurological effects of adult vitamin B_{12} deficiency, but so far none of these explanations has found any experimental support. Cynics have even claimed that one of the main effects of vitamin B_{12} deficiency on the human nervous system is its hypothesis-producing effect.

Vitamin B_{12} and nucleic acid metabolism

In human cells vitamin B_{12} is essential to the formation of nucleic acids, and especially to the formation of the DNA precursor thymidine monophosphate. Dividing cells (i.e. cells that have to synthesise chromosomal DNA rapidly) show the effects of vitamin B_{12} deficiency fairly early, in the form of macrocytic change. Macrocytes show enlargement both of nucleus and of cytoplasm. The cause of the nuclear enlargement is not known. It is probably not the result of an abnormality of mitotic division, for tetra- or polyploidy is not found, but may perhaps be a consequence of an alteration in the chemical composition of the nucleus, possibly related to a change in the rate of DNA synthesis. In vitamin B_{12} deficiency such macrocytosis has been reported in the buccal mucosa, in the mucosae of the tongue, nose, bronchi, urinary tract and vagina (Boddington and Spriggs, 1959) and in the gastric mucosa (Graham and Rheault, 1954).

In certain bacteria, vitamin B_{12} is involved in the operation of ribonucleotide reductases which catalyse the conversion of ribonucleotides to deoxyribonucleotides, the substrates necessary for DNA synthesis. Since the megaloblast is a cell with an increased RNA/DNA ratio, Beck (1968) suggested that a similar disorder might account for the impaired DNA synthesis in the bone marrow of vitamin B_{12}-depleted patients. The hypothesis, although attractive, has not so far been substantiated. In fact when vitamin B_{12} is added to cultures of bone marrow from patients with pernicious anaemia, there is no stimulation of ribonucleotide reductase activity (Silber et al, 1970).

That vitamin B_{12} deficiency impairs DNA synthesis seems well established.

* It is doubtful whether cyanocobalamin, which is the form in which vitamin B_{12} was first crystallised, and which is the most stable form of the vitamin, ever occurs in normal human tissues. It probably represents an isolation artefact, due to the presence of traces of cyanide in the charcoal used during the purification process.

While this may explain such concomitants of vitamin B_{12} deficiency as megaloblastic anaemia, leucopenia and glossitis, it is not helpful in relation to the nervous system. The neurones of the adult nervous system do not divide. Neuronal mitoses are never seen, while innumerable autoradiographic studies over the last 15 years have demonstrated an insignificantly low level of incorporation of ^{3}H-thymidine, and hence of DNA synthesis. It would, in fact, be hard to imagine any tissue where a theory linking vitamin B_{12} deficiency to rapid cell division would be less likely to be relevant than the human nervous system.

Vitamin B_{12} deficiency and methylmalonic acid excretion

In 1955 Flavin, Ortiz and Ochoa showed that propionic acid in animal tissues was metabolised to succinic acid via an intermediary compound: methylmalonic acid (MMA). The isomerisation of MMA to succinic acid involves a vitamin B_{12} cofactor. Cox and White (1962) and Kahn et al (1965) showed an increased urinary excretion of MMA in vitamin B_{12} deficiency and Gompertz, Jones and Knowles (1967) showed that this could be considerably increased following the oral administration of a 10 g valine load. An increased MMA excretion seems to be a fairly specific biochemical index of vitamin B_{12} deficiency. It is not a particularly sensitive index, however, since many patients with mild vitamin B_{12} deficiency (assessed by low serum vitamin B_{12} levels or even early megaloblastic anaemia due to vitamin B_{12} deficiency) may show no excretion of MMA, even after a valine load (Brozovic et al, 1967; Chanarin et al, 1973).

Although the administration of folic acid to patients with pernicious anaemia will produce a haematological response, it will not: (a) raise the serum B_{12} level; (b) diminish the excretion of MMA; or (c) improve the neurological complications, which it may in fact aggravate. From what has already been said it is obvious that some mechanism other than impaired DNA synthesis must be responsible for the neuropathology of vitamin B_{12} deficiency. Cox and White (1962) suggested that this mechanism might be related to MMA excretion. Vivacqua et al (1966) report that of 25 vitamin B_{12}-depleted patients without neurological symptoms, 24 excreted less than 150 mg of MMA per day, whereas two out of three patients with severe neurological complications excreted more than 450 mg/day. They argued that an accumulation of propionate or methylmalonate in nerve tissue might in some way impair the metabolism of neurones. Again, the hypothesis is attractive, but it could be argued that it is precisely the more severely B_{12}-depleted patients who would be likely to show both neurological complications and increased MMA excretion, without these two features being related in any directly causal sense. Moreover, considerable and persistent MMA excretion may be seen in some infants with methylmalonic acidurias who have no evidence of chronic neurological disease (Mahoney and Rosenberg, 1970; Rosenberg, 1972).

Vitamin B_{12} and the methylation of RNA

It has been claimed (Walerych, Venkataraman and Johnson, 1966) that methyl-B_{12} may take part in the methylation of transfer RNA in mammalian systems. This work has not been confirmed, but if corroborated could be of considerable significance. RNA turnover in neurones is, of course, very high. The Nissl substance in the neuronal perikaryon is RNA, and when the axon is damaged the ensuing chromatolysis, or 'axonal reaction', is a measure of the consequent disruption of RNA—and protein—synthesis. Survival of the axon, which in some neurones has a mass hundreds of times that of the perikaryon, is dependent upon maintenance (or restoration after such damage) of the normal high rate of RNA synthesis and the centrifugal transfer of proteins by axoplasmic flow. If lack of vitamin B_{12} were to lead to a disturbance of RNA synthesis, it is not surprising that the repercussions should be felt in those parts of the nervous system most at risk: long axons.

It is, of course, possible that the neurological repercussions of vitamin B_{12} deficiency are not due to any of these mechanisms but to a defect in some essential transport mechanism or enzyme reaction as yet unidentified. A recent review on the biochemistry of B_{12}-mediated reactions in man (Silber and Moldow, 1970) concluded that 'the pathogenesis of the neurological lesions in vitamin B_{12} deficiency remains obscure'. It is unlikely that either clinicians or pathologists will be able to throw much light upon this darkness.

Neurological effects in man

We consider the neurological picture of vitamin B_{12} deficiency to comprise, first, a mainly sensory peripheral neuropathy; secondly, a rather stereotyped myelopathy; and thirdly, somewhat variable cerebral manifestations (encephalopathy), including optic nerve involvement. In the subsequent sections of this chapter we will review these neurological symptoms and signs in some detail, stressing their more controversial aspects and seeking to define the diagnostic criteria we have adopted for including or rejecting cases previously described in the literature. We will also evaluate, again in detail, the significance to the neurologist of the various gastrointestinal causes of vitamin B_{12} deficiency.

We must emphasise that Addisonian pernicious anaemia, which is due to failure of intrinsic factor production consequent on autoimmune atrophic gastritis, is probably still the most frequent and important of these causes. We will not be discussing the disease itself in this monograph as we have nothing to add to the excellent reviews recently published on the subject (Chanarin, 1970; Hoffbrand, 1971). Although the pattern of recognised causes of vitamin B_{12} deficiency may be changing, the clinical features (and in particular the neurological features) clearly are not. They need looking at anew, however, in the light of modern neurophysiological concepts and of current investigative techniques. Our survey of the older cases will of necessity be largely an historical one. If not definitive, we hope it will at least be provocative.

In our discussion of the various disorders other than Addisonian pernicious anaemia that may be associated with vitamin B_{12} deficiency we will follow a certain pattern. Each section will comprise an explanation of the pathophysiology of the absorptive defect in the condition concerned, followed by a review of the relevant neurological literature and a short synopsis. The management of the primary conditions responsible for the B_{12} deficiency is beyond the scope of this monograph. The whole section on vitamin B_{12} will conclude with some general comments, in the course of which we will list some of the pitfalls encountered in the recognition of this condition.

PERIPHERAL NEUROPATHY IN VITAMIN B_{12} DEFICIENCY

It is remarkable how little is known about the peripheral neuropathy complicating vitamin B_{12} deficiency in man. Whereas hundreds of reports have been published about diabetic neuropathy, or concerning the neurological complications of thiamine deficiency, the hard facts about how vitamin B_{12} deficiency affects human peripheral nerves are confined to perhaps a dozen publications.

Today, in industrialised countries, vitamin B_{12} deficiency is usually recognised early by haematologists, gastroenterologists or general physicians. Appropriate therapy is prescribed before neurological complications have had time to appear. When neurological symptoms or signs develop they are seldom investigated by modern techniques of nerve biopsy or electromyography *before* specific therapy is instituted. Neurologists in fact seldom have a chance to study such patients in any depth. Their number, moreover, is unlikely to increase. On the contrary, as physicians become more aware of the various contexts in which vitamin B_{12} deficiency is to be anticipated the number of cases with neuropathy will probably diminish. Opportunities for necropsy studies in vitamin B_{12}-deficient patients are even less likely to occur. Between 1919 and 1943, 39 necropsies were performed on patients with 'subacute combined degeneration of the spinal cord' dying at a London teaching hospital dealing with nervous diseases. Between 1944 and 1972 the figure had fallen to three.

For many years the very existence of peripheral neuropathy in Addisonian pernicious anaemia was disputed. Many older authors attributed all the neurological complications of the disease to involvement of the spinal cord (Minnich, 1892; Nonne, 1895; Bramwell, 1915; Bremer, 1935) although there was always speculation as to the frequency and significance of an associated peripheral neuropathy (Woltmann, 1919; Hamilton and Nixon, 1921; McAlpine, 1929; Ungley, 1949; Victor and Lear, 1956).

In our opinion peripheral neuropathy is probably the commonest neurological complication of vitamin B_{12} deficiency. This statement, implicit in a number of reports, has not, to our knowledge, ever been made explicitly. The evidence is worth discussing in some detail. The emergence of this view has long been delayed because of the combined effects of two outdated clinical concepts, namely (a) that the main neurological impact of vitamin B_{12} deficiency is on the spinal cord, and (b) that lesions of the posterior columns can abolish tendon reflexes. Together, these beliefs created a conceptual straightjacket, now only gradually being discarded.

Clinical evidence

That sensory symptoms are common in patients with vitamin B_{12} deficiency is of course widely known. Woltmann (1919) reported sensory symptoms in

80 per cent of 150 patients with pernicious anaemia seen at the Mayo Clinic, 'regardless of whether or not involvement of the nervous system could be demonstrated objectively'. The prevalence of neurological signs is less clearly established, figures varying from 30 per cent (Grinker, 1926) to 80 per cent (Hurst, 1934).

Little is known of the aetiology of these paraesthesiae. Some may be related to the associated anaemia, particularly if it is severe. Discussing pernicious anaemia, James Collier (1925) warned that it was 'highly dangerous' to incriminate organic neurological changes as an explanation for peripheral subjective sensations in anaemic patients. He claimed that tingling and numbness were of common occurrence in every variety of anaemia and were not indications of pathological alterations in the nervous system, a viewpoint echoed by Grinker (1926) who emphasised that severe iron deficiency anaemia might be associated with distal paraesthesiae that subsided as the anaemia was corrected. The occurrence of tetany in some cases of malabsorption should not be forgotten and may occasionally lead to diagnostic confusion.

Neurologists will of course be familiar with patients in whom sensory symptoms precede the appearance of physical signs of peripheral neuropathy or myelopathy. But it is only when sensory symptoms are associated with abnormal physical signs that involvement of the nervous system can be accepted with that 'minimum' of certainty required if one is to attempt to estimate the prevalence of neurological complications in any given condition. We realise that the adoption of these rather strict criteria will result in an underestimation of the prevalence of such neurological complications, but have felt this to be a lesser evil than the inclusion of patients with neurological symptoms but no definite signs.

The immediate argument centres on whether these neurological symptoms and signs, whether in pernicious anaemia or in other forms of malabsorption of vitamin B_{12}, are of central (myelopathic) or of peripheral origin. Some of the earlier controversies were well summarised by Hamilton and Nixon (1921). McAlpine (1929), in a review of 24 cases of pernicious anaemia with neurological signs, stressed that two varieties of sensory loss might occur, with about equal frequency: (a) diminution or loss of vibration sense, either alone or occasionally accompanied by impaired postural sensibility in the fingers and toes, other forms of sensation being unaffected; (b) impairment of all forms of sensation in the periphery of the limbs, of 'glove and stocking' distribution. In over half the cases reviewed the tendon reflexes were absent in the lower limbs. McAlpine shrewdly criticised the notion, then widely held (and still propounded today in some quarters) that lesions of the posterior columns abolish reflexes. He stressed that pathological evidence did not support the occurrence of lesions in the posterior roots or posterior root entry zones, which might have explained the areflexia, and concluded that 'interruption of the reflex arc does not take place in the cord or posterior root, but in the peripheral nerve'.

In an excellent clinical study of 38 patients with pernicious anaemia and neurological symptoms, van der Sheer and Koek (1938) argued strongly for the existence of a peripheral neuropathy. While readily admitting that changes in the posterior and lateral columns of the spinal cord could account for many of the neurological findings in their cases, they concluded that it was seldom possible to explain the full clinical picture on the basis of myelopathy alone. Patients with pernicious anaemia were often found to have:

(a) superficial sensory impairment (i.e. deficits of tactile, pain and thermal senses) of distal distribution, in addition to the more 'classical' impairment of postural sense and of vibration sense;
(b) burning and painful dysaesthesiae, occasionally with hyperalgesia;
(c) a topographical distribution of sensory signs more in keeping with neuropathy than with either radiculopathy or myelopathy;
(d) tender peripheral nerves;
(e) early impairment or loss of ankle jerks;
(f) distal weakness out of proportion to any pyramidal deficit.

The authors pointed out that if the clinical picture was to be fully understood and an explanation found for the acroparaesthesiae, the pain, the impairment of cutaneous sensibility for all forms increasing distally, the pareses without pyramidal signs also increasing towards the periphery, the reflex reduction in the first stages of the disease, 'lesions in the peripheral nerves must be assumed, not as an exception but as a rule; they occur just as frequently as, and at the onset possibly more frequently than, the combined tract disease'. We concur with these views, with reservations concerning the frequency of lower motor neurone deficit which, in our experience, is rare.

If one accepts the view that peripheral neuropathy is often the cause of sensory disturbances in vitamin B_{12} deficiency, one should not of course forget that very similar symptoms may arise on a myelopathic basis. Older physicians will remember, for instance, the frequency with which similar paraesthesiae, in pernicious anaemia, might ascend from the feet and soon encircle the lower part of the trunk, sometimes with a definite upper level (Symonds, 1972). The differential diagnosis between myelopathy and peripheral neuropathy in patients with vitamin B_{12} deficiency may be difficult and is discussed in greater detail further on.

Dynes and Norcross (1943) defined the differential diagnostic problem in some detail. Using fairly strict criteria (tenderness on pressure over nerve trunks, a loss or diminution of tendon reflexes starting distally, distal impairment of tactile sense and of pain sense) they found unmistakable evidence of peripheral neuropathy in 23 per cent of 92 patients with pernicious anaemia. About the same proportion were thought to have evidence of combined system disease without peripheral neuropathy. Impaired vibration sense seems to have been taken as evidence of myelopathy and we feel that the figures therefore underestimate the prevalence of peripheral neuropathy. It is well known for instance that electrical evidence of peripheral neuropathy is often found (for instance, in conditions such as diabetes) without gross clinical signs, or in patients in whom the only clinical evidence of involvement of the nervous system consists of impaired vibration sense at the ankles and/or diminution of the ankle jerks.

Richmond and Davidson (1958) defined 'subacute combined degeneration' (SCD) as a disease of the spinal cord 'invariably associated with peripheral neuritis'. We accept this conception, which has wide implications. We would go even further and suggest that peripheral neuropathy due to vitamin B_{12} deficiency may occur without evidence of myelopathy.

In summary, the clinical evidence suggests that peripheral neuropathy is common in patients with vitamin B_{12} deficiency and sensory symptoms, and that recognition of its prevalence may long have been delayed as a result of faulty interpretation of physical signs.

Pathological evidence

In 1921, Hamilton and Nixon discussed at length the whole question of peripheral nerve involvement in pernicious anaemia. They wrote that in most of the reported cases 'the peripheral nerves had been studied either insufficiently or not at all'. Fifty years later there is little to add. The authors had reviewed the earlier literature. They described seven cases of their own in which histological evidence of peripheral neuropathy had been sought—and found. Commenting on the lack of parallelism that might be encountered between severe symptoms and signs during life and a relatively normal spinal cord at necropsy, they suggested that in these cases there were changes in the peripheral nerves.

Greenfield, an eminent neuropathologist, had written with Buzzard (1921) that the peripheral nerves were not involved in pernicious anaemia. This authoritative assertion was subsequently revised (Greenfield and Carmichael, 1935) when it was shown that peripheral neuropathy was in fact present in four patients with subacute combined degeneration of the spinal cord. The authors had examined biopsies of the terminal branch of the anterior tibial nerve in these four cases and found a reduction in the number of myelin sheaths, affecting predominantly the largest. These findings cannot be granted decisive significance, however, for it has since been shown (Swallow, 1966) that the fibre composition of this particular peripheral nerve is liable to wide variation in normal individuals. Van der Scheer and Koek (1938) also biopsied a cutaneous branch of the anterior tibial nerve in four of their patients with pernicious anaemia. They also found, in each instance, a great reduction in the amount of myelin compared with controls. In one patient the myelin had, in places, virtually disappeared.

Foster (1945) reported necropsy findings in three untreated and one treated case of pernicious anaemia with myelopathy and described biopsy data on one further case. All were found to have histological evidence of peripheral neuropathy manifested by reduction in the number of myelin sheaths and axis cylinders, degeneration of myelin, and increase in Schwann cells and endoneural connective tissue. Axonal reaction changes in the ganglion cells of the posterior root ganglia and degenerative changes in the intramedullary course of afferent posterior root fibres were also present, findings which today suggest that the peripheral neuropathy might have been in part a 'dying back' or axonal process. Foster (1945) shrewdly commented that the improvement of patients with SCD, when given specific therapy, was often stated to be most marked 'when there was a scarcity or absence of pyramidal signs, i.e. when manifestations commonly assigned to dysfunction of the posterior columns predominate'. He suggested that the improvement was in fact due to restoration of peripheral nerve function, a view with which we concur.

Pant, Asbury and Richardson (1968) reviewed the neuropathological data of 40 adequately documented cases of myelopathy complicating Addisonian anaemia seen between 1926 and 1966 at the Massachusetts General Hospital. The wealth of material and breadth of experience in this report is unlikely to be duplicated in the future and the study must in many respects be considered definitive. Unfortunately, however, the 'peripheral' material does not seem to have been processed in a manner that would enable it to be studied by modern neuropathological techniques. Portions of peripheral nerve were available for study in 11 cases, but in only eight patients had this material been systematically sampled. The authors commented that the distal nerves in the limbs were only rarely dissected. They rightly stressed that the interpretation of ordinary histological preparations of peripheral nerve was at best fraught with error. A definite change in the form of fibre loss was seen in only one case. In two other cases there was evidence of denervation atrophy in muscles taken from the leg, but no changes were recognised in the available sections of nerves. There was no comment about segmental demyelination having been either looked for or found. The authors concluded with the tantalising statement that their observations 'cannot be used as evidence either for or against the existence of a significant peripheral nerve lesion in patients with pernicious anaemia'.

In summary, the pathological evidence on the whole suggests that, when specifically sought for, evidence of peripheral neuropathy is usually found in patients with vitamin B_{12} deficiency and neurological symptoms.

Electrophysiological evidence

Gilliatt, Goodman and Willison (1961), in the course of their study of lateral popliteal nerve action potentials in man, investigated four patients with B_{12}-deficiency myelopathy (SCD). Stimulating the anterior tibial nerve at the ankle with a maximal or near maximal shock they failed to record any action potential from the lateral popliteal nerve at the head of the fibula in one case. In two cases the amplitude of the elicited potential was grossly reduced. These first three cases had presented 'mainly a picture of peripheral nerve involvement with flexor plantar responses and superficial sensory loss of stocking distribution'. Their observations would therefore seem to corroborate the existence of a peripheral neuropathy. In the fourth patient a potential of normal latency was recorded. This was the only patient in whom there was unequivocal evidence of spinal cord involvement with 'extensor plantar responses and with preservation of superficial sensation in spite of gross impairment of joint sense'.

Mayer (1965) reported his findings on 53 patients who at some stage or other had had serum vitamin B_{12} levels of less than 100 pg/ml or 'classical pernicious anaemia with histamine-fast achlorhydria that had improved as a result of treatment with liver extract'. Unfortunately only five of his patients were investigated prior to the administration of specific therapy (liver or vitamin B_{12}) and the author's presentation of his data makes it impossible to comment on this particular subgroup. Patients on maintenance therapy who had never had any symptoms or signs of neurological disorder all had normal conduction velocities in the fastest afferent ('sensory') and efferent (motor) fibres of the ulnar, median, deep peroneal and posterior tibial nerves. Patients on maintenance therapy who gave a past history of paraesthesiae but showed no neurological signs or symptoms at the time of examination also had normal conduction velocities.

Thirty-two patients with signs or symptoms 'secondary to central or peripheral nerve dysfunction' at the time of investigation, most of them receiving treatment, showed a reduction of mean conduction velocity in the distal sensory fibres in the median and ulnar nerves. Velocities in proximal motor and sensory fibres were normal, as were conduction velocities in sensory and motor fibres in the posterior tibial and deep peroneal nerves (ankle-to-knee segments). Distal afferent velocities in the lower limbs are more difficult to measure and were not investigated. Conduction velocities were normal in most patients with clinical signs attributed to peripheral neuropathy. Nine of the patients demonstrated defects in nerve conduction, localised to sites of potential chronic compression (wrist, elbow and knee). The study is probably the most extensive one reported to date, although we cannot endorse its underlying assumption that a reduction in conduction velocity is essential for the diagnosis of peripheral neuropathy. Experience with the neuropathies of predominantly 'axonal' type (Gilliatt, 1966) and knowledge of the fact that the nerve action potential may be diminished in patients with normal maximal conduction velocities refute this assumption.

In their review of the myelopathies following partial gastrectomy, Olivarius and Roos (1968) described five patients with clinical evidence of peripheral neuropathy. In two of the three patients in whom electromyography and studies of sensory and motor nerve conduction velocities were carried out there was evidence (unspecified) of 'peripheral neurogenic dysfunction'. The authors implied that vitamin B_{12} deficiency was responsible but as no values of serum vitamin B_{12} were given in these cases they cannot really be adduced as evidence in the discussion of whether B_{12} deficiency causes peripheral neuropathy in man. Some of the neuropathies complicating partial gastrectomy may have an entirely different aetiology (see p. 64).

In an interesting study of peripheral nerve function in proven pernicious anaemia, Lockner et al (1969) studied the size of the median nerve action potential in 27 patients using a carefully described technique. Fourteen of these patients had no sensory symptoms, six had symptoms and no signs and only seven had symptoms and signs. Nearly all the symptoms and signs were in the lower limbs. There was a highly significant reduction in the size of the nerve action potential in patients with pernicious anaemia, taken as a group, compared with that in 117 controls (even after taking into account the slightly higher mean age of the former). In 33 per cent of the patients the amplitude was outside the normal limits. Only 7 per cent of the patients, however, had had upper limb symptoms. Electrical evidence of neuropathy therefore seemed to be some five times as common as symptoms. The authors stressed that they tested an *upper* limb nerve in order to avoid having to use the more uncomfortable lower limb procedures which require the use of repeated stimulation and averaging. They then argued that in mild diffuse neuropathies electrical and clinical signs of neuropathy usually appeared earlier and were more pronounced in the lower limbs. 'If the factor of 5 could be applied to the legs also, where almost half the patients had subjective symptoms, *all* would have had objective signs of neuropathy'. The authors stressed that electrical signs of neuropathy were found in early cases of pernicious anaemia, suggesting that peripheral nerve involvement 'is not exceptional in pernicious anaemia and that neuropathy is not a late complication. It seems to be an early, intrinsic part of the disease'. So common in fact did the Swedish authors believe peripheral involvement to be that they suggested that in a patient with vitamin B_{12} deficiency and sensory symptoms in the legs, the presence of normal nerve action potentials in the arms might suggest a myelopathy as the cause of the patient's symptoms, rather than peripheral neuropathy. In Great Britain, where patients seem more stoical (or less informed) and where physicians seem to be less squeamish (or more rigorous) it should be possible to avoid this circuitous form of argument and to test the matter directly, by measuring the size of the nerve action potentials in the lower limbs!

In summary, the electrophysiological evidence is in keeping with a high prevalence of peripheral neuropathy in patients with vitamin B_{12} deficiency, whether or not they had sensory symptoms.

Animal experiments

It had been known since the early 1950s that demyelinating lesions of the nervous system might occur in vitamin B_{12} deficiency states in chicks, rats and calves (Alexander, 1956). Krohn, Oxnard and Chalmers (1963) and Oxnard (1964) then showed that primates maintained in captivity on strict vegetarian diets showed a rapid fall in serum B_{12} levels. Fed clean vegetables (i.e. vegetables without particles of soil), housed under optimum conditions of cage hygiene (which reduce the opportunities for coprophagy) and denied the insect ingredient of their 'normal' diet, some animals developed neurological signs. This led to a reinvestigation of the whole subject of 'cage paralysis', known for many years to affect captive monkeys and apes.

The condition had been originally described by Brooks (1903) and Rothmann (1906), amplified in the descriptions of Campbell and Cleland (1919), and well reviewed by Innes and Saunders (1962). In a crucial experiment, Oxnard and Smith (1966) studied 15 rhesus monkeys kept for variable but usually prolonged periods on a strict vegetarian diet. After many years on this regime five animals developed frank paralysis (group I). The account is worth reading if only as a description of how to carry out a neurological examination on *Macaca mulatta.* At postmortem these monkeys showed a spongiform demyelination of the posterior and lateral columns of the spinal cord without significant gliosis. In three of these five cases there was 'severe, patchy, active sudanophilic demyelination of the peripheral nerves', most marked distally. Seven of the original monkeys, also followed up for long periods, had shown no paralysis (group II) but four of them were found at necropsy to have qualitatively similar changes in both spinal cord and peripheral nerves, although of lesser severity. Even two of three captive monkeys, on the vegetarian diet for less than two years (group III) showed mild but unequivocal changes of a similar kind. All the monkeys developed low serum B_{12} levels, but no anaemia. Four additional paralysed monkeys were not sacrificed, but given parenteral cyanocobalamin. In all there was considerable objective improvement.

Subsequent studies (Oxnard, Smith and Torres, 1969, 1970; Torres, Smith and Oxnard, 1971) have amplified these findings and documented this experimental peripheral neuropathy in considerable detail. They confirmed that severe neuropathological lesions might be present not only in the few paralysed animals but also in functionally normal monkeys that had at some time or other been deficient in vitamin B_{12}. Using modern methods of staining and teasing individual nerve fibres, of measuring internodal lengths and fibre diameters, and of estimating mean fibre-densities they showed that segmental demyelination was the main lesion and that it was usually associated with evidence of remyelination. Lesions ranged in severity from random involvement of Schwann cells to axonal degeneration in the worst affected. There was no indication of selective distal involvement of axons ('dying back').

Conclusions

Peripheral neuropathy is common in patients with vitamin B_{12} deficiency who exhibit neurological symptoms or signs. This statement, never to our knowledge explicitly made before, is supported by clinical, pathological and electrophysiological evidence, and by the results of induced vitamin B_{12} deficiency in primates.

MYELOPATHY IN VITAMIN B_{12} DEFICIENCY

It is difficult to assess how often subacute combined degeneration of the spinal cord (SCD)—perhaps better referred to as myelopathy due to vitamin

Table 5.1

Vitamin B_{12} Deficiency Myelopathy in Conditions other than Addisonian Pernicious Anaemia

	Cases reported	Accepted	Inadequate data	Rejected	Necropsies in accepted cases
Nutritional	7	2	3	2	1
Total gastrectomy	8	3	4	1	2
Partial gastrectomy	71	16	39	16	0
Gastric carcinoma, gastritis	9	0	0	9	0
Congenital intrinsic factor deficiency	3	1	0	2	0
Diverticulosis	6	4	1	1	0
Gastroenterostomy	12	0	9	3	0
Fistulae, strictures, and stagnant loop	9	3	3	3	2
Enteritis, resection	2	2	0	0	1
Fish tapeworm	2	0	2	0	0
Congenital B_{12} malabsorption	2	2	0	0	0
TOTAL	131	33	61	37	6

Table 5.2

Published Cases of Myelopathy Attributed to Nutritional Vitamin B_{12} Deficiency

	Number of cases	Accepted	Inadequate data	Rejected	Lowest serum B_{12} (pg/ml)	Necropsy (spinal cord)	Comments on rejected cases
Badenoch (1954)	1		1				
Smith (1962)	2		2		142 176		
Connor and Pirola (1963)	1 (Case 2)			1			Cervical spondylosis with myelopathy not excluded
Riley (1966)	1			1	71		Multiple sclerosis plus dietary hypovitaminosis B_{12}
Verjaal and Timmerman-van den Bos (1967)	1	1			20	+	
Misra and Fallowfield (1971)	1	1			71		

Table 5.3

Published Cases of Myelopathy Attributed to Total Gastrectomy

	Number of cases	Accepted	Inadequate data	Rejected	Lowest serum B_{12} (pg/ml)	Necropsy (spinal cord)	Comments on rejected cases
Dennig (1929)	1	1				+	
Meyer et al (1941)	1	1					
MacDonald et al (1947) quoting S. F. Marshall	1		1				
Beebe and Meneely (1949)	1			1			No abnormal CNS signs
Paulson and Harvey (1954)	1		1				
MacLean and Sundberg (1956)	2		2				Cases 4 and 15
Pant et al (1968)	1	1				+ (Case 28)	

Table 5.4

Published Cases of Myelopathy Attributed to Partial Gastrectomy

	Number of cases	Accepted	Inadequate data	Rejected	Lowest serum B_{12} (pg/ml)	Necropsy spinal cord	Comments on rejected cases
Rowlands and Simpson (1932)	2	1 (Case 2)		1			Positive blood Wassermann CSF not examined
Schneider and Carey (1928)	2		2				
Salus (1932)	1	1 (Case 3)					
Hartfall (1934)	3	1	2				
Salus and Reiman (1934)	2	1		1			No sensory signs in lower limbs Ankle clonus
Ross et al (1948)	1			1 (Case 4)			No pyramidal signs Probably peripheral neuropathy
Bastrup–Madsen (1954)	1			1 (Case 1)			Time relationship incompatible with diagnosis
Badenoch et al (1953)	3		3		35 70		
Alexeieff (1957)	1			1			No pyramidal signs Probably peripheral neuropathy
Knox and Delamore (1960)	1	1			90		
Fone et al (1961)	1		1				
Deller and Witts (1962)	2		2		< 150 < 150		
Weir and Gattenby (1963)	2	1 (Case 2)		1 (Case 1)	87		No pyramidal signs Probably peripheral neuropathy
Cox et al (1963)	1		1		40		
Olivarius and Roos (1965)	28		28				
Olivarius and Roos (1968)	5	3		2	60 180 100		Case 3: Pyramidal signs probably of cerebral origin Case 5: Peripheral neuropathy plus radiculopathy from lumber spondylosis
Chanarin (1969)	1	1			40		
Williams et al (1969)	14	6		8	198 40 160 35		No pyramidal signs Probably peripheral neuropathy

Table 5.5

Published Cases of Myelopathy Attributed to Gastric Lesions other than Gastrectomy

	Number of cases	Accepted	Inadequate data	Rejected	Lowest serum B_{12} (pg/ml)	Necropsy (spinal cord)	Comments on rejected cases
Gastric carcinoma							
Brandes (1921)			1				
Waterfield and Shackle (1923)	1			1		+ (no data)	Wrong time relationships
Garvey and Stern (1924)	1			1		+	,, ,, ,,
Simpson (1931)	1			1		+	,, ,, ,,
Atrophic gastritis							
Wood et al (1964)	5			5			Probably peripheral neuropathy No pyramidal signs
Congenital intrinsic factor deficiency							
Reisner et al (1951)	3	1 (Case 3)		2			Case 1: peripheral neuropathy Case 4: SCD, but due to juvenile pernicious anaemia
Corrosive gastritis							
Alsted (1937)	1			1			No sensory signs in lower limbs Ankle clonus

Table 5.6

Published Cases of Myelopathy Attributed to Structural Lesions of the Small Bowel

	Number of cases	Accepted	Inadequate data	Rejected	Lowest serum B_{12} (pg/ml)	Necropsy (spinal cord)	Comments on rejected cases
Jejunal diverticulosis							
Krevans et al (1954)	1		1				
Badenoch et al (1955)	1 (Case 4)			1			CSF protein 300 mg/100 ml
Cooke et al (1963)	4	4					
Gastroenterostomy							
Glanvill and Hurst (1930)	1			1			No sensory signs No pyramidal signs
Salus (1932)	2			2		+ +	Case 1: No cord pathology Case 2: Bronchial carcinoma (?carcinomatous myelopathy)
Hurst (1934)	9		9				
Fistulae, strictures and stagnant loops							
Little et al (1929)	1			1			No abnormal physical signs
Taylor (1930)	1		1				
Hurst (1933)	1	1					
Woltman and Heck (1937)	1		1			+	
Naish and Kapper (1953)	1 (Case 2)	1				+	
Wilkinson (1955)	1	1					
Halsted et al (1956)	1		1				
Nicol (1960)	1			1			Patient had just completed course of isoniazid
Ragins and Oberhelman (1960)	1			1			Adhesive arachnoiditis at laminectomy

Table 5.7

Published Cases of Myelopathy Attributed to Other Intestinal Lesions Producing Vitamin B_{12} Deficiency

	Number of cases	Accepted*	Inadequate data	Lowest serum B_{12} (pg/ml)	Necropsy (spinal cord)
Intestinal tuberculosis					
Richmond and Davidson (1958)	1 (Case 1)	1			+
Gut resection					
Best (1959)	1	1		25	
Fish tapeworm					
Björkenheim (1966)	2		2		
Congenital B_{12} malabsorption					
François et al. (1967)	1 (Case 1)	1		10	
Brizard and Fraisse (1973)	1	1		40	

* No rejected cases.

B_{12} deficiency—complicates disorders of the gastrointestinal tract other than Addisonian pernicious anaemia. Bremer (1931) once claimed that 'even the greatest industry on the part of a reviewer would not permit a critical survey of this field'. We have, nonetheless, accepted the challenge, seeking to review both the subject as a whole (Table 5.1) and the various disorders that have been incriminated from time to time (Tables 5.2 to 5.7; references relating to the cases mentioned in these tables are not included in the bibliography of this section but will be found under the appropriate sectional headings).

Our search of the literature, mainly confined to that in the English language, yielded 131 cases of alleged 'SCD', 'funicular myelitis', or 'combined system disease' complicating disorders of the gastrointestinal tract, excluding sprue and coeliac disease. Neurological data were totally lacking in 61 cases—bald statements being made that the patient had 'obvious' or 'classical' SCD (we have listed these cases, but cannot comment on them). We have accepted 33 cases on clinical or pathological grounds (or both). Thirty-seven cases were rejected: the data given, far from being 'classical', were so atypical as to allow of a number of alternative and, in our opinion, more probable interpretations. Many of these cases were reported before the significance of cervical spondylosis as a cause of myelopathy in middle or late life was fully appreciated, and before carcinomatous myelopathic syndromes of a non-metastatic nature had been described. To illustrate the uncritical nature of some of these case reports, we have found myelopathy attributed to vitamin B_{12} deficiency when:

(a) there were no abnormal neurological signs during life (Little, Zerfas and Trusler, 1929; Beebe and Meneely, 1949), or just before death (Simpson, 1931);

(b) there were no pathological changes in the cord at post-mortem (Salus, 1932, Case 1);
(c) lumbar laminectomy had shown evidence of adhesive arachnoiditis (Ragins and Oberhelman, 1960);
(d) the blood Wassermann reaction was positive but the CSF had not been examined (Rowlands and Simpson, 1932);
(e) the CSF had been examined, and the protein concentration found to be 300 mg! (Richmond and Davidson, 1958, commenting on the patient described by Badenoch, Bedford and Evans, 1955);
(f) increased (sic!) abdominal reflexes had been taken as evidence of spinal cord disease (Simpson, 1931);
(g) the patient had just completed a course of isoniazid (Nicol, 1960), a drug well known to produce peripheral neuropathy;
(h) the patient was found, at necropsy, to have a bronchial carcinoma and changes confined to the posterior columns of the spinal cord (Salus, 1932, Case 2);
(i) review articles had attributed physical signs of spinal cord disease to various authors, but a survey of the original papers had shown that the original authors had made no such claims (Olivarius and Roos, 1968, commenting on the cases of Welbourn, Hughes and Wells, 1951, and of MacLean, 1957).

It will be seen that only about 25 per cent of the reported cases are sufficiently well-documented to stand up to critical examination. We are aware of the fact that our figures certainly underestimate the prevalence of SCD in these patients. A number of authors mention having seen 'several' or 'many' cases. These have not been included: clinical data were lacking and we were unable to give numerical expression to the claims. We have also excluded reports specifying the number of cases seen, but giving no clinical details.

We must now define our own concept of what may legitimately be covered by the terms 'subacute combined degeneration of the spinal cord' or 'combined system disease'. We have already stated that in our opinion the commonest neurological complication of vitamin B_{12} deficiency is a peripheral neuropathy, that this neuropathy has a predilection for afferent fibres and that it often causes symptoms. We have also mentioned that the main diagnostic problem was to determine whether the patient had peripheral neuropathy or disease of the posterior columns, or both. There were heated controversies in the past as to whether clinical differentiations of this kind were possible. Hyperalgesia of the calves was stated to imply peripheral neuropathy, whereas a 'disproportionate loss of postural sensibility' in the feet, or loss of vibration sense extending to the trunk, were said to imply a lesion of the posterior columns. A positive Lhermitte sign ('electric' dysaesthesiae shooting down the back or into the lower limbs on flexing the neck) would have the same significance. Areflexia, strange as it may seem, was repeatedly claimed to be compatible with disease confined to the posterior columns (Salus, 1932; Wilson, 1954; Victor and Lear, 1956; Davidson, 1957), a view we consider untenable in the light of modern concepts relating to the monosynaptic reflex arc.

The attempt at differentiation between neuropathy and myelopathy on the basis of *sensory* symptoms or signs is rather academic, first because there is probably an associated peripheral neuropathy in virtually every case of myelopathy due to vitamin B_{12} deficiency, and secondly because if there is myelopathy, it will usually reveal its presence in the form of pyramidal insufficiency. James Collier, who had an unrivalled experience of SCD, claimed (1941) that an extensor plantar response was 'almost always present', a statement corroborated by Wilson (1954) who stated that extensor plantar responses were 'not only almost invariable, but appear soon and stay to the finish'. Moreover, some of the earlier controversies seem in part a question of semantics: the axons in the dorsal columns are, after all, as integral a part of the bipolar cells of the dorsal root ganglia as are their peripherally-directed extensions.

If we are correct in our view (a) that vitamin B_{12} deficiency has early 'peripheral' repercussions, and (b) that when B_{12} deficiency affects the spinal cord there will usually be evidence of a lesion of the pyramidal tracts, two main conclusions must follow. These are that one cannot accept the diagnosis of B_{12} deficiency myelopathy as *proven:*

(a) in patients presenting with pure pyramidal syndromes, without sensory symptoms or signs (or, for instance, in patients with ankle clonus);
(b) in patients presenting with exclusively sensory symptoms or signs, without evidence of pyramidal deficit. Such patients may well be suffering from peripheral neuropathy due to vitamin B_{12} deficiency, but cannot be claimed to be cases of B_{12} deficiency myelopathy.

We hold that the combination of depressed or absent ankle jerks (due to peripheral neuropathy) and extensor plantar responses (or other evidence of an upper motor neurone lesion in the lower limbs) is not only 'classical' but necessary for a fairly confident diagnosis of SCD. We appreciate that 'atypical' cases occur, but feel that in the presence of such atypical pictures alternative diagnoses were seldom excluded with the necessary rigour. We are also aware of the differing clinical pictures that may result from the admixture, in varying proportions, of peripheral neuropathy and lesions of the posterior and lateral columns. We are, finally, familiar with the changing neurological signs that may be encountered as the disease progresses, or as its peripheral component regresses, under the influence of treatment. Nevertheless, we feel that unless rather strict diagnostic criteria are adopted, the understanding of the neuropathies and myelopathies complicating gastrointestinal disease is likely to be impeded rather than helped.

ENCEPHALOPATHY AND OPTIC NEURITIS

Diagnostic problems

The diagnosis of encephalopathy in vitamin B_{12} deficiency is beset with inferential fallacies and other difficulties, of which the high incidence of psychiatric disease in the elderly (pernicious anaemia itself being a disease of middle and old age), and the frequent occurrence of depressive reactions in response to insidiously developing ill-health, are but two. It is hardly surprising that current psychiatric textbooks should describe mental changes in vitamin B_{12} deficiency as being both 'rare' (Slater and Roth, 1969) and as 'not at all rare' (Noyes and Kolb, 1963): there are contradictory statistics which reflect not only divergent views on what constitutes a causal relationship—as distinct from mere association—but also the varying criteria deemed necessary for the diagnosis of psychiatric disease.

The reported incidence of psychosis in patients with pernicious anaemia varies between 4 per cent (Woltman, 1924) and 16 per cent (Herman, Most and Jolliffe, 1937). Lesser mental changes are more common, reports as to their prevalence again varying widely, from 25 per cent (Ahrens, 1932) to 64 per cent (Goldhamer et al, 1934). The significance of these differing figures is uncertain, in view of the necessarily subjective clinical assessment involved.

When seeking to evaluate the role of vitamin B_{12} deficiency in the genesis of psychiatric abnormality in patients with pernicious anaemia, further problems arise. Uncritical attitudes will lead to an overestimation of the importance of vitamin deficiency, while excessively rigid criteria will undoubtedly exclude some genuine cases of B_{12}-deficiency encephalopathy. Eilenberg (1960) employed such ultra-rigid yardsticks when discussing whether mental illness in patients with pernicious anaemia could be attributed to the cerebral effects of vitamin B_{12} deficiency. His criteria included: (a) no past history of psychiatric illness; (b) no evidence of disturbed premorbid personality; (c) absence of psychologically or socially disturbing events preceding the illness; (d) unequivocal presence of mental illness; (e) associated and proven pernicious anaemia; (f) resolution of the mental illness with vitamin B_{12} treatment. He examined the records of 20 patients admitted with combined diagnoses of pernicious anaemia and a psychiatric illness to a well-known psychiatric hospital, but could find only four cases that satisfied his criteria. Causes other than hypovitaminosis B_{12} were, in his view, responsible for psychiatric symptoms in the remaining 16.

It can be seen that the true incidence of encephalopathy in vitamin B_{12} deficiency is undetermined (and possibly indeterminable). It is likely that when both a psychiatric illness and vitamin B_{12} deficiency coexist, the latter is seldom responsible for the former.

B_{12} deficiency encephalopathy: pathological and EEG correlates

The pathological basis of B_{12} deficiency encephalopathy was firmly established by Adams and Kubik (1944) who reviewed the earlier literature. The main pathological changes consist of multifocal, often perivascular foci of demyelination in the cerebral white matter, generally occurring with little axonal destruction or reactive gliosis.

Cerebral oxygen uptake is frequently impaired in patients with vitamin B_{12} deficiency (Scheinberg, 1951) and the EEG is often abnormal (Romano and Engel, 1944; Samson et al, 1952). The whole subject is well reviewed by Walton et al (1954). As the EEG is usually normal in other chronic anaemias, at least until the haemoglobin falls to a very low level, the occurrence of a very abnormal EEG in an only mildly anaemic patient may at one time have been a hint that there was more to the anaemia than just iron deficiency, but now that serum vitamin B_{12} can be directly assayed such considerations are only of historical interest. Samson et al (1952) claimed that EEG improvement following specific therapy might antedate changes in red cell count. In vitamin B_{12} deficiency neither the degree of anaemia nor the presence or absence of neurological signs appear to be significant correlates of an abnormal EEG. The severity of the mental disturbance bears no close relation to the degree of abnormality of the EEG (Walton et al, 1954).

An interesting point, first stressed by Adams and Kubik (1944) is that in all authentic reports of 'subacute degeneration of the brain' there had always been lesions of the spinal cord. Pathologically, this may well be true. The observations are in general keeping with the clinical findings of Herman et al (1937) who reported that over 70 per cent of 40 patients with pernicious anaemia and cerebral symptoms also had physical signs of spinal cord disease, and with the more recent observations of Holmes (1956), whose 14 patients with pernicious anaemia and 'well marked cerebral symptoms' all showed signs of spinal cord or peripheral nerve involvement, although cerebral symptoms had preceded those of more peripheral origin in several instances.

Patterns of psychiatric disorder

The type of mental disturbance that might be attributed to vitamin B_{12} deficiency is uncertain. McAlpine (1929) reported disorders ranging from states of depression, accompanied by loss of mental energy, to definite psychoses. Herman et al (1937) stated that the mental picture 'did not show any characteristic or diagnostic content'. In order of decreasing frequency they had encountered acute confusional states, paranoid conditions, affective disorders and organic mental deterioration. Although the authors could not accept the psychiatric symptoms of a number of their patients as being causally related to the pernicious anaemia, they nevertheless found patients with causally related symptoms to constitute the majority.

Holmes (1956) also found that the mental symptoms were extremely variable and included 'mild disorders of mood, mental slowness, memory defect which may be gross confusion, severe agitation and depression, delusions and paranoid behaviour, visual and auditory hallucinations, urinary and faecal incontinence in the absence of overt spinal lesions, dysphasia, violent maniacal behaviour and epilepsy'. Slowness of mental reactions, confusion and memory defect were present in all 14 of his cases, 12 of whom responded satisfactorily to intensive therapy with vitamin B_{12}.

Shulman (1967), in a study of the psychiatric status of 27 patients with pernicious anaemia compared with 21 patients with other types of anaemia, found that approximately one third of both groups had 'moderate' or 'severe' psychiatric symptoms. Of the symptoms encountered, only memory impairment appeared to be specifically related to vitamin B_{12} deficiency. When depression accompanied pernicious anaemia it was 'related less to the direct effect of vitamin B_{12} deficiency than to the uncovering of a constitutional predisposition to depressive illness precipitated by the anxiety of unexplained fatigue and physical incapacity'.

A number of reports have alleged that mental changes in patients with pernicious anaemia may precede the characteristic haematological changes by months or even years (Langdon, 1905; Strachan and Henderson, 1965). Another point originally made in Langdon's once-controversial paper on 'nervous and mental manifestations of pre-pernicious anaemia' was the occurrence of spontaneous variation in the mental state of the patient. However, in some of the reported cases in which mental symptoms antedated the recognition of vitamin B_{12} deficiency by long periods one cannot help suspecting the concurrence of two independent conditions, while in other cases the 'intermittent' nature of the psychiatric disturbance suggests only that more than one aetiological factor may have been operative.

That organic mental deterioration may be due to vitamin B_{12} deficiency is sometimes recognised after its precipitation by folic acid, as in the case of Smith and Oliver (1967).

Vitamin B_{12} deficiency in patients with mental illness

While the incidence of pernicious anaemia in patients admitted to mental hospitals is no greater, and possibly less, than in the population at large (Henderson et al, 1966; Murphy et al, 1969), low serum vitamin B_{12} levels in such patients are found relatively frequently (Edwin et al, 1965; Nielsen, 1966). This does not necessarily imply a deficiency state.

Edwin et al (1965) reported levels below 100 pg/ml in 5·8 per cent of 396 patients aged over 30 admitted in one year to a hospital in Norway. They stressed that these patients presented no clinical or haematological manifestations of vitamin B_{12} deficiency. Nielsen (1966) found that 11·8 per cent of 127 consecutive patients over the age of 65 admitted to a Danish mental hospital had serum B_{12} levels below 165 pg/ml. With one exception all the values were above 100 pg/ml and no correlation could be detected between low plasma concentrations of vitamin B_{12} and the presence of either paraesthesiae or reduced vibration sense. A group of younger patients, admitted during the same period, had a significantly higher mean plasma B_{12} level. This report raises interesting problems, originally hinted at by Gaffney et al (1957) who suggested that there was a physiologically unimportant decline in serum vitamin B_{12} due to age alone, regression lines indicating that the values approached 100 pg/ml in extreme old age.

Psychiatric manifestations due to vitamin B_{12} deficiency in patients with gastrointestinal disorders

Hunter, Jones and Matthews (1967) reviewed 2000 patients admitted to a London mental hospital over a four-year period. Twenty (1 per cent) had had a partial gastrectomy. Five were admitted within five years of operation and five each 6–10, 11–15 and 16–20 years after surgery. Five of the patients who had had a gastrectomy were found to have serum levels of vitamin B_{12} below 100 pg/ml. Vitamin B_{12} deficiency was considered to be the cause of the psychiatric illness in four of these five. The 25 per cent prevalence of vitamin B_{12} deficiency in this small group of psychiatrically disturbed patients far exceeded that reported in any unselected group of mental hospital admissions, and the authors made the point that psychiatric case-taking could be regarded as incomplete without specific inquiry for a history of gastric surgery; if this was obtained, a serum vitamin B_{12} estimation was necessary.

Visual impairment

Optic nerve involvement is well known, both pathologically (Bickel, 1914; Adams and Kubik, 1944) and clinically, as a complication of vitamin B_{12} deficiency. Optic neuritis in pernicious anaemia is today of great rarity, though in the past it was claimed that 6 per cent of cases of retrobulbar neuritis were due to this cause (Benedict, 1933). The onset of visual symptoms is more often gradual than acute, the patient complaining of increasing difficulty in reading small print. The disturbance is usually bilateral but may be more marked in one eye than in the other. Examination reveals disc pallor and centrocaecal scotomata with peripheral constriction of visual fields (Benham, 1951). Anaemia is usually severe, only one third of the cases reviewed by Hamilton, Ellis and Sheets (1959) having a red cell count greater than $10^6/mm^3$.

Optic atrophy may rarely be the presenting feature of pernicious anaemia (Cohen, 1936). It is said to occur in 3 per cent of patients with vitamin B_{12} deficiency myelopathy (Young, 1932; Benham, 1951), and to occur almost exclusively in males (Hamilton et al, 1959). The visual defect sometimes antedates other manifestations of pernicious anaemia, but usually accompanies myelopathy and peripheral neuropathy.

Optic neuropathy is rare in vitamin B_{12} deficiency due to causes other than pernicious anaemia, but is well documented in relation to fish tapeworm infestation (Björkenheim, 1966). The role of vitamin B_{12} deficiency in 'nutritional amblyopia' is uncertain and is reviewed, on the basis of a wide experience, by Wadia and Swami (1970).

Among other causes of visual impairment in patients with vitamin B_{12} deficiency, macular haemorrhage might be mentioned. This occurs with severe anaemia and thrombocytopenia (Smith, Smith and Fletcher, 1962).

Other neurological features of vitamin B_{12} deficiency

Cerebellar ataxia and proximal muscle weakness were reported in Indian patients with vitamin B_{12} deficiency of dietary origin by Wadia and Swami (1970). Two of their 14 cases had well-marked cerebellar ataxia, dysarthria and nystagmus, while five had proximal muscle weakness of the lower limbs. The cerebellar deficit was unresponsive to thiamine but diminished promptly following the administration of vitamin B_{12}. The relationship of proximal muscle weakness to hypovitaminosis B_{12} appeared much less definite in view of the occurrence of this feature in pellagra and of its resolution, in Wadia and Swami's cases, on a ward diet alone.

Nystagmus is seen occasionally in Western patients with SCD, as was noted by Kinnier Wilson (1954).

THE NERVOUS SYSTEM AND NUTRITIONAL VITAMIN B_{12} DEFICIENCY

It is impossible to discuss the relation of a low serum B_{12} to disorders of the gastrointestinal tract without prior reference to the vexed question of reduced vitamin B_{12} intake. This has been incriminated as a contributory cause of neuropathy in a number of the conditions to be discussed. In our view it seldom plays a significant role.

Pathophysiology

Vitamin B_{12} is unique among vitamins, in that it has to be synthesised by microorganisms. These live in water, soil, sewage and the intestines of man and animals. Almost all products of animal origin contain deoxyadenosyl-B_{12}, the major dietary form of the vitamin. Vitamin B_{12} is only present in negligible amounts in *clean* foods of vegetable origin. Daily requirements probably exceed 2 μg. They may in fact exceed 5 μg (Chanarin, 1969). It is difficult to consume a diet defective in vitamin B_{12}. Contamination of water supplies by *Escherichia coli* may be an important source of vitamin B_{12} in some parts of the world.

Man is entirely dependent on his food for vitamin B_{12}. Although the vitamin is synthesised in appreciable amounts in the human caecum and colon, and although human beings excrete far more vitamin B_{12} than they ingest, this autogenous B_{12} cannot be absorbed because the specific receptors involved in the process are situated too proximally: in the terminal ileum. Man gets around this problem by including meat and dairy products in his diet. Other species (such as the rat and rabbit) get around it by practising coprophagy. For other species (such as ruminants) there is no problem: they synthesise vitamin B_{12} in the foregut and absorb it further down.

Vitamin B_{12} deficiency of dietary origin is rare. It may occur in certain very strict vegetarians termed 'vegans' (Hill, 1952) who will eat neither eggs nor milk products. Wokes, Badenoch and Sinclair (1955a, b) found low serum vitamin B_{12} levels in such people. Vegetarianism, widely practised in India on both religious and economic grounds, is also associated with a low mean serum B_{12} (Mehta, Rege and Satoskar, 1964; Dastur et al, 1972).* In interpreting data from India it is important to keep in mind the fairly wide prevalence of B_{12} malabsorption in certain areas. It has been shown that structural intestinal lesions similar to those of sprue may be encountered in patients with no clear-cut history of gastrointestinal disorder (Baker, 1957; Jeejeebhoy, Wadia and Desai, 1967). The problem is even further complicated by the fact that folate deficiency, of nutritional origin, may affect ileal function and interfere with the absorption of vitamin B_{12} (Lees, 1961; Mollin and Waters, 1968; Scott et al, 1968). Iron deficiency may also impede the absorption of

* Veganism is never practised, in India, on purely religious grounds: even those sects to whom eggs are forbidden will drink milk, if they can afford it. Much so-called 'veganism' in India is due to sheer economic necessity and not to religious or cultural influences. The latter, however, may influence the definition of vegetarianism. For instance many Bengali 'vegetarians' eat fish, getting around the problem by defining it as the 'fruit of the sea'.

vitamin B_{12} (Cox et al, 1959). Vitamin B_{12} deficiency itself may have the same effect (Lawrence, 1966; Carmel and Herbert, 1967). With regard to veganism, the important question is not why some people develop B_{12} deficiency but why so many do not.

The prevalence of nutritional vitamin B_{12} deficiency cannot be judged by the prevalence of megaloblastic anaemia. Most megaloblastic anaemia of dietary origin is due to folate deficiency. Proof that an anaemia is due to dietary deficiency of vitamin B_{12} would require the demonstration of (a) a megaloblastic marrow; (b) a low serum vitamin B_{12}; (c) the absence of complicating factors such as pregnancy, a gastric operation or the taking of anticonvulsant drugs; (d) normal vitamin B_{12} absorption; (e) normal fat absorption; (f) free acid in the gastric juice; and (g) improvement of the anaemia (with restoration of normoblastic erythropoiesis) by small oral doses of vitamin B_{12}, of the order of 5 to 10 μg/day which is the amount of vitamin B_{12} contained in a normal mixed diet. That such a condition in fact exists was only finally proven quite recently when Stewart, Roberts and Hoffbrand (1970) provoked an excellent haematological response in an anaemic Hindu lady by the daily oral administration of 1 μg cyanocobalamin.

Neurological complications

Neurological complications of vitamin B_{12} deficiency of dietary origin are very rare. It is interesting to speculate whether 'intentional' Western vegans may be more liable to such complications than 'unintentional' Indian vegans, whose diet is also poor in folate (a high folate intake is known to predispose to the neurological complications of vitamin B_{12} deficiency). There are a few references to myelopathy due to nutritional B_{12} deficiency but a paucity of adequately documented cases. An unusual syndrome with encephalopathic features has been described in Indian infants, brought up on breast milk from vitamin B_{12}-deficient mothers (see p. 56).

Myelopathy. Badenoch (1954) mentions a boy of 15, a strict vegetarian, who developed a dietary deficiency of vitamin B_{12}. He suffered from classical SCD which responded dramatically to treatment with vitamin B_{12} alone. Gastric biopsy was normal, as was the absorption of radioactive vitamin B_{12}. The serum B_{12} was not given and no further clinical details provided.

In a survey of vitamin B_{12} deficiency in 235 British, Dutch and American vegans, Wokes et al (1955a) state that 'nervous symptoms were common'. They give no further details, except that many of their subjects had experienced paraesthesiae. The mean serum vitamin B_{12} was 111 pg/ml, the figures ranging from 45 to 195 pg/ml. In over 50 per cent of cases the serum B_{12} was below 120 pg/ml. Wokes (1956) later stated that dietary deficiency of vitamin B_{12} did not lead to the classical blood picture of pernicious anaemia—or indeed to any pronounced macrocytosis—but that it may be accompanied by 'marked changes in the nervous system, extending in some instances as far as subacute combined degeneration of the cord'. Again no details are given.

Smith (1962) carefully investigated a group of 12 Western vegans who had been living for periods from 4 to 50 years on a diet *totally* lacking in animal protein. Their heights and weights were within normal limits for age and sex.

Haemoglobin values ranged from 80 to 100 per cent. Serum B_{12} levels ranged from 48 to 220 pg/ml (in only five instances were they below 120 pg/ml). 'The notable feature of the histories lay in the paucity of symptoms.' The EEG was abnormal in nine of the 11 instances in which information on this point was sought. (These abnormalities were considered the result rather than the cause of the dietary fad!) Two patients were stated to have 'unequivocal subacute combined degeneration of the cord'. No clinical details were given but the serum B_{12} levels (142 and 176 pg/ml respectively) were considerably higher than is usually found in myelopathy due to B_{12} deficiency. It may be relevant that these two patients were the only two smokers in the whole group.

An obvious warning should be uttered at this stage. The association of a myelopathy and a low serum B_{12} does not necessarily imply a causal relation. There is no reason why vegans or other food faddists should not develop any of a number of neurological diseases characterised by myelopathy. If a low serum vitamin B_{12} is found under these circumstances, there will be a natural temptation to attribute the neurological signs to vitamin B_{12} deficiency. The following two cases illustrate this error in two very different age groups. Both were originally claimed as cases of SCD due to dietary deficiency and have found their way into review articles under this heading.

Connor and Pirola (1963). A man aged 76 had been a strict vegan for 18 years—and a vegetarian before that! He had developed a spastic paraparesis, with exaggerated knee and ankle jerks and extensor plantar responses. There had been no sensory symptoms. Postural sense was found to be impaired in the toes and there was 'generalised impairment of vibration sense considered within normal limits for his age'. The peripheral blood and marrow were normal, but the serum vitamin B_{12} was 45 pg/ml. There was normal absorption of labelled B_{12}, without the addition of intrinsic factor. There were considerable radiographic changes of cervical and dorsal spondylosis. The CSF protein was 60 mg/100 ml. No myelogram was performed. We feel this may well have been a case of spondylotic myelopathy in an elderly vegan.

Riley (1966). A youth aged 17 developed paraesthesiae in both hands, aggravated by neck flexion. No abnormal signs were found and the symptoms subsided. Three years later he complained of increasing weakness and stiffness of the legs and difficulty with micturition. He was found to have a spastic paraparesis with ankle clonus, extensor plantar responses, loss of vibration sense below the iliac crests and impaired postural sense in the toes. It was then discovered that he had subsisted, since early childhood, on a diet of bread, chips and fruit. He was polycythaemic. Marrow normoblasts were said to show 'megaloblastic tendencies'. There was free HCl in the gastric juice. The serum vitamin B_{12} was 71 pg/ml and absorption of labelled vitamin B_{12} was normal. He was said to have SCD but we suggest a more likely diagnosis would be disseminated sclerosis in a patient with a low serum B_{12} of dietary origin. The presenting complaint (Lhermitte sign) and the early remission—without change in dietary habits—would be consistent with this diagnosis.

We have found only two adequately documented cases in which we are prepared to accept the diagnosis of myelopathy due to dietary vitamin B_{12} deficiency. They are worth quoting in some detail as they provide a model of the sort of information needed—and so often lacking—before such a causal relation can be accepted.

Verjaal and Timmermans-van den Bos (1967). A woman aged 68 was admitted to a Dutch hospital in a confused and wasted condition, with a large bedsore. She died five months later. She had lived in Indonesia for many years. At the age of 50, after a short psychotic illness, she had become a Seventh Day Adventist and strict vegetarian. Her marriage broke up a few years later and she came to Holland where she lived alone, eating a grossly inadequate diet. Three years before admission her gait gradually deteriorated and she became bedridden.

In hospital she was found to have a paraplegia in flexion, with brisk upper limb reflexes, absent knee and ankle jerks and extensor plantar responses. There was a severe disturbance of deep sensibility in the lower limbs. Radiographs of the skull and spine were normal. There was free HCl in the gastric juice and no steatorrhoea. She was anaemic with a megaloblastic marrow, an MCV of 137 μm^3 (normal: 82–96 μm^3) and hypersegmented polymorphs. The serum B_{12} was very low (20 pg/ml) and the the serum folate normal (4 ng/ml). Liver function tests and serum albumen were normal. Despite large doses of vitamin B_{12} her condition deteriorated as a result of bladder infections, bedsores and broncho-pneumonia. A detailed necropsy showed signs of SCD, classical in both nature and distribution. The pathological appearances were fully described (with photographs). The only unusual feature was the finding of 12 cells/mm^3 in the spinal fluid. (The CSF protein was 57 mg/100 ml and colloidal gold curves were normal.)

Misra and Fallowfield (1971). A spinster aged 62 had been a vegan for five years and, prior to that, a vegetarian for more than a decade. Over a period of three years she had developed paraesthesiae in the hands and feet and an increasingly ataxic gait. She was found to have a spastic paraparesis with diminished ankle jerks and extensor plantar responses. There was hypalgesia and hypoesthesia of glove and sock distribution, vibration sense being absent below the costal margins and postural sense grossly impaired in both legs. She was anaemic with a megaloblastic marrow, low serum vitamin B_{12} (71 pg/ml), free acid in the gastric juice, normal barium meal and follow through, and normal CSF. She absorbed labelled vitamin B_{12} normally. Following specific therapy with vitamin B_{12} the marrow became normoblastic, the anaemia cleared up and there was a marked improvement in the neurological signs.

Encephalopathy. In 1962 Jadhav et al reported from Vellore (South India) six cases of an unusual syndrome, seen in breast-fed infants, when the mother herself was vitamin B_{12}-deficient. The milk of such mothers is vitamin B_{12}-deficient (Baker et al, 1962). The syndrome consisted of apathy, developmental regression, pallor of the mucous membranes, hyperpigmentation of the skin (usually affecting the hands and feet) and, in the fully developed form, involuntary movements of the head, trunk and limbs. The movements affecting the head were described as 'side-to-side tossing movements', those affecting the limbs as 'purposeless jerky movements of external rotation', and those affecting the trunk as 'twisting or wriggling'. The infants, all less than a year old, were well nourished, but all had megaloblastic marrows, low serum B_{12} levels (64, 29, 56, 35, 62, and 25 pg/ml respectively) and normal vitamin B_{12} absorption. They all responded well to very small doses of oral vitamin B_{12}. Clinically similar cases had previously been described from other parts of India but this is the first series in which serum B_{12} levels were estimated on both mothers and infants, and the B_{12} concentration estimated in the maternal milk.

Conclusions

Vegetarians, as a group, have lower serum vitamin B_{12} levels than non-vegetarians. This, however, is of doubtful clinical significance. Except in vegans, vitamin B_{12} *deficiency* is always due to malabsorption. The association of a low serum vitamin B_{12} and of a neurological disorder does not necessarily imply a causal relationship. Myelopathy due to dietary B_{12} deficiency is extremely rare and only two cases have been adequately documented. Encephalopathy may occur in the breast-fed infants of vitamin B_{12}-deficient mothers.

TOTAL GASTRECTOMY

Pathophysiology

As far as is known, intrinsic factor (IF) is only produced by the parietal cells in the body of the stomach (the same cells as produce acid). The upper two thirds of the human stomach have been found to be most active from the haematopoietic point of view (Fox and Castle, 1942; Landboe-Christensen, Berk and Castle, 1952). IF is a glycoprotein (molecular weight about 50 000) which combines (molecule for molecule) with dietary B_{12} to form complexes which are absorbed by specialised cells in the terminal ileum (Booth and Mollin, 1957, 1959; Cooke et al, 1957). One unit of IF is defined as the amount combining with 1 ng of vitamin B_{12}.

In fact *two* mechanisms exist for the absorption of vitamin B_{12}. One is inefficient, passive, occurs equally throughout the jejunum and ileum and does not require IF. It only accounts for the absorption of about 1 per cent of a large oral dose (Hoffbrand, 1971). The second is efficient, occurs in the human ileum, and requires the mediation of IF.

Total gastrectomy, by removing the cells which produce IF, abolishes the major mechanism involved in the absorption of vitamin B_{12}. Glass, Pack and Mersheimer (1955) showed that eight patients who had undergone total gastrectomy were completely unable to absorb labelled vitamin B_{12} and that the defect could be corrected by the concurrent administration of IF. Unless IF is given by mouth to such patients (or vitamin B_{12} by injection) they will sooner or later *all* show evidence of B_{12} deficiency. Paulson and Harvey (1954) and MacLean and Sundberg (1956) showed that megaloblastic anaemia would occur in every case, if oral IF or parenteral vitamin B_{12} were not given. In the various series reviewed by Cox, Williams and Jones (1963) the time interval between total gastrectomy and the patient's presentation with megaloblastic anaemia ranged from $2\frac{1}{2}$ to 14 years.

The body stores of vitamin B_{12} are relatively large (3000 to 5000 μg). The liver may contain up to 1500 μg. Daily body losses of vitamin B_{12} probably amount to some 0·1 per cent of the total B_{12} pool, whatever the size of that pool (Heyssel et al, 1966). The size of these stores (in relation to daily requirements) accounts for the delay before evidence of depletion manifests itself in totally gastrectomised patients.

Neurological complications

The neurological complications of total gastrectomy are not well documented. Paraesthesiae are said to have occurred on several occasions. We have found eight cases of alleged myelopathy (see Table 5.3). Three of these cases are acceptable, including two in whom necropsy findings are reported. One case is unacceptable. Data are inadequate for us to comment on the alleged cases of myelopathy following total gastrectomy reported by

MacDonald, Ingelfinger and Belding (1947), Paulson and Harvey (1954) and MacLean and Sundberg (1956).

Dennig (1929). Nine years after total gastrectomy for gastric ulcer, a man aged 41 developed glossitis, a severe megaloblastic anaemia, paraesthesiae and pains in the legs, and an ataxic gait. The knee and ankle jerks were absent. After an initial response to liver the patient died of bronchopneumonia. Necropsy confirmed the diagnosis of pernicious anaemia. Examination of the spinal cord showed degeneration of the central part of the posterior columns. The clinical findings are equivocal but the pathological findings in keeping with SCD.

Meyer, Schwartz and Weissman (1941). A patient aged 23 underwent total gastrectomy for 'linitis plastica', the histological findings, however, being those of a severe non-specific chronic interstitial gastritis. Six years after operation he developed pallor, glossitis, and increasing numbness of the hands and feet. The knee and ankle jerks were exaggerated but the plantar responses were flexor. Vibration sense was diminished at the ankles. The marrow was megaloblastic. There was good clinical response to injection of liver extract. The case is acceptable.

Beebe and Meneely (1949). A woman aged 46, after several months of gastrointestinal symptoms, underwent a total gastrectomy for what turned out to be ulcerative syphilitic gastritis. Six years later she developed numbness and tingling in the sole of one foot. Her tongue was 'smooth, magenta-coloured and tender' and she had a hyperchromic, macrocytic anaemia. There were no abnormal neurological signs. Her symptoms improved on liver. On this very scanty evidence she was claimed to have had 'combined system disease'. The claim is unacceptable.

Pant, Asbury and Richardson (1968), in their excellent neuropathological reappraisal of the whole subject of myelopathy complicationg pernicious anaemia, mention a man aged 67 (Case 28) who had had a gastrectomy for carcinoma 18 years previously. He had developed progressive neurological symptoms over a period of 12 years, at the end of which time he was barely able to walk. He was found to have a spastic paraplegia with absent postural sense and vibration sense in the legs. Necropsy showed characteristic findings in the posterior and lateral columns of the spinal cord.

Conclusions

The absorption of vitamin B_{12} is virtually abolished following total gastrectomy, due to lack of IF. Vitamin B_{12} deficiency will inevitably develop, although the onset may be delayed for several years. Myelopathy has been recorded in this context and there are two acceptable necropsies. In none of the reported cases with neurological complications are data available concerning the serum vitamin B_{12} levels.

PARTIAL GASTRECTOMY

Pathophysiology

If patients who have undergone partial gastrectomy are followed up over a number of years, low serum vitamin B_{12} levels will be found in about 15 per cent of cases (Chanarin, 1969; Hoffbrand, 1971). In a detailed study of 265 such patients, Deller and Witts (1962) recorded a progressive decline in the serum B_{12} level, the steepest fall occurring during the first six years. Levels below 150 pg/ml were found in 14 per cent of the cases, and frank megaloblastic anaemia in 1·5 per cent. Hines, Hoffbrand and Mollin (1967) found megaloblastic anaemia due to vitamin B_{12} deficiency in 4 per cent of such cases. Jones et al (1962) reported on 100 unselected patients who had undergone gastric operations five or six years previously for peptic ulceration. No fewer than 57 had serum vitamin B_{12} levels of 150 pg/ml or less. Several factors are involved in the pathogenesis of this abnormal state.

Lous and Schwartz (1959) studied the absorption of labelled vitamin B_{12} in 119 patients who had undergone gastrectomy. A third had impaired absorption, in all cases improved—and usually completely corrected—by the simultaneous administration of IF. Similar figures were given by Jones et al (1962). The results strongly suggested that the defective absorption of vitamin B_{12} was due to a reduced production of IF. Theoretically this could have been due either to resection of too large a part of the IF-producing area of the stomach, or to postoperative changes in the gastric remnant, interfering with IF synthesis. According to Lous and Schwartz (1959) the extent of the resection does not appear to be decisive, although in other studies (Johnson and Hoffbrand, 1970) the prevalence of vitamin B_{12} deficiency increased with the size of the resected area. Absorption of labelled vitamin B_{12} is unimpaired, however, in the *immediate* postgastrectomy period (Cox, Williams and Jones, 1963) clearly showing that resection per se is not the main factor.

The severity of inflammatory and atrophic changes in the gastric remnant is probably of great importance. The nature of these changes is discussed in detail by Jones and Williams (1963). In some studies impaired absorption of vitamin B_{12} is found more often in patients whose partial gastrectomy has been performed for gastric ulcer than in those in whom it has been done for duodenal ulcer (Lous and Schwartz, 1959; Deller, Richards and Witts, 1962). These findings are what might have been anticipated from the biopsy study of the gastric mucosa undertaken by Joske, Finckh and Wood (1955) who demonstrated atrophic gastritis (see p. 66) in 30 per cent of 65 patients with gastric ulcer, as against only 5 per cent of 98 patients with duodenal ulcer.

Deller et al (1962) confirmed the frequent finding of impaired B_{12} absorption following partial gastrectomy and the fact that the defect was nearly always correctable by the administration of IF. Biopsy of the gastric remnant was invariably abnormal following partial gastrectomy. They stressed that whereas removal of IF-secreting tissue, combined with gastritis and atrophy of the remaining mucosa, were the main factors responsible, other factors might also be involved. Among these they listed inadequate intake of vitamin B_{12}, inadequate proteolytic activity in the stomach (resulting in incomplete splitting-off of vitamin B_{12} from complexes in food), inadequate stimulation to the secretion of IF because of removal of the gastric antrum and of over-rapid emptying, and faulty complexing of IF and dietary vitamin B_{12}, as a result of loss of the reservoir function of the stomach. Temperley et al (1969) suggested that duodenal juice might inhibit IF.

Yet other mechanisms have been suggested to explain vitamin B_{12} deficiency in these patients. Iron deficiency is common following partial gastrectomy and it has been shown (Badenoch, Evans and Richards, 1957) that such deficiency per se may impair the secretion of IF, and hence, by implication, the absorption of vitamin B_{12}. Cox et al (1959) showed that vitamin B_{12} absorption is in fact defective in a number of patients with iron deficiency anaemia and was correctable by iron therapy.

It has also been suggested that following certain types of partial gastrectomy the duodenal stump might act as a large diverticulum (Ogg, 1959; Goldstein, Wirts and Kramer, 1961). Colonisation of the jejunum by colonic bacteria (Tabaqchali et al, 1966) might further impede the absorption of vitamin B_{12}, despite a normal dietary intake and a normal production of IF.

Defective dietary intake of vitamin B_{12} may also conceivably play a role. The prime concern of some patients following gastrectomy is to avoid 'dumping' rather than to ensure their own adequate nutrition. Jones et al (1962) have shown that low serum B_{12} levels in postgastrectomy patients is occasionally associated with normal B_{12} absorption.

Following partial gastrectomy megaloblastic anaemia takes several years to develop. So do most of the neurological complications. This is not surprising in view of the fact that the biological half-life of hepatic vitamin B_{12} is 12 months (Schloesser, Deshpande and Schilling, 1958).

Neurological complications

It is not known how often these occur. In some large series of gastrectomised patients followed up over long periods (Wells and MacPhee, 1954; Bistrom, 1961), neurological complications are not even mentioned. They were not alluded to in a recent revision article dealing with postgastrectomy problems (Williams, 1967). Our review of the literature suggests that the mean delay before neurological symptoms develop may be as long as 10 years, a period exceeding the duration of follow-up in many of the reported series.

Paraesthesiae. The general problem presented by this symptom has already been discussed. Patients with minor sensory symptoms and no objective neurological signs are frequently seen. We have carried out motor and sensory nerve conduction studies in the lower limbs of six such patients but failed to find any abnormalities. The serum B_{12} levels were all above 130 pg/ml. If there are definite physical signs (i.e. if there is an unequivocal organic basis for the complaint) this is more likely to be neuropathy than myelopathy.

Myelopathy. While some reports of myelopathy in gastrectomised patients are immediately acceptable, others should be viewed with caution. In several of the alleged cases there were no pyramidal signs and—as previously explained (see p. 48)—we prefer to consider the sensory abnormalities in such patients as due to peripheral neuropathy rather than to myelopathy. In other instances the occurrence of pyramidal signs could well have been of cerebral (and not spinal) origin. Finally, even when the diagnosis of myelopathy seems firmly established it does not always follow that the myelopathy is *due to* vitamin B_{12} deficiency. We will stress some of these points in our discussion of the relevant literature.

Schneider and Carey (1928) were probably the first to report the occurrence of SCD in partially gastrectomised patients. Their two reported cases cannot be adequately assessed, however, because no data were provided.

Rowlands and Simpson (1932) also described two patients in whom SCD was alleged to have occurred after partial gastrectomy.

Case 1. A woman aged 32 underwent partial gastrectomy for a large gastric ulcer. The resected portion showed changes in keeping with syphilis and the patient was subsequently found to have a positive Wassermann reaction. Six years later, she developed paraesthesiae, first in one foot then in the other, and progressive ataxia. She was found to have an anaemia with a high colour index, and a spastic paraplegia with brisk ankle jerks. Vibration sense was impaired in the legs but there was normal perception to pin and cotton wool. Romberg's sign was positive. The CSF was not examined. The gastric juice lacked free HCl and had a 'low total acidity'. She was given liver, and both the anaemia and the disorder of gait improved. The brisk ankle jerks, the presence of a positive WR, and the failure to examine the spinal fluid lead us to reject this as a case of SCD.

Case 2. A man aged 42 had had a partial gastrectomy and posterior gastrojejunostomy performed for gastric carcinoma 15 years earlier. After remaining symptom-free for many years, he developed sensory symptoms in hands and feet, and an ataxic gait. He was found to be wasted and anaemic, with glossitis, absent knee and ankle jerks, extensor plantar responses and absent vibration sense in the legs. The haematological findings suggested pernicious anaemia and a test meal showed absence of free HCl and a low total acidity. He died a few months later. There was no necropsy. The clinical features are in keeping with SCD but the relation to surgery remains conjectural.

Salus (1932). Eight years after a partial gastrectomy, a man aged 55 (Case 3) developed sensory symptoms in the lower limbs and ataxia of gait. Examination revealed a paraparesis with brisk knee jerks, absent ankle jerk, and extensor plantar responses. Romberg's sign was positive. The CSF was normal. There was no free HCl in the gastric juice. No abnormalities were found in the peripheral blood. The clinical data, although scanty, are compatible with a diagnosis of SCD.

Hartfall (1934) mentions three cases of SCD occurring after partial gastrectomy, but himself queries two of them. Data on the remaining patient were meagre but probably just sufficient to warrant acceptance. The author claims the diagnosis to be 'beyond dispute, with spasticity, extensor plantar responses and absent vibration and position sense suggesting posterior column loss'.

Salus and Reimann (1934) described two cases. The first cannot be accepted. There were no sensory signs in the lower limbs and ankle clonus was a prominent feature. We have accepted their second case, despite doubts concerning the asymmetric clinical picture.

Ross, Belding and Paegel (1948) in their classic paper on the deleterious effects of folate on SCD mention a man aged 67 (Case 4) who had developed neurological symptoms following partial gastrectomy. He experienced paraesthesiae and was found (before being given folic acid) to have impaired vibration sense in the lower limbs and absent ankle jerks. The plantar responses were flexor. Postural sense was normal and the Romberg sign negative. Although the case is mentioned in some reviews (Chanarin, 1969) as an instance of SCD, we feel peripheral neuropathy to be a more probable diagnosis.

Bastrup-Madsen (1954). Two months after a partial gastrectomy for duodenal ulcer, a man aged 60 developed numbness and clumsiness of the hands. Examination a year later revealed a gross sensory deficit affecting all modalities in both upper and lower limbs. Power and tone were normal. Coordination was said to be slightly impaired. The Romberg sign was positive. The upper limb reflexes were depressed, those in the lower limbs being normal. No plantar responses could be elicited. There was a histamine-fast achlorhydria but no abnormalities in blood or marrow. The WR was negative in blood and CSF. He improved following injections of B_{12}, the paraesthesiae subsiding within a fortnight. A year later there were no residual neurological signs. The author suggests this was a case of myelopathy due to B_{12} deficiency, precipitated by surgery, adducing the time relationship as evidence in favour of his claim. In our opinion it is this very time relationship that renders a diagnosis of SCD unlikely. The diagnosis is also suspect because of the absence of pyramidal involvement and because of the predominance of sensory signs and symptoms in the *upper* limbs.

Badenoch et al (1955) found symptoms suggestive of SCD in three out of six patients with postgastrectomy megaloblastic anaemia. No clinical details were given. The serum B_{12} levels were 35 and 70 pg/ml in the two cases in which this was estimated.

Alexeieff (1957), reviewing the experience of a large clinic in Moscow, reported a further case who, within a year of a subtotal gastrectomy, developed 'un tableau de pseudotabes'.

Knox and Delamore (1960) report the case of a mentally defective male aged 32 admitted to hospital because of the recent development of paraesthesiae, weakness and unsteadiness of the legs. Ten years earlier he had had a Polya gastrectomy for gastric ulcer. He was found to have a megaloblastic anaemia with a low serum B_{12} (90 pg/ml) and malabsorption of labelled B_{12}, correctable by intrinsic factor but not by antibiotics. An augmented histamine-secretion test showed achlorhydria and a gastric biopsy features of chronic atrophic gastritis. The jejunal mucosa was normal. A barium meal showed a normal mucosal pattern. The neurological signs consisted of generalised weakness and hypotonia, hyporeflexia (including absent ankle jerks) and an extensor plantar response on one side. Vibration sense was lost below the iliac crests and postural sense severely impaired in the legs. The WR was negative and the cervical spine radiologically normal. There was a good haematological response to parenteral cyanocobalamin and the neurological disability lessened considerably. Short of necropsy, this is as well-documented a case of SCD as can be found, and the exclusion of intestinal causes of impaired B_{12} absorption makes the association with gastrectomy highly plausible.

Deller and Witts (1962) in a very full study of haematological changes occurring in 265 patients following partial gastrectomy, mention two cases of SCD. Both were men who had been operated on by the Polya technique for duodenal ulcer. The neurological symptoms appeared 10 years after operation. No clinical details were given. Serum B_{12} levels were in the 'subnormal' range (i.e. < 150 pg/ml).

Weir and Gatenby (1963), reviewing 257 patients who had undergone partial gastrectomy in three Dublin hospitals, reported two cases of SCD. The first, a man aged 41, had had a gastroenterostomy for duodenal ulcer 14 years previously, and a Polya gastrectomy for stomal ulcer four years later. He presented with paraesthesiae of the feet, weakness and ataxia. The calves were tender and he was areflexic. Postural sense was reduced in the legs, where vibration sense was absent. There was no comment about pyramidal signs. The patient was anaemic, the marrow being megaloblastic. A histamine test meal showed achlorhydria. A gastric biopsy showed gastritis and jejunal biopsy a normal mucosal pattern. There was malabsorption of orally administered labelled B_{12}, correctable by simultaneous ingestion of IF. The WR was negative and the CSF normal. The patient improved following injections of vitamin B_{12}. B_{12} deficiency seems adequately established in this case. The neurological features suggest a diagnosis of peripheral neuropathy rather than SCD.

The second patient reported by Weir and Gatenby (1963) was a housewife aged 56 who, 15 years after a Polya gastrectomy for chronic gastric ulcer, was found to be mildly anaemic with a megaloblastic marrow. The ankle jerks were absent and the other tendon reflexes depressed. One plantar response was extensor. Vibration sense was impaired at the malleoli and Romberg's sign was positive. There was achlorhydria on the histamine test meal. Serological tests for syphilis were negative. The serum B_{12} level was 87 pg/ml and the Schilling test showed malabsorption of B_{12}, correctable by IF. Blood picture and neurological status both improved following injections of cyanocobalamin.

Cox et al (1963), in a useful discussion of the pathogenesis of vitamin B_{12} deficiency following partial gastrectomy, described a man aged 68 who, 13 years after a Billroth II operation, developed a megaloblastic anaemia and 'a classical picture of SCD'. The serum vitamin B_{12} was 40 pg/ml. The neurological signs were not reported.

Until less than a decade ago, these cases (numbering less than two dozen) were the main instances of alleged myelopathy complicating partial gastrectomy. In a brief communication, Olivarius and Roos (1965) suggested that systematic, long-term follow-up of gastrectomised patients would reveal a much higher figure. They surveyed the Scandinavian literature and mention

23 previously described cases of 'myelopathy' to which they added five from their own experience. Unfortunately, no clinical details were provided. They also mentioned having seen three patients with peripheral neuropathy complicating partial gastrectomy. Neurological complications occurred on average 10·3 years after surgery. The authors stressed that although all patients had 'subnormal values of serum B_{12}', only one had megaloblastic anaemia. Four had no anaemia whatsoever (the authors attributed the absence of megaloblastic anaemia, in several other cases, to the associated iron deficiency). The absorptive defect, in all but one case, was confirmed by a Schilling test. Many of the patients had for years suffered from symptoms such as irritability, apathy and excessive fatigue. Several further cases were discovered in the course of a prospective study of all patients seeking incapacity pensions following partial gastrectomy. The authors recommend the routine determination of serum B_{12} levels in all gastrectomised patients. They suggested that a special watch be kept on patients with low B_{12} levels, to ensure early detection of neurological disease.

Three years later the same authors (Olivarius and Roos, 1968) reviewed in greater depth the whole subject of these myelopathies. It is difficult to comment on this survey because the authors did not specify which sensory symptoms or signs they took to imply myelopathy (as distinct from peripheral neuropathy). Their review of the literature included several cases we have deliberately rejected, for reasons already mentioned. It also included other patients to whom the authors attribute pyramidal signs, where none are recorded in the original reports. In addition, the authors described five personally observed cases. Three of these are acceptable (Cases 1, 2 and 4) as cases of myelopathy. The serum vitamin B_{12} levels in these three cases were 60, 180 and 100 pg/ml respectively. Case 3 suffered from seizures and cerebral arteriosclerosis, and had an upper motor neurone facial weakness. His pyramidal signs could well have been of cerebral origin. The diagnosis of myelopathy is unacceptable, although the patient almost certainly had a peripheral neuropathy. Case 5 probably also suffered from peripheral neuropathy, complicated by what sounds like a bilateral radiculopathy from lumbar spondylosis (limitation of spinal movements, tenderness over the lumbar spinous processes, etc.). The confident diagnosis of myelopathy is unacceptable. The authors made the interesting comment that the haematological findings were normal in all their cases and stressed that this might have delayed recognition of the real nature of the neurological disorder in a number of instances. While this may at times be true, we feel that the finding of *normal* serum B_{12} levels in some of these cases suggests that the myelopathies had arisen on the basis of disorders *other than* vitamin B_{12} deficiency.

In one of the largest documented series to date, Williams and his co-workers (1969) described 14 patients who developed neurological disease between five and 16 years after partial gastrectomy (performed for gastric ulcer in nine instances, for duodenal ulcer in five). The authors stressed the severity and at times irreversible nature of the neurological disorder. All patients had difficulty in walking, with unsteadiness and muscular weakness. Most had experienced paraesthesiae or numbness. All had abnormal neurological signs in the legs. Most exhibited gross wasting with loss of vibration sense below the costal margins. Only six of the patients had extensor plantar responses, however. In these patients (i.e. in the small group in which the diagnosis of myelopathy is tenable) pre-treatment serum B_{12} levels were available in four instances. They were 198, 40, 160 and 35 pg/ml respectively. Electromyography and nerve conduction studies were normal in half the cases.

The neurological deficits in these patients may not have been of uniform aetiology. Half the patients, for instance, had serum B_{12} levels of above 150 pg/ml when first seen (only two had previously received injections of B_{12}). Over a third of the patients in whom it was tested had normal absorption of radioactive B_{12}. Eight patients had osteomalacia proved by bone biopsy or biochemical response to vitamin D therapy, and part at least of their neurological signs could have been myopathic. The response to therapy with vitamin B_{12} was variable. This series is of considerable interest in that it suggests that neurological syndromes very similar, if not clinically indistinguishable from SCD, may follow partial gastrectomy and yet *not* be associated with B_{12} deficiency. What some of these cases resemble most are the neurological syndromes seen in patients with coeliac disease, to which we will be referring later.

Encephalopathy. Cerebral manifestations may first draw attention to the vitamin B_{12} deficiency state complicating partial gastrectomy. Hunter and Jones (1967) reported on 2000 consecutive admissions to a mental hospital. Twenty (1 per cent) patients had had a previous partial gastrectomy and of these a quarter had serum levels below 100 pg/ml. In four of these five patients the vitamin B_{12} deficiency was considered the primary cause of the psychiatric illness. The authors stressed that psychiatric case-taking should include specific enquiry for a history of gastric surgery. If this is obtained, serum B_{12} estimations should be performed routinely, irrespective of the psychiatric picture or of the presence or absence of physical signs.

Other complications. Welbourn, Hughes and Wells (1951) claimed that vitamin deficiencies (other than vitamin B_{12} deficiency) were common in gastrectomised patients, laying particular stress on thiamine deficiency. The claim is considered more fully under the appropriate heading.

Metabolic bone disease is not uncommonly encountered after partial gastrectomy. It is considered more fully on p. 157 as it may itself entail neurological complications. Myopathy complicating partial gastrectomy was first stressed by Ekbom et al (1964) and further cases reported by Jensen (1965) and d'Eramo (1965). These are reviewed more fully under the heading of osteomalacia. A disorder with features of motor neurone disease has also been described (Jensen, 1965; Kniffen and Quick, 1969) and is discussed further on p. 165.

Conclusions

Low vitamin B_{12} levels are encountered in up to 15 per cent of gastrectomised patients. Some of these patients may present with neuropathy, myelopathy or mental disturbance, often many years after their surgical operation. Confirmation of these diagnoses has seldom been established pathologically. Estimation of serum B_{12} should be mandatory in any gastrectomised patient suffering from any neurological or mental disorder. Gastrectomised patients may also develop neurological complications unrelated to vitamin B_{12} deficiency.

GASTRIC LESIONS OTHER THAN GASTRECTOMY

The commonest gastric disorder to be associated with malabsorption of vitamin B_{12} is of course Addisonian pernicious anaemia. A full discussion of the non-neurological aspects of the condition is beyond the scope of this monograph. The reader is referred to useful reviews by Chanarin (1970) and Hoffbrand (1971).

Gastric carcinoma

Confronted with a patient with gastric carcinoma and neurological signs the first problem is to exclude spinal or cerebral metastases. If the patient has a macrocytic anaemia, the clinical problem might be thought to be one of deciding whether he was suffering from Addisonian pernicious anaemia and had developed both subacute combined degeneration of the spinal cord and a gastric carcinoma, or whether the gastric carcinoma, by interfering with a sufficiently large area of the stomach, had induced a deficiency of IF and hence a disorder of vitamin B_{12} absorption. A little reflection will show that the latter occurrence is most unlikely, in view of the fact that carcinoma of the stomach tends to be a rapidly lethal disease, whereas SCD only develops several years after destruction of the IF-producing area of the stomach.

Carcinoma of the stomach complicates pernicious anaemia in from 3 to 5 per cent of cases, although it has been claimed that up to 10 per cent of patients with pernicious anaemia may develop this complication (Jandl, 1971). Symptoms of myelopathy have been said to occur, sooner or later, in from 30 to 85 per cent of patients with untreated pernicious anaemia (Grinker, 1926; Hurst, 1934; Dreyfus, 1971).* It is therefore scarcely surprising that the two complications may at times be associated.

The diagnostically crucial investigation in such cases would be the search for antibodies against IF, which one would expect to find in over 50 per cent of patients with pernicious anaemia (Ardeman and Chanarin, 1963; Chanarin, 1969) but in hardly any other condition. This IgG immunoglobulin would not be found in the blood of non-Addisonian patients developing carcinoma of the stomach. Most of the recorded cases of myelopathy associated with gastric carcinoma were recorded long before these sophisticated immunological aids to diagnosis were available. The following cases illustrate some of the traps in which earlier authors were ensnared:

Waterfield and Shackle (1923). A man aged 52 had recently developed paraesthesiae in the hands and feet, some ataxia of gait and indigestion. He had been losing weight. He was found to be pale, with a subicteric tint, glossitis and a slightly enlarged spleen. The only abnormal neurological signs were extensor plantar responses, impaired vibration sense in the lower limbs and some tactile impairment over the feet. The WR was negative and the CSF normal. There was complete achlorhydria and an anaemia of high colour

* These widely differing estimates depend on the criteria used for making a diagnosis of myelopathy.

index. A mass was felt in the epigastrium, which at laparotomy was found to be a large gastric neoplasm. He died 10 days later. Necropsy by Dr C. P. Symonds was stated to have shown the typical changes of subacute combined degeneration of the spinal cord. It is possible that, in this case, both gastric carcinoma and myelopathy developed in a patient with preexisting pernicious anaemia, although it is intriguing that the two complications appeared simultaneously. We do not question the pathological findings but the case is not acceptable as an instance of SCD *due to* carcinoma of the stomach because of the incompatible time relationships.

Garvey and Stern (1924). A 50-year-old man presented with distal paraesthesiae of recent onset. The tongue was smooth and the skin lemon-tinted. There was no paresis and the reflexes were all normally brisk. There were no pyramidal signs. Postural sense and the appreciation of deep pain were lost at the ankles but vibration sense was normal. Tactile sense was unimpaired. There was anaemia with a high colour index but 'no noteworthy changes in the red cells indicative of pernicious anaemia'. There was no free acid in the gastric juice and the total acidity was very low. Six weeks after admission to hospital he developed abdominal symptoms. At laparotomy he was found to have an extensive gastric carcinoma. A posterior gastroenterostomy was performed. He deteriorated a few weeks later during which time he lost both knee jerks and ankle jerks. At necropsy the spinal cord showed 'marked postero-lateral degeneration of the type seen in pernicious anaemia'. The marrow was hyperplastic but there was no haemosiderosis of liver or spleen. The state of the gastric mucosa, beyond the confines of the tumour, is not mentioned. The case is again unacceptable because of the time relationships.

Simpson (1931) mentions some earlier cases (Brandes, 1921; Porges, 1929) and describes a patient of his own, as follows. A man aged 53 developed anorexia, epigastric pain and anaemia, at the same time as tingling and numbness, primarily affecting the hands and fingers. The only abnormal neurological signs were an exaggerated left ankle jerk and an extensor left plantar response. There were no sensory abnormalities. Slight improvement was recorded following the administration of hog's stomach. He died a few weeks after an exploratory operation which confirmed the presence of a gastric neoplasm. At necropsy the spinal cord presented a swollen, gelatinous appearance. There was no neuroglial proliferation. We are told that 'sections prepared from this cord fully justified diagnosing "subacute combined degeneration" '. Myelin was irregularly lost in the posterior and lateral columns and lipid débris were present in large compound granular corpuscles. Although the diagnosis of SCD seems well-documented, its relationship to the carcinoma is unacceptable in view of the time relationships. Both conditions were probably complications of underlying Addisonian pernicious anaemia.

Atrophic gastritis and gastric atrophy not associated with pernicious anaemia

In *chronic atrophic gastritis*, the thickness of the gastric mucosa is reduced, the mucosa is diffusely infiltrated with chronic inflammatory cells, and there is a variable loss of specialised glands together with overgrowth of glands of intestinal type. In *gastric atrophy* the mucosa is very thin, shows little or no inflammatory change, is composed largely of a mucus-secreting or intestinal-type epithelium, and lines a thinned muscular wall. One or other of these changes is invariably seen in the stomach of patients with Addisonian pernicious anaemia. However, this disease is not the only cause of gastric atrophy or indeed the major cause of atrophic gastritis, which may be associated with a wide variety of conditions, including partial gastrectomy, iron-deficiency anaemia, and old age (Joske, Finckh and Wood, 1955; Morson, 1966).

Whatever their cause, these pathological changes in the stomach may sometimes lead to a vitamin B_{12} deficiency state. The reason, of course, is that the production of IF is reduced; it is low in patients with the more severe degrees of atrophic gastritis and very low in patients with gastric atrophy (Ardeman and Chanarin, 1966). The absorption of vitamin B_{12} is not interfered with, however, until the production of IF falls to less than 1 per cent of its normal 50 000 units/24 h (Ardeman and Chanarin, 1965). The serum B_{12} is normal in patients with superficial gastritis, but about 25 per cent of patients with the more severe degrees of atrophic gastritis have a subnormal serum B_{12} level. This is seldom in the severely deficient range, i.e. below 100 pg/ml (Hoffbrand, 1971).

The documentation of neurological disease associated with atrophic gastritis or gastric atrophy due to conditions other than pernicious anaemia is minimal. One report, that of Wood et al (1964), is of interest in this respect. This study reported the long-term (mean duration: nine years) follow-up of 30 middle-aged or elderly patients, mostly women, originally presenting with vague dyspeptic symptoms, and diagnosed, on gastric biopsy, as suffering from chronic atrophic gastritis of moderate or severe degree. In the majority of patients, serial serum B_{12} estimations showed a downward trend, the lowest levels recorded ranging from 20 to 270 pg/ml (the levels were below 150 pg/ml in 18 cases). The patients did not complain of major distressing or debilitating symptoms which could definitely be attributed to B_{12} deficiency. However, increasing weakness, loss of memory and mental depression were frequently recorded, together with the flatulent dyspepsia of which they had originally complained. Paraesthesiae were often experienced. Four patients are recorded as having signs of peripheral neuritis and five as having signs of SCD. The latter cases cannot be uncritically accepted as such without further information in view of the unambiguous statement that 'no patient had abnormal plantar reflexes'. Minor haematological abnormalities were detected but no patient developed frank pernicious anaemia, probably because of an adequate folate intake. Some of these 30 patients plainly had vitamin B_{12} deficiency related to decreased production of IF. Nevertheless, it would be foolhardy to attribute their neurological symptoms and signs to this cause: alternative explanations (such as Alzheimer's disease) for their loss of memory and depression would seem at least plausible.

Other forms of gastritis

Older authors considered an 'alcoholic gastritis' to be indirectly responsible for some of the neurological effects of chronic alcoholism. Nonne (1906) published a very detailed clinical and pathological account of six cases of chronic alcoholism who developed SCD. In four there was a hyperchromic anaemia. It is impossible, in retrospect, to say whether these were alcoholics who happened to develop pernicious anaemia and myelopathy, or whether the high alcohol intake itself induced sufficient changes in the gastric mucosa sufficient to interfere with IF production and hence with vitamin B_{12} absorption. It should be pointed out that chronic 'alcoholic gastritis'—whatever its clinical status—has no distinctive histopathological existence. Most chronic alcoholics have normal stomachs.

A *corrosive gastritis* may occasionally be followed by megaloblastic anaemia and neurological symptoms. The following case is of interest:

Alsted (1937). A 29-year-old woman had attempted suicide by drinking nitric acid. She recovered but developed fibrosis of the stomach. Eight years later, radiographic examination revealed a gastric lumen reduced to an 'orange-sized space in the fundus'. Evacuation into the duodenum took place through a canal 10 cm long and 'with a width hardly that of a pencil'. Gastroenterostomy was performed to relieve vomiting. The walls of the pylorus were 1 cm thick. The mucosa, submucosa and parts of the muscularis had been converted into fibrous tissue. She was found to have a megaloblastic anaemia. Two years later she developed acroparaesthesiae and her gait became unsteady. There was a paraparesis with ankle clonus and extensor plantar responses, but no sensory signs. Her general condition improved following liver therapy but the neurological signs remained unchanged.

Congenital intrinsic factor deficiency

This is a rare gastric disorder, transmitted through an autosomal recessive gene. The gastric mucosa is histologically normal and the gastric juice contains normal amounts of hydrochloric acid and pepsin but, in the homozygote, IF is only produced in minute amounts, if at all. Labelled vitamin B_{12} is very poorly absorbed, the defect being correctable by concurrent administration of IF. The condition usually presents early in the second year of life and progresses steadily until recognised and treated. There is megaloblastic anaemia and loss of weight, associated with diarrhoea or constipation, vomiting, listlessness, and refusal to walk or stand. Stomatitis, glossitis and splenomegaly may be found. The condition is well reviewed by Chanarin (1969). The main differential diagnosis is from juvenile pernicious anaemia (a term best used to designate *acquired* 'auto-immune' pernicious anaemia occurring in the first decade of life), in which condition there is achlorhydria and severe atrophy of the gastric mucosa, and from congenital malabsorption of vitamin B_{12} (see p. 81).

The nervous system may be involved in congenital intrinsic factor deficiency. Unfortunately it is difficult to assess how often this occurs as some early cases were almost certainly reported under the title of 'juvenile pernicious anaemia'. One group of authors (Reisner et al, 1951) went so far as to say that in juvenile pernicious anaemia 'I.F. deficiency may occur without achlorhydria' (despite the fact that most authorities believed at the time—and still believe—that achlorhydria is essential for a diagnosis of pernicious anaemia). This attitude epitomises the difficulty experienced before a novel concept can emerge, people preferring to believe they are witnessing an exception to an established rule rather than the first example of something new.

Reisner et al (1951). Of the four cases of 'juvenile pernicious anaemia' reported by Reisner and his colleagues three had neurological signs attributed to spinal cord disease.

Case 1 was a girl with recurrent megaloblastic anaemia and free hydrochloric acid in the gastric juice (even without histamine) who at the age of 9 developed physical signs suggestive of *peripheral neuropathy* (absent knee and ankle jerks and depressed vibration sense in the toes). Therapy with oral vitamin B_{12} was ineffective, unless given with normal gastric juice. This combination resulted in an excellent response. The patient clearly had peripheral neuropathy but the claim that she had SCD is unacceptable.

Case 3 was that of a boy who between the ages of 15 months and seven years had had several episodes of profound macrocytic anaemia associated with glossitis. These responded to parenteral liver extract and to parenteral vitamin B_{12} but not to the same substances administered by mouth. At the age of three, at which time there was free hydrochloric acid in the gastric juice, he developed a disorder of gait and was found to have depressed knee and ankle jerks and extensor plantar responses. He improved markedly following therapy with parenteral liver but then gradually deteriorated when given oral folic acid. Over a period of several months, he became increasingly lethargic, gradually lapsing into an incontinent, stuporous state, with a recurrence of his earlier neurological signs. He improved dramatically when liver injections were substituted for oral folate. The case is documented in some detail, and the absence of albuminuria makes it unlikely the authors were dealing with a case of congenital malabsorption of vitamin B_{12} (see p. 81). The claim that the patient had SCD is acceptable and it would seem that at a later date he also developed an encephalopathy related to B_{12} deficiency.

Case 4 had achlorhydria and was probably the only genuine case of juvenile pernicious anaemia in the series. Her neurological disturbance, although compatible with SCD, does not warrant discussion under the present heading.

Pearson, Vinson and Smith (1964) also reported a case of 'pernicious anaemia with neurologic involvement in childhood' which was almost certainly a case of congenital intrinsic factor deficiency. A premature child had developed normally until the age of seven months, when he gradually became lethargic. By the age of a year and a half a megaloblastic anaemia had been diagnosed and the child given folic acid, which improved the anaemia. Shortly before his third birthday the child again became increasingly lethargic and this time ataxic as well. He was found to have sluggish reflexes but flexor plantar responses. He gradually lapsed into a profound stupor with Cheyne–Stokes respiration, hypothermia and hypotension. Dramatic improvement followed cessation of folic acid therapy and parental injections of vitamin B_{12}. The child regained consciousness and eventually became ambulant again, but with nerve deafness and some impairment of cerebration as permanent sequelae. The interesting comments are made that there was free hydrochloric acid but no IF (even after a carbachol injection) in the gastric aspirate, and that the serum contained no antibodies against IF. Although there was no albuminuria (see p. 81) the Schilling test performed with and without IF only improved the absorption of radioactive vitamin B_{12} from 0·7 to 4·2 per cent, suggesting an additional absorptive defect.

Gastric by-pass

Oesophagojejunostomies are now seldom performed. In this operation the stomach was left in situ and gastric secretions allowed to drain into the jejunum. Follow-up studies have revealed low serum B_{12} levels and impaired absorption of vitamin B_{12} only partially improved by IF (Callender et al, 1961). Five of 12 patients in this series had paraesthesiae in the hands and feet. There were no cases of myelopathy.

Conclusions

Although on theoretical grounds 'chronic gastritis' and carcinoma of the stomach might be expected to interfere with IF production, there are no adequately recorded instances of such disorders being associated with myelopathy *due to* B_{12} deficiency. All the formerly reported cases of gastric neoplasm complicated by SCD are suspect in view of the time now known to be necessary between the destruction or removal of the IF-producing area of the stomach and the development of neurological complications due to B_{12} deficiency. The only 'chronic gastritis' to give rise to myelopathy is the gastric atrophy of Addisonian pernicious anaemia. Congenital IF deficiency, a rare hereditary disorder, may give rise to neurological complications.

STRUCTURAL LESIONS OF THE SMALL BOWEL

Structural lesions of the small bowel such as diverticulosis, strictures, blind loops and anastomoses are well-recognised causes of malabsorption of vitamin B_{12}. Both megaloblastic anaemia and neurological symptoms may occur in this setting. Considerable advances have been made, in the last few years, in our understanding of how vitamin B_{12} deficiency may arise in this context.

Direct involvement of area concerned in vitamin B_{12} absorption

Some structural disorders involve the vitamin B_{12} absorbing area (i.e. the distal ileum) directly. Malabsorption of vitamin B_{12} will occur, for instance, following resection of the last few feet of the small intestine. Tropical sprue, regional ileitis, Whipple's disease, coeliac disease and systemic sclerosis may all interfere with vitamin B_{12} absorption by affecting this area. In most of the conditions to be discussed, however, the defect in B_{12} absorption is more complex and is thought to arise, at least in part, as a result of colonisation of the small bowel by bacteria, normally resident in the large bowel.

Bacterial overgrowth of the small intestine

Under ordinary conditions the human stomach, duodenum and upper ileum contain relatively few bacteria (less than 10^5 organisms per millilitre of fasting aspirate). These are mainly Gram-positive aerobes, probably of dietary origin. Their growth is usually inhibited by the low pH in the stomach, by intestinal peristalsis (Dack and Petran, 1934), by the presence of bile (Floch et al, 1970), and by secretory immunoglobulins (Hersh et al, 1970). If any of these factors is deficient, the bacterial population of the small bowel may reach a density of 10^{10}/ml. Although variable from individual to individual this population explosion will consist mainly of anaerobic organisms of faecal type. The presence of such 'bacterial overgrowth in the small intestine' has profound metabolic and nutritional consequences, recently reviewed by Neale et al (1972).

Dietary vitamin B_{12} linked to intrinsic factor (IF) is poorly absorbed in patients with blind loops, strictures, jejunal diverticulosis, or various other lesions predisposing to stasis. Absorption may also be impaired when there is free communication between large and small bowel, as in patients with gastrocolic or enterocolic fistulae. This malabsorption can often be corrected if the patient is treated with broad-spectrum antibiotics administered by the oral route, particularly if the ileum is intact and has not been short circuited (Halsted, Lewis and Gasster, 1956; Mollin, Booth and Baker, 1957). The striking response to antibiotics suggests that the malabsorption is, in some way, related to bacterial overactivity. The ecology of the intestinal microflora has been the subject of intensive investigation in the last few years (Dubos, 1966; Gall, 1970). Numerous studies, well reviewed by Tabaqchali (1970), have shown the profound changes that may occur in various pathological conditions.

It is not known for certain how bacterial 'colonisation' of the small intestine interferes with vitamin B_{12} absorption. Although some intestinal bacteria readily take up free vitamin B_{12}, the IF–B_{12} complex is relatively resistant to bacterial action in vitro. In vivo there is probably some form of competitive uptake of the vitamin by certain enteric bacteria, even though IF provides a considerable degree of protection. Previously suggested mechanisms, such as bacterial damage to enterocyte receptors for vitamin B_{12}, or bacterial destruction of IF (resulting in the release of free IF and its subsequent uptake by bacteria) are not now considered clinically significant. Giannella, Broitman and Zamcheck (1971) have shown that certain bacteria have an avidity for vitamin B_{12} approaching that of human intrinsic factor, B_{12} bound to IF being interchanged with that bound to the surface of the bacterial cell.

The presence of bacterial colonisation of the small bowel can usually be recognised by evidence other than malabsorption of vitamin B_{12}. There is often *steatorrhoea*. This is due to changes in bile salt metabolism as originally suggested by Dawson and Isselbacher (1960). As already described in an earlier chapter, conjugated bile salts are normally present in the small intestine at concentrations adequate to promote micelle formation. Deconjugation and hydroxylation of conjugated bile salts by certain bacteria reduces their concentration enough to interfere with micelle formation, thereby leading to steatorrhoea. Bacteria such as *Bacteroides*, *Veillonella*, *Clostridia* and *Bifidobacteria* seem to be predominantly responsible (Midtvedt and Norman, 1967; Hill and Drasar, 1968).

Indicanuria was long considered a useful index of excessive bacterial metabolism (Tabaqchali et al, 1966) but many factors are involved in its production (Neale, Lambert and Gorbach, 1969) and failure to take these into account may lead to gross errors of interpretation. Among such factors reviewed by Neale et al (1972) are diet, intraluminal pH, available substrate, inhibition by certain monosaccharides and the presence of certain absorptive disorders even in the absence of bacterial overgrowth. Despite these limitations it is felt that a high indican excretion (i.e. over 200 mg/day) in the absence of marked steatorrhoea (less than 20 g fat/day) is almost diagnostic of stagnant loop (Neale et al, 1972).

The most recently described method of recognising bacterial contamination of the small bowel consists in *estimating volatile fatty acids in jejunal fluid.* These acids, which have to be estimated by gas–liquid chromatography, represent the major end-product of the anaerobic fermentation of many intermediate metabolites, derived not only from carbohydrate but also from fatty acids and amino-acids. In a recently reported study (Chernov, Doe and Gompertz, 1972) patients with stagnant loops showed several times more acetate, propionate and butyrate than did normal controls, the abnormal values falling to normal following the administration of antibiotics. More recently still the ^{14}C-glycocholic acid breath test has been described (James, Agnew and Bouchier, 1973) which may prove useful in the detection of bacterial deconjugation of bile acids.

Improvement in vitamin B_{12} absorption following a course of broad-spectrum antibiotics (tetracycline is widely used for this purpose) remains, however, the sheet anchor of the diagnosis of bacterial colonisation of the small bowel.

Types of anatomical defect

Stagnant areas of bowel are particularly prone to such bacterial overgrowth. The simplest examples are probably the large 'blind' pouches of *jejunal or ileal diverticulosis.* These herniations of intestinal mucosa through the submucosa and muscularis occur on the mesenteric side of the gut, at the point of entrance of blood vessels. As pointed out by Cooke et al (1963) they lack a muscular component. As a result they are completely atonic. The peristaltic activity of the small intestine tends to fill them with fluid chyme, after which they empty only very sluggishly.

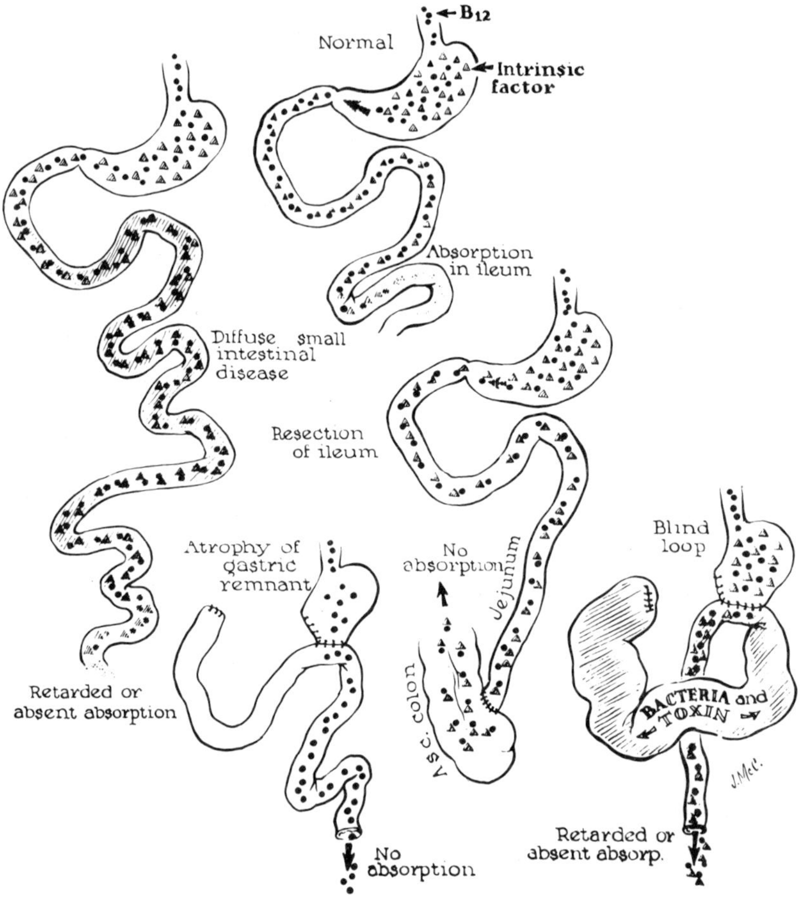

Figure 5.1. Structural changes in small intestine producing vitamin B_{12} malabsorption. (Slightly adapted from Starzl, Butz and Hartman, 1961, *Surgery*, **50,** 849–858.)

Other structural defects include gastrojejunal, gastrocolic and jejunocolic *fistulae*, or entero-entero-anastomoses. In many cases the 'stagnant' loop develops spontaneously, following perforation due to peptic ulcer, regional or tuberculous ileitis, or diverticulitis. Such perforations establish communications through which food may pass, but as a result of which an area of bowel becomes a stagnant or 'blind' loop.

In other instances the structural abnormality has been produced by abdominal surgery. Poorly functioning gastroenterostomies are particularly important in this respect. The long, non-emptying, afferent loop is 'blind' as far as bacterial colonisation is concerned. Of the 78 patients with macrocytic anaemia of gastrointestinal origin reviewed by Halsted, Lewis and Gasster (1956), no fewer than 32 had developed their blind loops following abdominal surgery.

Intestinal strictures may also lead to malabsorption of vitamin B_{12}. Bacterial colonisation is particularly prone to occur just proximal to such a lesion. In the series reported by Barker and Hummel (1939) such strictures affected the small intestine in 25 instances and the large intestine in seven. Most were located in the ileum. About a third were tuberculous but in the majority the aetiology was obscure. They were often multiple.

Some common causes of malabsorption of vitamin B_{12} are shown diagrammatically in Figure 5.1. The abnormalities found at laparotomy may be extremely complex and prove baffling to abdominal surgeons, let alone to those more used to dealing with the tracts of the spinal cord. The defects are, however, usually compounded of these basic ingredients. The effects of orally administered IF and of antibiotics on such 'prototype' conditions as (a) pernicious anaemia, (b) partial gastrectomy, (c) diverticulosis, blind loop or stricture, and (d) regional ileitis or distal gut resection sare shown schematically in Table 5.8.

Table 5.8

Effect of Oral IF and of Antibiotics on the Absorption of Vitamin B_{12}

	IF	Antibiotics
Pernicious anaemia	Enhanced	Unaltered
Partial gastrectomy	Enhanced	Unaltered
Diverticulosis, blind loop or stricture	Unaltered	Enhanced
Regional ileitis or distal gut resection	Unaltered	Unaltered

Diverticulosis of the small bowel. The relation of jejunal and ileal diverticulosis to malabsorption of vitamin B_{12} is well reviewed by Chanarin (1969). Defects of this type are now considered the commonest structural lesion of the small bowel to be associated with malabsorption of vitamin B_{12}. This in itself reflects a remarkable change of opinion. For many decades no special significance was attached to their presence. For instance, in 1933 Harvey and Murphy described a patient with 'pernicious anaemia' and SCD who had acid in his gastric juice. They remarked on the radiographic demonstration of multiple diverticula, but did not associate them with the anaemia. As late as 1958 Lee and Finby could write 'in most cases these diverticula are incidental findings detected radiographically, at operation or on post mortem examination. Patients with diverticula may have signs and symptoms, but co-existing organic processes or functional states are in most cases the cause of the complaints rather than the diverticula'.

It is now known that jejunal diverticulosis is commonly associated with anaemia, weight loss and abdominal symptoms, and that neurological complications are not infrequent (Cooke et al, 1963).

Neuropathy. Blachford and Dawson (1956), Townsend and Cameron (1957) and Scudamore et al (1958) all reported patients with diverticulosis, megaloblastic anaemia and signs or symptoms suggestive of peripheral neuropathy. There were no electrophysiological or biopsy data but the documentation is adequate on clinical grounds.

The most detailed report to date dealing with the neurological complications of jejunal diverticulosis is that of Cooke and his co-workers (1963) from Birmingham. In a comprehensive study of 33 patients with jejunal diverticulosis, over a third (13) were found to have such complications. In five instances it was the neuropathy that had driven the patient to seek medical advice. Four of the 13 patients were stated to have 'subacute combined degeneration of the spinal cord with objective signs of both posterior and lateral column disease and of peripheral neuritis'. In this particular subgroup the serum B_{12} was subnormal in the two patients tested and absorption of labelled vitamin B_{12} was impaired. The four patients all showed neurological improvement following B_{12} therapy. Five other patients had 'objective evidence of peripheral neuropathy and posterior column disease confined to the lower limbs'. They had complained of paraesthesiae in the feet and were found to have reduced or absent ankle jerks, blunting of peripheral sensation, a positive Romberg sign and a widely based gait. From the data presented, it is not clear what the serum B_{12} levels were in this second subgroup. The response to B_{12} therapy was disappointing. Two further patients suffered from paraesthesiae in the feet, lightning pains and heaviness of the legs but had no objective neurological signs.

This well-documented study is of particular significance in that it establishes that there is probably more to some of these neuropathies than B_{12} deficiency based on impaired absorption. In the five patients with neuropathy on whom pretreatment serum vitamin B_{12} levels were available, the readings were 135, 135, 60, 110 and 100 pg/ml respectively. Five (Cases 1, 4, 27, 28 and 32) of the patients with neuropathy were found to have normal absorption of labelled B_{12}.

Myelopathy. Krevans, Conley and Sachs (1954) mentioned a patient with megaloblastic anaemia, SCD, normal gastric acidity and jejunal diverticulosis. There was markedly impaired vitamin B_{12} absorption, which became normal during the administration of aureomycin. No clinical details were given relating to the myelopathy.

In the classic paper which firmly established jejunal diverticulosis as a cause of steatorrhoea and megaloblastic anaemia, Badenoch, Bedford and Evans (1955) described in some detail a patient with florid neurological signs and symptoms. Further details concerning this patient were published by Richmond and Davidson (1958) who claimed the neurological condition to have been SCD, a statement widely quoted in the subsequent literature. We do not believe such a diagnosis to be tenable, on either clinical or pathological grounds.

A woman aged 46 had gradually developed loss of weight, tiredness, abdominal pain and diarrhoea. On admission to hospital, two years later, she was found to be anaemic with a megaloblastic marrow and free HCl in the gastric juice. She improved slightly following the administration of folic acid and vitamin B_{12}. A year later the diarrhoea became worse. She became febrile and developed a rapidly progressive neurological disorder from which she died within a month. The disease was heralded by paraesthesiae in the limbs and weakness of the legs, which very soon became flaccid and areflexic. There was initially sensory loss of stocking distribution which later ascended to the groins The CSF protein was 300 mg/100 ml. Extensive diverticulosis of the small bowel was shown on barium meal. She was referred to a neurosurgical centre where a myelogram proved negative. No studies of B_{12} absorption were undertaken but she failed to respond to oral folic acid and injected vitamin B_{12}. Necropsy revealed patchy demyelination in all columns of the spinal cord, and some demyelination of the peripheral nerves. The nature of the spinal cord changes was described as 'uncertain' by the original authors. In a review of the neuropathological data, Richmond and Davidson (1958) provided the additional information to the effect that the foci of demyelination 'did not correspond to anatomical tracts', that there were haemorrhages in several posterior root ganglia, and that there were 'groups of inflammatory cells in their dural sheaths'. We cannot accept this as a case of B_{12} deficiency myelopathy and would prefer to attribute the clinical and pathological findings to a myeloradiculopathy of unknown aetiology. It is interesting that in a review of the effects of jejunal diverticulosis (Cooke et al, 1963) this particular patient is listed as a case of peripheral neuropathy.

Gastroenterostomy. A poorly functioning gastroenterostomy is a common cause of a 'blind loop' situation. Although macrocytic anaemia is well documented in such a context, neurological symptoms seem to be rare—at least among those patients in whom gastroenterostomy was the *only* operation performed. Myelopathy following uncomplicated gastroenterostomy has been reported in several instances but none of these reports will stand up to critical examination.

The patient described by Glanvill and Hurst (1930) is unacceptable as a case of myelopathy. The only evidence of neurological disorder consisted of paraesthesiae of the feet and absent ankle jerks. Peripheral neuropathy seems the probable diagnosis. Two further cases of alleged SCD were reported by Salus (1932). These are not acceptable either. In Case 1 there was no spinal cord disorder at necropsy. In Case 2 an unexpected bronchial carcinoma was discovered and both the clinical and the pathological findings suggest a carcinomatous myelopathy, a condition of course unknown at the time.

In 1934 Hurst claimed to have seen nine cases of subacute combined degeneration of the spinal cord following gastroenterostomy. He gave no clinical details but stressed that the operation was often followed by gastritis and loss of acid secretion. Loss of intrinsic factor, due to the gastritis, was felt to be the main factor responsible. Palmer (1953) has certainly confirmed a very high prevalence of gastritis following gastroenterostomy.

Strictures and anastomoses. In a review of 51 patients with intestinal strictures and anastomoses associated with macrocytic anaemia, Barker and Hummel (1939) found reported involvement of the nervous system in 10 cases. In 12 there was said to be no involvement of the nervous system. No mention of neurological symptoms or signs is made in the other 29 reports. Six patients had complained of paraesthesiae of the extremities but had shown no objective signs. One patient (Fairley and Kilner, 1931) had had signs of peripheral neuropathy. Three patients (Little, Zerfas and Trusler, 1929; Taylor, 1930; Hurst, 1933) had allegedly 'presented signs of combined degeneration of the spinal cord'. Examination of the original protocols revealed no abnormal physical signs in the first report—and no comment about the nervous system in the second! The third case (Hurst, 1933) is acceptable as SCD on clinical grounds. The harvest of hard neurological facts is meagre indeed. Barker and Hummel point out that these cases, taken as a whole, can be distinguished from cases in which there is a coincidental association of pernicious anaemia and intestinal lesion by (a) the frequent presence of free HCl in the gastric juice, and (b) the number of cases in which the anaemia responded to correction of the structural defect, without resort to liver injections.

Barker and Hummel's series (1939) does not include the case reported by Woltman and Heck (1937). A woman aged 60 developed multiple intestinal fistulae and a faecal fistula following appendicectomy. 'Later the haematologic and neurologic picture of pernicious anaemia developed and typical subacute combined degeneration was verified at necropsy'. No further details are given. According to the criteria outlined on p. 47–48 attention is drawn to this report, which cannot, however, be accepted as a proven case of SCD. Some further cases with neurological complications have since been reported.

Naish and Capper (1953). A man aged 62 had had a gastroenterostomy more than 30 years earlier, an entero-entero-anastomosis being carried out between a long afferent loop and the jejunum. He was found to be wasted with steatorrhoea, glossitis, hypoproteinaemia, a macrocytic anaemia and peripheral neuritis. There was no free HCl in the gastric juice. The plantar responses later became extensor. No mention is made of sensory signs or symptoms. He improved following injections of vitamin B_{12} but died a few months later from a carcinoma of the stoma. The spinal cord is said to have shown 'considerable' degeneration of the posterior columns. The case is acceptable.

Wilkinson (1955). A 25-year-old woman had an ileocolic fistula of obscure aetiology, possibly related to a perforated diverticulum. She developed a macrocytic anaemia and classical SCD, with absent knee and ankle jerks, extensor plantar responses, grossly reduced vibration sense in the lower limbs and a positive Romberg sign. There was free acid in the gastric juice. Slight improvement took place following the administration of liver, further improvement occurred after surgical correction of the defect. The case is acceptable.

Halsted et al (1956). Three years after surgical treatment of an intestinal obstruction, a boy aged 19 was found to have a macrocytic anaemia and signs (unspecified) of 'combined system disease'. There was free acid in the gastric juice. There was impaired absorption of labelled vitamin B_{12} transiently correctable by a course of aureomycin but not by intrinsic factor. The case is not acceptable, due to inadequate data.

Other cases of neuropathy occurring in the context of intestinal blind loop or strictures cannot be accepted as due to B_{12} deficiency, despite the demonstration of impaired absorption of vitamin B_{12}. In the patient reported by Nicol (1960) there was an alternative explanation for some at least of the neurological signs, namely an isoniazid-induced neuropathy. In the patient reported by Ragins and Oberhelman (1960) a lumbar laminectomy had revealed evidence of adhesive arachnoiditis.

REGIONAL ENTERITIS, INTESTINAL TUBERCULOSIS AND GUT RESECTION

Pathophysiology

Vitamin B_{12} is absorbed by active transport in the terminal ileum (McIntyre et al, 1956; Booth and Mollin, 1957, 1959; Allcock, 1961). The complex mechanisms involved in the attachment of the IF–B_{12} complex to the ileal mucosa and subsequent entry of B_{12} (possibly with IF or a portion of IF) into the mucosal cell are reviewed by Hoffbrand (1971). The absorptive mechanism is readily saturated. In fact man can only absorb some 2 to 4 μg of vitamin B_{12} per day. This remarkable lack of reserve capacity accounts for the frequent occurrence of malabsorption with lesions at this site. Patients with distal ileal lesion tend to have gross or total malabsorption of vitamin B_{12}.

The effects of gut resection on the intestinal absorption of vitamin B_{12} are reviewed by Chanarin (1969). In one study the absorption of vitamin B_{12} was found to be normal with resections involving less than 60 cm of ileum, but impaired when 180 cm or more had been removed (Booth, 1963). The characteristic feature in these cases is that the malabsorption cannot be corrected either with IF or following the administration of antibiotics.

Regional enteritis is the commonest condition to involve this part of the bowel. Data on serum vitamin B_{12} levels in *Crohn's disease* are scanty. Megaloblastic anaemia in regional enteritis was first described by Plum and Warburg (1939). Low levels of serum B_{12} were recorded by Meynell et al (1957) in 23 out of 43 patients and by Hoffbrand et al (1968) in 6 out of 54 patients. Many patients with Crohn's disease are treated surgically because of stenosing lesions of the terminal ileum and it is often difficult to distinguish between the effects on vitamin B_{12} absorption of (a) the disease process itself; (b) the resection or by-pass operation performed; and (c) abnormal bacterial colonisation of the small bowel. Tuberculosis may affect the terminal ileum and impair the absorption of vitamin B_{12}.

Neurological complications

We are not aware of any adequately documented cases of neuropathy or myelopathy complicating Crohn's disease but there are single reports of myelopathy, possibly due to vitamin B_{12} deficiency, complicating tuberculous enteritis and distal gut resection.

Richmond and Davidson (1958). A naval fireman aged 43 developed diarrhoea, abdominal distention, a sore tongue and burning sensations in the soles of the feet. He had very brisk knee and ankle jerks and bilaterally extensor plantar responses. There was loss of vibration sense in one leg and contralateral hypoaesthesia of stocking distribution. He had a megaloblastic anaemia, steatorrhoea and free HCl in the gastric juice. He was thought to be suffering from tropical sprue. Treatment with iron, folic acid and liver improved his anaemia but the diarrhoea persisted and the neurological signs were unaltered. A few months later he developed subacute intestinal obstruction and widespread abdominal tuberculosis was found at laparotomy. He died a few months later. At necropsy he was found to have many large tuberculous ulcers in the intestine, many of them completely encircling the lumen, but no stenosis. The spinal cord showed demyelination at all levels in the gracile tracts of the dorsal columns. There was only slight involvement of the lateral columns, and little or no gliosis.

Best (1959). A man aged 56 had developed a faecal fistula 18 years previously following appendicectomy for what had turned out to be Crohn's disease. The diseased area of bowel had later been excised and an end-to-end anastomosis performed. Two further operations were performed a few years later on account of recurrent abscesses in the right groin and subacute intestinal obstruction, more ileum being removed on each occasion. Sixteen years after the original operation he developed macrocytic anaemia and two years later paraesthesiae of the hands and feet, some visual deterioration and personality change. He was found to be ataxic with brisk knee and angle jerks, extensor plantar responses, absent vibration sense over the malleoli and bilateral loss of light touch with hyperalgesia in a sock distribution. He was slightly anaemic and the marrow was megaloblastic. There was free acid in the gastric juice and steatorrhoea. The serum B_{12} was very low (25 pg/ml). The absorption of labelled vitamin B_{12} was grossly impaired whether given alone, with intrinsic factor, or following a course of oral chlortetracycline. Haematological and neurological improvement followed the parenteral administration of vitamin B_{12}.

Intestinal involvement in scleroderma may interfere with gut motility and be associated with bacterial colonisation and megaloblastic anaemia (Salen, Goldstein and Wirts, 1966; Kahn, Jeffries and Sleisenger, 1966). We are not aware of any neurological complications developing in this particular context; nor have neurological complications been reported following vagotomy, whether surgical or medical (produced by hexamethonium bromide), although these procedures may result in a low serum B_{12} level (Cox, quoted by Chanarin, 1969), possible impairment of IF secretion (Bitsch et al, 1966), and bacterial overgrowth of the small intestine (Tabaqchali, 1970).

INTESTINAL HELMINTHIASIS

Pathophysiology

Probably every medical student remembers the 'fish tapeworm' as a cause of megaloblastic anaemia, but few doctors except those practising in Finland or in certain parts of the United States or Canada are ever likely to see a case. The fish tapeworm, *Diphyllobothrium latum*, is harboured by people in several parts of the world. Megaloblastic anaemia from this cause is common only in Finland, possibly due to the existence in that country of a particular variety of the worm.

Man becomes the host of the adult tapeworm through eating raw, cured or insufficiently cooked freshwater fish. The adult worm develops in the human intestine within a few weeks, its scolex usually attached to the middle or distal ileum. It may reach a length of 30 feet. Up to a million eggs may be evacuated daily from the mature proglottids (Faust and Russell, 1964). The ciliated embryos, developing from the ova, are ingested by a minute crustacean (*Diaptomus vulgaris*) in whose body a precercoid larva develops. When freshwater fish eat these infected crustaceans, the larva enters their muscles. There the 'cycle' ends unless the fish itself is eaten, raw, by man or dog.

In Finland, probably over a million people are carriers of the fish tapeworm. Nyberg et al (1961) found that in East Finland 27 per cent of the 'normal' subjects studied excreted tapeworm ova. By the age of 70, 45 per cent of those studied were excreting ova. The mean serum vitamin B_{12} level in 366 carriers was 116 pg/ml (as compared with 274 pg/ml among the controls). Over 50 per cent of carriers had serum B_{12} levels below 100 pg/ml. Frank megaloblastic anaemia was present in only 3 per cent of carriers. Palva (1962) showed that early changes in the marrow might be found in 8 per cent of carriers. Low serum B_{12} levels were shown to be associated with impaired absorption of labelled B_{12} (Nyberg, Grasbeck and Sippola, 1958; Palva, 1962).

The fish tapeworm is an avid consumer of vitamin B_{12}. In five patients with megaloblastic anaemia Nyberg (1958a, b) showed that between 83 and

100 per cent of an administered dose could be recovered from the worm (usually from its proximal portion) after its expulsion by an anthelminthic. Von Bonsdorf (1956) had shown that if the worm had attached itself high up in the gut of the host, it competed more effectively with the host for dietary B_{12}. Unlike man, the fish tapeworm does not need intrinsic factor to absorb vitamin B_{12}, as shown by the occurrence of infestation in patients with previously proven pernicious anaemia.

Neurological complications

Neurological signs are common in patients with tapeworm anaemia. Minnich (1892) and Woltman and Heck (1937) mention the occurrence of myelopathy but give no clinical details. The early literature on this subject is well reviewed by Björkenheim (1951) who also described a detailed neurological survey of 95 such patients. Seventy five (79 per cent) had either symptoms or signs referable to the nervous system. The commonest by far were paraesthesiae, experienced by 55 patients. Sixty-five of the 95 patients had abnormal physical signs. Vibration sense was impaired in the legs in 37 patients, 19 had an ataxic gait, 17 impaired sense of passive movement in the fingers or toes, and 15 a positive Romberg sign. The lower limb reflexes were diminished or absent in 15 cases. Pyramidal signs were found in 11 instances and were frequently unilateral. There was distal impairment of superficial sensibility in 10 patients. The overall prognosis was fairly good. Expulsion of the worm followed by injections of liver extract or vitamin B_{12} resulted in improvement in the majority of cases. Improvement also followed mere expulsion of the worm. Treatment with liver injections (without expelling the worm) was also beneficial.

The neurological complications of tapeworm anaemia were clinically indistinguishable from those due to 'cryptogenetic' (Addisonian) pernicious anaemia, although as a group the latter patients were more severely disabled and included a larger proportion of older patients. Remission of both anaemia and neurological symptoms and signs following a worm cure was taken as proof of the helminthic aetiology of a neuropathy or myelopathy. Minor neurological symptoms and signs were encountered in 10 of 30 patients who were harbouring fish tapeworms but had no evidence of anaemia. The haematological investigation of these cases does not seem to have been very thorough, however. In many respects the situation resembled the onset of SCD in certain patients, who only develop obvious haematological evidence of Addisonian pernicious anaemia at a later stage.

This excellently documented study was unfortunately carried out before estimations of serum vitamin B_{12} or studies of the absorption of labelled B_{12} had become widely practised. The clinical evidence suggests, however, that neurological complications in patients harbouring *Diphyllobothrium latum* are mainly, if not entirely, due to a conditioned deficiency of vitamin B_{12}. A surprising fact, about which Björkenheim makes no comment, is that achlorhydria was encountered in 58 of the 81 patients in whom a fractional test meal was performed. Neurological complications were, however, encountered in 15 of the 23 patients who had a normal secretion of gastric acid. This surprisingly high prevalence of achlorhydria in patients with tapeworm anaemia suggests, to us at least, that the pathogenesis of the neurological complications might have been multifactorial. It is interesting that a recent study from Finland (Salokannel, 1970) has shown that IF deficiency is not uncommon in patients with tapeworm anaemia. As the reduced production of IF persisted following expulsion of the worm it must have been a factor predisposing to the development of anaemia, rather than a consequence of the infestation.

Optic neuropathy is well documented in the B_{12} deficiency state associated with fish tapeworm (Björkenheim, 1966). It may take the form of a bilateral centrocaecal scotoma, greater to red than to white, and may occur with or without other evidence of neurological disease (Björkenheim, 1966). Many patients may show less obvious signs and merely complain of symptoms of asthenopsia (fatigue on reading, overlapping of letters, print becoming indistinct, etc.). Expulsion of the worm will result in spontaneous improvement. The pre-mentioned study is of particular interest in that it stresses the fact that in infestation with the fish tapeworm very low serum B_{12} levels may occur *without anaemia*. The four patients with definite optic neuropathy had serum B_{12} levels of 16, 21, 25 and 72 pg/ml respectively, with associated haemoglobin levels of 13·4, 14·5, 15·3 and 15 g/100 ml.

OTHER CAUSES OF MALABSORPTION OF VITAMIN B_{12}

The absorption of the IF–B_{12} complex may be considered to occur in three phases (Mackenzie and Donaldson, 1969):

1. Attachment of IF–B_{12} complex to the ileal mucosa.
2. Entry of B_{12}, possibly with IF (or a portion of IF) into the ileal cell.
3. Entry of B_{12} into the portal blood.

The first stage takes place rapidly, does not require the expenditure of energy, requires a neutral pH, and is calcium-dependent. Uptake can be blocked by a specific antibody to ileal brush-border membrane (Mackenzie et al, 1968). The second stage takes place more slowly and requires the expenditure of energy. During this process the B_{12} is localised and concentrated in mitochondria (Peters and Hoffbrand, 1970), in which it is very firmly protein-bound (Rosenthal, Cutler and Sobieszczanka, 1970). During this stage there may be some conversion of vitamin B_{12} from one form to another, for instance from cyanocobalamin to coenzyme B_{12} (Latner, Hodson and Smith, 1962). Evidence is contradictory as to whether IF enters the mucosal cell (or whether only part of it does). It is widely agreed that IF does not enter the portal blood, where vitamin B_{12} is only found bound to its various 'carrier' proteins.

Intrinsic factor bound to vitamin B_{12} is relatively resistant to digestion whereas free IF is rapidly destroyed by enzymic proteolysis. It is not known for certain how B_{12} is released from IF–B_{12} complex. In vitro, extracts of intestine and other tissues can release IF bound to radioactive B_{12}. A specific ileal 'releasing factor' has been postulated. It is possible that this is in part endogenous B_{12}, which can be shown to exchange with radioactive B_{12} bound to IF (Donaldson and Katz, 1963).

Congenital malabsorption of vitamin B_{12}

Congenital malabsorption of vitamin B_{12} is a rare autosomal recessive disease described a few years ago (Imerslund, 1960; Gräsbeck et al, 1960; Mohamed, McKay and Galloway, 1966) in which affected individuals seem to lack the specific ileal receptors for the IF–B_{12} complex or the appropriate ileal transport mechanism for vitamin B_{12} (Mackenzie et al, 1972). Children suffering from this condition present with megaloblastic anaemia, usually during the first or second year of life. Gastric biopsy reveals a normal mucosa and the production of gastric juice and IF are normal. There is an associated proteinuria, in most cases persistent, and often a non-specific aminoaciduria, which persists after vitamin B_{12} therapy. This unusual association suggests a failure of protein transport across cell membranes, involving both ileum and renal tubule.

Central nervous system disease has occasionally been described in this context. Imerslund (1960) in her original account of 10 children with 'idiopathic chronic megaloblastic anaemia' mentioned that three had 'slight, doubtful and transient neurological signs'.

François et al (1967), in an excellent review of the whole subject, report the case of a boy, known to have had proteinuria since the age of two, who at the age of 12 developed neurological signs and symptoms compatible with SCD. His gait had become unsteady and examination revealed a positive Romberg sign with absent tendon reflexes, and bilateral extensor plantar responses. Myelography having proved negative an estimation of the serum B_{12} was carried out, revealing a level of only 10 pg/ml. The child was then found to have a mild anaemia with a megaloblastic marrow. The patient's gastric juice contained normal amount of IF. A Schilling test showed impaired absorption of labelled vitamin B_{12}, whether administered alone or with a commercial preparation of IF. Three siblings were found to have proteinuria and one suffered, in addition, from a megaloblastic anaemia.

Brizard and Fraisse (1973) describe the case of a mentally rather retarded boy of unrelated parents who had been known to have had proteinuria since the age of 7. Renal biopsy had shown no abnormalities. At the age of 14 he developed a fairly severe megaloblastic anaemia and an unsteady gait. Examination revealed pathologically brisk tendon reflexes with extensor plantar responses and absent ankle jerks. There was no significant posterior column deficit. There were also other signs more difficult to fit into the picture of SCD such as mild bilateral cerebellar signs, slight wasting of the small muscles of the hand, marked lordosis and bilateral pes cavus. The serum B_{12} was 40 pg/ml. A Schilling test showed grossly impaired absorption both of labelled vitamin B_{12} and of labelled B_{12} complexed to intrinsic factor. After three months of treatment with parenteral vitamin B_{12} the gait had become normal and the plantar responses flexor: however, the other signs were unchanged. Although one cannot help feeling that part of the neurological disturbance might have been due to a spino-cerebellar degeneration, the abolition of the presenting neurological symptom following specific therapy was striking and the case has been accepted as a possible instance of SCD.

Vitamin B_{12} malabsorption due to biologically inert IF

Another condition has recently been described which is likely to be confused both with the disease described by Imerslund and Gräsbeck, and with congenital intrinsic factor deficiency (see p. 68), namely vitamin B_{12} malabsorption due to the production of biologically inert intrinsic factor (Katz, Sook and Cooper, 1972). A child presenting with megaloblastic anaemia due to vitamin B_{12} deficiency did not absorb free vitamin B_{12} given orally but absorbed normal quantities if the vitamin B_{12} was given bound to normal human gastric juice. Gastric biopsy was normal. The child's own gastric juice was acid and contained normal quantities of immunologically identifiable IF, which could not be shown to differ from normal IF by standard chromatographic procedures. All tests of small bowel function were normal. To our knowledge neurological complications have not so far been described in this condition.

The relationship between these various conditions is outlined in Table 5.9.

Table 5.9

Juvenile Pernicious Anaemia and Congenital Disorders Associated with a Low Serum B_{12}

	Achlorhydria and gastric atrophy	Anti-IF antibodies	Effect of oral IF on B_{12} absorption	Albuminuria	Reported neurological complications
Juvenile pernicious anaemia	Yes	Yes (in > 50% of cases)	Enhanced	No	Yes
Congenital IF deficiency	No	No	Enhanced	No	Yes
Congenital production of biologically inert IF	No	No	Enhanced	No	No
Congenital selective B_{12} malabsorption	No	No	Unaltered	Yes	Yes
Transcobalamin II deficiency	No	No	Unaltered	No	No

Other rare causes of malabsorption of vitamin B_{12}

Malabsorption of vitamin B_{12} may complicate severe pancreatic disease (Perman et al, 1960), the Zollinger–Ellison syndrome (Shimoda, Saunders and Rubin, 1968), the administration of potassium chloride (Salokannel, Palva and Takkunen, 1970), anticonvulsants (Reynolds et al, 1965), para-aminosalicylic acid (Heinivaara and Palva, 1964), colchicine (Webb et al, 1968) or neomycin (Jacobson, Chodos and Faloon, 1960). Neurological complications due to B_{12} deficiency have not, to our knowledge, been reported in these various contexts.

PRACTICAL PROBLEMS AND PITFALLS

In this final section we would like to draw attention to certain pitfalls that may confront the unwary physician as he seeks to interpret certain laboratory results relating to vitamin B_{12}.

Great care is needed in assessing the significance of a low reading. The first step should probably consist in getting the estimation repeated. Chanarin (1969), reviewing the reproducibility of the *Euglena* assay for serum B_{12}, reported coefficients of variation, on the same sample, ranging from 4·2 to 25 per cent. The physician should next bear in mind the effects of the technique used on the results obtained (Raven et al, 1972). Assays involving

Euglena gracilis are most sensitive at low levels of serum B_{12}. They tend to give lower readings than assays using *Lactobacillus leichmanii*. The microbiological tests, taken as a whole, give lower readings than the newer isotope dilution techniques.

A low serum B_{12} does not always imply a deficiency state, although it usually does. The term 'deficiency' is most usefully used to describe an abnormal state of affairs which has detectable clinical or biochemical repercussions. In practice, this will mean disturbances of haemopoietic or neural function, or biochemical effects detectable on examination of the urine (increased methylmalonic acid excretion).

A low serum B_{12} without evidence of deficiency will usually be in the range 100 to 160 pg/ml. As so often in contemporary clinical medicine, it is important to enquire what drugs the patient is receiving. Low readings may result from the ingestion of drugs which inhibit the growth of the test organism. Antibiotics and antimitotic agents are the most important in this respect, although tranquillisers such as chlorpromazine have also been found to inhibit the growth of *Euglena gracilis* (Herbert, Gottlieb and Altschule, 1965).

A low serum B_{12} without evidence of B_{12} deficiency is also encountered in some pregnant women and in about a third of patients with severe folate deficiency. The explanation for this phenomenon is unknown. It may represent an altered distribution of vitamin B_{12} in the presence of severe folate deficiency. In most of these cases the absorption of vitamin B_{12} is normal, although in a few cases folate deficiency may itself possibly interfere with vitamin B_{12} absorption (Lees, 1961; Mollin and Waters, 1968; Scott et al, 1968). In deciding whether a megaloblastic anaemia is primarily due to folate or to B_{12} deficiency an absent or impaired haematological response to vitamin B_{12} may be of more help than the finding of a low serum level of vitamin B_{12}.

The earliest clinical effects of vitamin B_{12} deficiency are on haemopoiesis. Megaloblastic changes occur in the marrow and abnormalities are found at about the same time or a little later in the peripheral blood. Among the earliest peripheral effects are the appearance of oval macrocytes (macro-ovalocytosis) and hypersegmented polymorphs. A shift in the 'lobe average' is very suggestive (Herbert, 1964), as is a mean corpuscular volume of over 100 μm^3. With modern methods of automatic counting this is relatively easy to determine.

These haematological changes are sensitive and usually precede the appearance of methylmalonic acid (MMA) in the urine, and even its appearance after valine loading. Neurological complications only appear when the deficiency is more severe.

There has been a lot of confusion about the occurrence of peripheral neuropathy and subacute combined degeneration of the spinal cord in patients without anaemia. This has been reported many times and was in fact the subject of many heated controversies in the past, of which there have been more recent echoes (Edwin et al, 1966). Three points need stressing:

(a) The evidence of anaemia may not be obvious. As in most fields of medicine the experienced clinician will first want to know who looked at the film—and what was looked for. The essentially macrocytic nature of the anaemia may be difficult to ascertain in the presence of concomitant iron deficiency.

(b) The ingestion of large amounts of folate, either in the diet or in the form of tablets, may ensure normal haemopoiesis, while not of course preventing (and possibly even enhancing) the development of the neurological complications of vitamin B_{12} deficiency.

(c) Whether patients with neuropathy due to vitamin B_{12} deficiency have anaemia or not they will always have a low serum B_{12}. *The attribution of a neuropathy or of a myelopathy to vitamin B_{12} deficiency is probably impermissible when the serum B_{12} is above* 100 *pg/ml* on the *Euglena* assay. But there are two important provisos. The first is that the patient should not have received an injection of vitamin B_{12} prior to the estimation of the serum level (the commonest mistake here is to estimate the serum B_{12} level after the performance of a Schilling test). The second is that the B_{12} assay should be an accurate one. False 'normal' levels may be found if the blood sample or apparatus have been contaminated with either bacteria or with vitamin B_{12} itself.

Anaemia and neuropathy, in B_{12} deficiency, should be thought of as developing 'in parallel' and not 'in series'. B_{12}-deficient patients may have anaemia and no neuropathy, neuropathy and no anaemia, or both neuropathy and anaemia. Whatever the clinical findings however they will always have a low serum B_{12}.

Recent advances promise to render this complicated field even more confusing. Vitamin B_{12} is carried on two carrier proteins: transcobalamin I and transcobalamin II. Only the vitamin B_{12} attached to the latter seems to be readily available for use by the bone marrow or nervous system. Congenital deficiency of transcobalamin II has recently been reported in two infants who presented with megaloblastic anaemia, failure to thrive, repeated infections and systemic signs (Hakami et al, 1971). If we may finish this whole section on vitamin B_{12} on a Kafkaesque note it would be by pointing out that the serum B_{12} levels in these severely B_{12}-deficient children may be *normal* (Scott et al, 1972) as most of the B_{12} is then carried on transcobalamin I!

References

Biological considerations

Barker, H. A. (1968). Vitamin B_{12}—biochemical systems. In *The Vitamins: Chemistry, Physiology, Pathology, Methods*, ed. Sebrell, W. H. & Harris, R. S., 2nd edition, Vol. 2. p. 184. New York: Academic Press.

Beck, W. S. (1968). Deoxyribonucleotide synthesis and the role of vitamin B_{12} in erythropoiesis. *Vitamins and Hormones*, **26,** 413–442.

Boddington, M. M. & Spriggs, A. I. (1959). The epithelial cells in megaloblastic anaemia. *Journal of Clinical Pathology*, **12,** 228–234.

Brozovic, M., Hoffbrand, A. V., Dimitriadou, A., & Mollin, D. L. (1967). The excretion of methylmalonic acid and succinic acid in vitamin B_{12} and folate deficiency. *British Journal of Haematology*, **13,** 1021–1032.

Chanarin, I. (1970). Pernicious anaemia and other vitamin B_{12} deficiency states. *Abstracts of World Medicine*, **44,** 73–85.

Chanarin, I., England, J. M., Mollin, C. & Perry, J. (1973). Methylmalonic acid excretion studies. *British Journal of Haematology*, **25,** 45–53.

Cox, E. V. & White, A. M. (1962). Methylmalonic acid excretion: An index of vitamin B_{12} deficiency. *Lancet*, **2,** 853–856.

Flavin, M., Ortiz, P. J. & Ochoa, S. (1955). Metabolism of propionic acid in animal tissues. *Nature*, **176**, 823–826.

Gompertz, D., Jones, J. H. & Knowles, J. P. (1967). Metabolic precursors of methylmalonic acid in vitamin B_{12} deficiency. *Clinica chimica acta*, **18**, 197–204.

Graham, R. M. & Rheault, M. H. (1954). Characteristic changes in epithelial cells in pernicious anaemia. *Journal of Laboratory and Clinical Medicine*, **43**, 235–245.

Hoffbrand, A. V. (1971). The megaloblastic anaemias. In *Recent Advances in Haematology*, ed. Brain, M. C. & Goldberg, A. London: Churchill.

Hogenkamp, H. P. C. (1968). Enzymatic reactions involving corrinoids. *Annual Review of Biochemistry*, **37**, 225–245.

Kahn, S. B., Williams, W. J., Barness, L. A., Young, D., Shafer, B., Vivacqua, R. J. & Geaupre, E. M. (1965). Methylmalonic acid excretion, a sensitive indicator of vitamin B_{12} deficiency in man. *Journal of Laboratory and Clinical Medicine*, **66**, 75–83.

Mahoney, M. J. & Rosenberg, L. E. (1970). Inherited defects of B_{12} metabolism. *American Journal of Medicine*, **48**, 584–593.

Minot, G. R. & Murphy, W. P. (1926). Treatment of pernicious anemia by a special diet, *Journal of the American Medical Association*, **87**, 470–476.

Moore, H. W. & Folkers, K. (1968). Vitamin B_{12}—chemistry. In *The Vitamins: Chemistry, Physiology, Pathology, Methods*, ed. Sebrell, W. H. & Harris, R. S., 2nd edition, Vol. 2, p. 121. New York: Academic Press.

Rickes, E. L., Brink, N. G., Koniuszy, F. R., Wood, T. R., Folkers, K. (1948). Crystalline vitamin B_{12}. *Science*, **107**, 396–397.

Rosenberg, L. E. (1972). Disorders of propionate, methylmalonate and vitamin B_{12} metabolism. In *The Metabolic Basis of Inherited Disease*, ed. Stanbury, J. B., Wyngaarden, J. B. & Fredrickson, D. S., Ch. 22. New York: McGraw-Hill.

Silber, R., Fujioka, S., Moldow, C. F. & Cox, R. (1970). Altered regulation of deoxyribonucleotide synthesis in B_{12} or folate deficiency. *Clinical Research*, **18**, 416.

Silber, R. & Moldow, C. F. (1970). The biochemistry of B_{12} mediated reactions in man. *American Journal of Medicine*, **48**, 549–554.

Smith, E. L. (1965). *Vitamin B_{12}*. 3rd edition. London: Methuen.

Smith, E. L. & Parker, L. F. J. (1948). Purification of antipernicious anaemia factor. *Biochemical Journal*, **43**, VIII-IX.

Vivacqua, R. J., Myerson, R. M., Prescott, D. J. & Rabinowitz, J. L. (1966). Abnormal propionic-methylmalonic-succinic acid metabolism in vitamin B_{12} deficiency and its possible relationship to the neurologic syndrome of pernicious anemia. *American Journal of Medical Sciences*, **251**, 507–515.

Walerych, W. S., Venkataraman, S. V. & Johnson, B. C. (1966). The methylation of transfer RNA by methylcobamide. *Biochemical and Biophysical Research Communications*, **23**, 368–374.

Weissbach, H. & Taylor, R. T. (1968). Metabolic role of vitamin B_{12}. *Vitamins and Hormones*, **26**, 395–412.

Peripheral neuropathy

Alexander, W. F. (1956). Pathomorphology of the nervous system in vitamin B_{12} deficiency. In *Vitamin B_{12} und Intrinsic Factor*, ed. Heinrich, H. D., pp. 372–383. Stuttgart: Enke.

Bramwell, B. (1915). Clinical studies. II. On the association of pernicious anaemia with subacute combined degeneration of the spinal cord. *Edinburgh Medical Journal*, **14**, 260–276.

Bremer, F. W. (1935). Funikuläre Spinalerkrankung. In *Handbuch der Neurologie*, ed. Bumke, O. & Foerster, O., pp. 941–986. Berlin: Springer.

Brooks, H. (1903). Cage paralysis, with a preliminary pathological study of five cases. In *8th Annual Report of the New York Zoological Society*, p. 115.

Buzzard, E. F. & Greenfield, J. B. (1921). *Pathology of the Nervous System*. London: Constable.

Campbell, A. W. & Clelland, J. B. (1919). Cage paralysis in monkeys. *Journal of Comparative Pathology and Therapeutics*, **32**, 95–104.

Collier, J. (1925). Discussion on the aetiology and treatment of subacute combined degeneration of the spinal cord. *Proceedings of the Royal Society of Medicine*, **18**, 21–27.

Dynes, J. B. & Norcross, J. W. (1943). Peripheral neuritis as a complication of pernicious anemia and combined system disease. *Journal of the American Medical Association*, **122**, 586–588.

Foster, D. B. (1945). Degeneration of peripheral nerves in pernicious anemia. *Archives of Neurology and Psychiatry*, **54**, 102–109.

Gilliatt, R. W. (1966). Applied electrophysiology in nerve and muscle disease. *Proceedings of the Royal Society of Medicine*, **59**, 989–993.

Gilliatt, R. W., Goodman, H. V. & Willison, R. E. (1961). The recording of lateral popliteal nerve action potentials in man. *Journal of Neurology, Neurosurgery and Psychiatry*, **24**, 305–318.

Greenfield, J. G. & Carmichael, E. A. (1935). The peripheral nerves in cases of subacute combined degeneration of the cord. *Brain*, **58**, 483–491.

Grinker, R. R. (1926). Pernicious anemia, achylia gastrica and combined cord degeneration and their relationship. *Archives of Internal Medicine*, **38**, 292–302.

Hamilton, A. S. & Nixon, C. F. (1921). Sensory changes in the subacute combined degeneration of pernicious anemia. *Archives of Neurology and Psychiatry*, **6**, 1–31.

Hurst, A. F. (1934). The clinical importance of achlorhydria. *British Medical Journal*, **2**, 665–669.

Innes, J. R. M. & Saunders, L. Z. (1962). *Comparative neuropathology*, pp. 67 and 688. New York and London: Academic Press.

Krohn, P. L., Oxnard, C. E. & Chalmers, J. N. M. (1963). Vitamin B_{12} in the serum of the rhesus monkey. *Nature*, **197**, 186.

Lockner, D., Reizenstein, P., Wennberg, P. & Widen, L. (1969). Peripheral nerve function in pernicious anaemia before and after treatment. *Acta haematologica*, **41**, 257–263.

McAlpine, D. (1929). A review of nervous and mental aspects of pernicious anaemia. *Lancet*, **2**, 643–647.

Mayer, R. F. (1965). Peripheral nerve function in vitamin B_{12} deficiency. *Archives of Neurology*, **13**, 355–362.

Minnich, W. (1892). Zur Kenntniss der im Verlaufe der perniciösen Anämie beobachteten Spinalerkrankungen. *Zeitschrift für klinische Medizin*, **21**, 264–314.

Nonne, M. (1895). Weitere Beiträge zur Kenntniss der im Verlaufe letaler Anämien beobachteten Spinalerkrankungen. *Deutsche Zeitschrift für Nervenheilkunde*, **6**, 313–368.

Olivarius, B. de F. & Roos, D. (1968). Myelopathy following partial gastrectomy. *Acta neurologica scandinavica*, **44**, 347–362.

Oxnard, C. E. (1964). Some variations in the amount of vitamin B_{12} in the serum of the rhesus monkey. *Nature*, **201**, 1188–1191.

Oxnard, C. E. & Smith, W. T. (1966). Neurological degeneration and reduced serum vitamin B_{12} levels in captive monkeys. *Nature*, **210**, 507–509.

Oxnard, C. E., Smith, W. T. & Torres, I. (1969). Peripheral neuropathy and hypovitaminosis B_{12} in captive monkeys. In *Proceedings of the 2nd International Congress Primatology*, Vol. 3, pp. 162–168. Basel & New York: Karger.

Oxnard, C. E., Smith, W. T. & Torres, I. (1970). Vitamin B_{12} deficiency in captive monkeys and its effect on the nervous system and the blood. *Laboratory Animals*, **4**, 1–12.

Pant, S. H., Asbury, A. K. & Richardson, E. P. (1968). The myelopathy of pernicious anemia. A neuropathological reappraisal. *Acta neurologica scandinavica*, **44**, Supplement 35.

Richmond, J. & Davidson, S. (1958). Subacute combined degeneration of the spinal cord in non-Addisonian megaloblastic anaemia. *Quarterly Journal of Medicine*, **N.S. 27**, 517–531.

Rothmann, M. (1906). Über eine Tabes-artige Erkrankung beim Affen. *Monatsschrift für Psychiatrie und Neurologie*, **20** (Supplement) 204–221.

Swallow, M. (1966). Fibre size and content of the anterior tibial nerve of the foot. *Journal of Neurology, Neurosurgery and Psychiatry*, **29**, 205–213.

Symonds, C. P. (1972). Personal communication.

Torres, I., Smith, W. T. & Oxnard, C. E. (1971). Peripheral neuropathy associated with vitamin B_{12} deficiency in captive monkeys. *Journal of Pathology*, **105**, 125–146.

Ungley, C. C. (1949). Subacute combined degeneration of the cord. *Brain*, **72**, 382–427.
van der Sheer, W. N. & Koek, H. C. (1938). Peripheral nerve lesions in cases of pernicious anaemia. *Acta psychiatrica et neurologica*, **13**, 61–92.
Victor, M. & Lear, A. A. (1956). Subacute combined degeneration of the spinal cord. *American Journal of Medicine*, **20**, 896–911.
Woltmann, H. W. (1919). The nervous system in pernicious anemia: an analysis of one hundred and fifty cases. *American Journal of Medical Sciences*, **157**, 400–409.

Myelopathy

Badenoch, J., Bedford, P. D. & Evans, J. R. (1955). Massive diverticulosis of the small intestine with steatorrhoea and megaloblastic anaemia. *Quarterly Journal of Medicine*, **N.S. 24**, 321–330.
Beebe, R. T. & Meneely, J. K. (1949). Pernicious anemia following gastrectomy. *New York State Journal of Medicine*, **49**, 2437–2438.
Bremer, F. W. (1931). Zentralnervensystem und perniziöse Anämie. *Ergebnisse der inneren Medizin und Kinderheilkunde*, **41**, 143–201.
Collier, James (1941). *Price's Textbook of the Practice of Medicine* 6th edition, p. 1741. London: Oxford University Press.
Davidson, L. S. P. (1957). Clinical picture of pernicious anaemia prior to introduction of liver therapy in 1926 and in Edinburgh subsequent to 1944. *British Medical Journal*, **1**, 241–243.
Little, W. D., Zerfas, L. G. & Trusler, H. M. (1929). Chronic obstruction of the small bowel; result of 2 enteroenterostomies and apparently the cause of pernicious anemia. *Journal of the American Medical Association*, **93**, 1290–1291.
MacLean, L. D. (1957). Incidence of megaloblastic anemia after subtotal gastrectomy. *New England Journal of Medicine*, **257**, 262–265.
Nicol, W. A. (1960). Non-Addisonian megaloblastic anaemia complicated by subacute combined degeneration of the cord. *British Medical Journal*, **1**, 322–324.
Olivarius, B. de F. & Roos, D. (1968). Myelopathy following partial gastrectomy. *Acta neurologica scandinavica*, **44**, 347–362.
Ragins, H. & Oberhelman, H. A. Jr. (1960). Anemia associated with a stagnant ('blind') jejunal loop. *Archives of Surgery*, **80**, 524–527.
Richmond, J. & Davidson, S. (1958). Subacute combined degeneration of the spinal cord in non-Addisonian megaloblastic anaemia. *Quarterly Journal of Medicine*, **N.S. 27**, 517–531.
Rowlands, R. A. & Simpson, S. L. (1932). Addisonian anaemia following gastrectomy and gastrojejunostomy. *Lancet*, **2**, 1202–1209.
Salus, F. (1932). Zur Entstehung der funikulären Myelitis. *Klinische Wochenschrift*, **11**, 237–240.
Simpson, C. K. (1931). A case of Addison's anaemia with subacute combined degeneration of the cord associated with carcinoma of the stomach. *Guy's Hospital Reports*, **11**, 392–406.
Victor, M. & Lear, A. A. (1956). Subacute combined degeneration of the spinal cord. *American Journal of Medicine*, **20**, 896–911.
Welbourn, R., Hughes, R. & Wells, C. (1951). Vitamin B deficiencies after gastric operations. *Lancet*, **1**, 939–945.
Wilson, S. A. K. (1954). *Neurology*. 2nd edition. London: Butterworth.

Encephalopathy and optic neuritis

Adams, R. D. & Kubik, C. S. (1944). Subacute degeneration of the brain in pernicious anemia. *New England Journal of Medicine*, **231**, 1–9.
Ahrens, R. S. (1932). Neurologic aspects of primary anemia. *Archives of Neurology and Psychiatry*, **28**, 92–111.
Benedict, W. L. (1933). Retrobulbar neuritis and disease of the nasal accessory sinuses. *Proceedings of the Staff Meetings of the Mayo Clinic*, **8**, 147–149.
Benham, G. H. H. (1951). Visual field defects in subacute combined degeneration of spinal cord. *Journal of Neurology, Neurosurgery and Psychiatry*, **14**, 40–46.

Bickel, H. (1914). Funikuläre Myelitis mit bulbären und polyneuritischen Symptomen. *Archiv fur Psychiatrie und Nervenkrankheiten*, **53**, 1106–1117.

Björkenheim, B. (1966). Optic neuropathy caused by vitamin-B_{12} deficiency in carriers of the fish tapeworm, Diphyllobothrium latum. *Lancet*, **1**, 688–690.

Cohen, H. (1936). Optic atrophy as presenting sign in pernicious anaemia. *Lancet*, **2**, 1202–1203.

Edwin, E., Holten, K., Norum, K. R., Schrumpf, A. & Skaug, O. E. (1965). Vitamin B_{12} hypovitaminosis in mental diseases. *Acta medica scandinavica*, **177**, 689–699.

Eilenberg, M. D. (1960). Psychiatric illness and pernicious anemia: a clinical re-evaluation. *Journal of Mental Science*, **106**, 1539–1548.

Gaffney, G. W., Horonick, A., Okuda, K., Meier, P., Chow, B. F. & Shock, N. W. (1957). Vitamin B_{12} serum concentrations in 528 apparently healthy human subjects of ages 12–94. *Journal of Gerontology*, **12**, 32–38.

Goldhamer, S. M., Bethell, F. H., Isaacs, R. & Sturgis, C. S. (1934). The occurrence and treatment of neurologic changes in pernicious anemia. *Journal of the American Medical Association*, **103**, 1663–1667.

Hamilton, H. E., Ellis, P. P. & Sheets, R. F. (1959). Visual impairment due to optic neuropathy in pernicious anaemia: report of case and review of the literature. *Blood*, **14**, 378–385.

Henderson, J. G., Strachan, R. W., Beck, J. S., Dawson, A. A. & Daniel, M. (1966). The antigastric-antibody test as a screening procedure for vitamin B_{12} deficiency in psychiatric practice. *Lancet*, **2**, 809–813.

Herman, M., Most, H. & Jolliffe, N. (1937). Psychoses associated with pernicious anemia. *Archives of Neurology and Psychiatry*, **38**, 348–361.

Holmes, J. M. (1956). Cerebral manifestations of vitamin-B_{12} deficiency. *British Medical Journal*, **2**, 1394–1398.

Hunter, R., Jones, M. & Matthews, D. M. (1967). Postgastrectomy vitamin B_{12} deficiency in psychiatric practice. *Lancet*, **1**, 47.

Langdon, F. W. (1905). Nervous and mental manifestations of pre-pernicious anaemia. *Journal of the American Medical Association*, **45**, 1635–1638.

McAlpine, D. (1929). A review of the nervous and mental aspects of pernicious anaemia. *Lancet*, **2**, 643–647.

Murphy, F., Srivastava, P. C., Varadi, S. & Elwis, A. (1969). Screening of psychiatric patients for hypovitaminosis B_{12}. *British Medical Journal*, **3**, 559–560.

Nielsen, B. (1966). Mental symptoms in vitamin B_{12} deficiency. *Lancet*, **1**, 985.

Noyes, A. P. & Kolb, L. C. (1963). *Modern Clinical Psychiatry*. London: Saunders.

Romano, J. & Engel, G. L. (1944). Delirium: electroencephalographic data. *Archives of Neurology and Psychiatry*, **51**, 356–377.

Samson, D. C., Swisher, S. N., Christian, R. M. & Engel, G. L. (1952). Cerebral metabolic disturbance and delirium in pernicious anemia. *Archives of Internal Medicine*, **90**, 4–14.

Scheinberg, P. (1951). Cerebral blood flow and metabolism in pernicious anemia. *Blood*, **6**, 213–227.

Shulman, R. (1967). Psychiatric aspects of pernicious anaemia: a prospective controlled investigation. *British Medical Journal*, **3**, 266–270.

Slater, E. & Roth, M. (1969). *Mayer-Gross, Slater* & *Roth; Clinical Psychiatry*, Third edition. London: Bailliere, Tindall & Cassell.

Smith, M. D., Smith, D. A. & Fletcher, M. (1962). Haemorrhage associated with thrombocytopenia in megaloblastic anaemia. *British Medical Journal*, **1**, 982–985.

Smith, R. & Oliver, R. A. M. (1967). Sudden onset of psychosis in association with vitamin B_{12} deficiency. *British Medical Journal*, **3**, 34.

Strachan, R. W. & Henderson, J. G. (1965). Psychiatric syndromes due to avitaminosis B_{12} with normal blood and marrow. *Quarterly Journal of Medicine*, **34**, 303–317.

Wadia, N. H. & Swami, R. K. (1970). Pattern of nutritional deficiency disorders of the nervous system in Bombay. *Neurology (India)*, **18**, 203–219.

Walton, J. N., Kiloh, L. G., Osselton, J. W. & Farrall, J. (1954). The electroencephalogram in pernicious anaemia and subacute combined degeneration of the cord. *Electroencephalography and Clinical Neurophysiology*, **6**, 45–64.

Wilson, S. A. K. (1954). *Neurology*, Second edition. London: Butterworth.

Woltman, H. W. (1924). The mental changes associated with pernicious anemia. *American Journal of Psychiatry*, **80**, 435–449.

Young, R. H. (1932). Neurologic features of pernicious anemia. *Journal of the American Medical Association*, **99**, 612–614.

The nervous system and nutritional vitamin B_{12} deficiency

Badenoch, J. (1954). The use of labelled vitamin B_{12} and gastric biopsy in the investigation of anaemia. *Proceedings of the Royal Society of Medicine*, **47**, 426–427.

Baker, S. J. (1957). Idiopathic tropical steatorrhoea, a report of 60 cases. *Indian Journal of Medical Science*, **11**, 687–703.

Baker, S. J., Jacob, E., Rajan, K. T.& Swaminathan, S. P. (1962). Vitamin B_{12} deficiency in pregnancy and the puerperium. *British Medical Journal*, **1**, 1658–1661.

Carmel, R. & Herbert, V. (1967). Correctable intestinal defect of vitamin B_{12} absorption in pernicious anemia. *Annals of Internal Medicine*, **67**, 1201–1207.

Chanarin, I. (1969). *The Megaloblastic Anaemias*. Oxford & Edinburgh: Blackwell.

Connor, P. M. & Pirola, R. C. (1963). Nutritional vitamin B_{12} deficiency. *Medical Journal of Australia*, **2**, 451–453.

Cox, E. V., Meynell, M. J., Gaddie, R. & Cooke, W. T. (1959). Inter-relation of vitamin B_{12} and iron. *Lancet*, **2**, 998–1001.

Dastur, D. K., Quadros, E. V., Wadia, N. H., Desai, M. M. & Bharucha, E. P. (1972). Effect of vegetarianism and smoking on vitamin B_{12}, thiocyanate and folate levels in the blood of normal subjects. *British Medical Journal*, **3**, 260–263.

Hill, C. (1952). Food and fads. *Journal of the Royal Society of Arts*, **100**, 181–190.

Jadhav, M., Webb, J. K. G., Vaishnava, S. & Baker, S. J. (1962). Vitamin B_{12} deficiency in Indian infants. A clinical syndrome. *Lancet*, **2**, 903–907.

Jeejeebhoy, K. N., Wadia, N. H. & Desai, H. G. (1967). Role of vitamin B_{12} deficiency in tropical 'nutritional' neuromyelopathy. *Journal of Neurology, Neurosurgery, and Psychiatry*, **30**, 7–12.

Lawrence, C. (1966). B_{12} binding protein deficiency in pernicious anemia. *Blood*, **27**, 389–394.

Lees, F. (1961). Radioactive vitamin B_{12} absorption in the megaloblastic anaemia caused by anticonvulsant drugs. *Quarterly Journal of Medicine*, **30**, 231–248.

Mehta, B. M., Rege, D. V. & Satoskar, R. S. (1964). Serum vitamin B_{12} and folic acid activity in lacto-vegetarian and non-vegetarian healthy adult Indians. *American Journal of Clinical Nutrition*, **15**, 77–84.

Misra, H. N. & Fallowfield, J. M. (1971). Subacute combined degeneration of the spinal cord in a vegan. *Postgraduate Medical Journal*, **47**, 624–626.

Mollin, D. L. & Waters, A. H. (1968). Nutritional megaloblastic anaemia. *Symposium of the Swedish Nutritional Foundation*, **6**, 121–134.

Riley, C. J. (1966). Unusual case of subacute combined degeneration of spinal cord. *British Medical Journal*, **2**, 566.

Scott, R. B., Kammer, R. B., Burgher, W. F. & Middleton, F. G. (1968). Reduced absorption of vitamin B_{12} in two patients with folic acid deficiency. *Annals of Internal Medicine*, **69**, 111–114.

Smith, A. D. M. (1962). Veganism: a clinical survey with observations on vitamin-B_{12} metabolism. *British Medical Journal*, **1**, 1655–1658.

Stewart, J. S., Roberts, P. D. & Hoffbrand, A. V. (1970). Response of dietary, vitamin B_{12} deficiency to physiological oral doses of cyanocobalamin. *Lancet*, **2**, 542–545.

Verjaal, A. & Timmermans-van den Bos, A. H. (1967). Combined degeneration of the spinal cord due to deficiency of alimentary vitamin B_{12}. *Journal of Neurology, Neurosurgery and Psychiatry*, **30**, 464–467.

Wokes, F. (1956). Diet and anaemia; anaemia and vitamin B_{12} dietary deficiency. *Proceedings of the Nutrition Society*, **15**, 134–141.

Wokes, F., Badenoch, J. & Sinclair, H. M. (1955a). Human dietary deficiency of vitamin B_{12}. *Voeding*, **16**, 590–602.

Wokes, F., Badenoch, J. & Sinclair, H. M. (1955b). Human dietary deficiency of vitamin B_{12}. *American Journal of Clinical Nutrition*, **3**, 375–382.

Total gastrectomy

Beebe, R. T. & Meneely, J. K. (1949). Pernicious anemia following gastrectomy. *New York State Journal of Medicine*, **49**, 2437–2438.
Booth, C. C. & Mollin, D. L. (1957). Importance of ileum in the absorption of vitamin B_{12}. *Lancet*, **2**, 1007.
Booth, C. C. & Mollin, D. L. (1959). The site of absorption of vitamin B_{12} in man. *Lancet*, **1**, 18–21.
Cooke, W. T., Cox, E. V., Meynell, M. J. & Gaddie, R. (1957). The ileal absorption of vitamin B_{12}. *Lancet*, **2**, 1231.
Cox, E. V., Williams, J. A. & Jones, C. T. (1963). Anaemia and the post-gastrectomy state. In *Partial Gastrectomy*, ed. Stammers, F. A. R. & Williams, J. A., p. 175. London: Butterworth.
Dennig, H. (1929). Perniziöse Anämie nach Magenresektion. *Münchener medizinische Wochenschrift*, **76**, 633.
Fox, H. J. & Castle, W. B. (1942). Observations on the etiologic relationship of achylia gastrica to pernicious anemia. IX. Difference in site of secretion of intrinsic factor in the hog and in the human stomach. *American Journal of Medical Sciences*, **203**, 18–28.
Glass, G. B. J., Pack, G. T. & Mersheimer, W. L. (1955). Uptake of radioactive vitamin B_{12} by the liver in patients with total and subtotal gastrectomy. *Gastroenterology*, **29**, 666–683.
Heyssel, R. M., Bozian, R. C., Darby, W. J. & Bell, M. C. (1966). Vitamin B_{12} turnover in man. *American Journal of Clinical Nutrition*, **18**, 176–184.
Hoffbrand, A. V. (1971). The Megaloblastic Anaemias. In *Recent Advances in Haematology*, ed. Goldberg, A. & Brain, M. C., Ch. 1. Edinburgh & London: Churchill Livingstone.
Landboe-Christensen, E., Berk, L. & Castle, W. B. (1952). Observations on the etiologic relationship of achylia gastrica to pernicious anemia. XIV. Intrinsic factor activity of desiccated and defatted fundus, duodenum and jejunum. *American Journal of Medical Sciences*, **224**, 1–8.
MacDonald, R. M., Ingelfinger, F. J. & Belding, H. W. (1947). Late effects of total gastrectomy in man. *New England Journal of Medicine*, **237**, 887–896.
MacLean, L. D. & Sundberg, R. D. (1956). Incidence of megaloblastic anemia after total gastrectomy. *New England Journal of Medicine*, **254**, 885–893.
Meyer, K. A., Schwartz, S. O. & Weissman, L. H. (1941). Pernicious anemia following total gastrectomy. *Archives of Surgery*, **42**, 18–24.
Pant, S. H., Asbury, A. K. & Richardson, E. P. (1968). The myelopathy of pernicious anemia. A neuropathological reappraisal. *Acta neurologica scandinavica*, **44**, Supplement 35.
Paulson, M. & Harvey, J. C. (1954). Hematological alterations after total gastrectomy. *Journal of the American Medical Association*, **156**, 1556–1560.

Partial gastrectomy

Alexeieff, G. (1957). Sur le problème des anémies chirurgicales. *Le Sang*, **28**, 305–315.
Badenoch, J., Evans, J. R. & Richards, W. C. D. (1957). The stomach in hypochromic anaemia. *British Journal of Haematology*, **3**, 175–185.
Badenoch, J., Evans, J. R., Richards, W. C. D. & Witts, L. J. (1955). Megaloblastic anaemia following partial gastrectomy and gastroenterostomy. *British Journal of Haematology*, **1**, 339–344.
Bastrup-Madsen, P. (1954). Non-anaemic neuropathy caused by deficiency of the anti-pernicious-anaemia principle following subtotal gastrectomy. *Acta medica scandinavica*, **147**, 399–404.
Biström, O. (1961). Ten years of surgical treatment of peptic ulcer at the Maria Hospital, Helsinki. *Annales chirurgiae et gynaecologiae Fenniae*, **50**, 1–39.
Chanarin, I. (1969). *The Megaloblastic Anaemias*. Oxford & Edinburgh: Blackwell.
Cox, E. V., Meynell, M. J., Gaddie, R. & Cooke, W. T. (1959). Inter-relation of vitamin B_{12} and iron. *Lancet*, **2**, 998–1001.

Cox, E. V., Williams, J. A. & Jones, C. T. (1963). Anaemia and the post-gastrectomy state. In *Partial Gastrectomy*, ed. Stammers, F. A. R. & Williams, J. A. p. 175. London: Butterworth.

Deller, D. J., Richards, W. C. D. & Witts, L. J. (1962). Changes in the blood after partial gastrectomy with special reference to vitamin B_{12}. II. The cause of the fall in serum vitamin B_{12}. *Quarterly Journal of Medicine*, **31**, 89–102.

Deller, D. J. & Witts, L. J. (1962). Changes in the blood after partial gastrectomy with special reference to vitamin B_{12}. I. Serum vitamin B_{12}, haemoglobin, serum iron and bone marrow. *Quarterly Journal of Medicine*, **31**, 71–88.

D'Eramo, N. (1965). Progressive myopathic muscular atrophy after gastric resection. *Lancet*, **1**, 1277–1278.

Ekbom, K., Hed, R., Kirstein, L. & Aström, K. E. (1964). Weakness of proximal limb muscles probably due to myopathy after partial gastrectomy. *Acta medica scandinavica*, **176**, 493–496.

Fone, D. J., Cooke, W. T., Meynell, M. J. & Harris, E. L. (1961). Co^{58} B_{12} absorption (hepatic surface count) after gastrectomy, ileal resection and in coeliac disorders. *Gut*, **2**, 218–224.

Goldstein, F., Wirts, C. W. & Kramer, S. (1961). The relationship of afferent limb stasis and bacterial flora to the production of post-gastrectomy steatorrhea. *Gastroenterology*, **40**, 47–55.

Hartfall, S. J. (1934). Gastrectomy and gastro-enterostomy anaemia. *Guy's Hospital Reports*, **84**, 448–467.

Hines, J. D., Hoffbrand, A. V. & Mollin, D. L. (1967). The hematologic complications following partial gastrectomy. A study of 292 patients. *American Journal of Medicine*, **43**, 555–569.

Hoffbrand, A. V. (1971). The megaloblastic anaemias. In *Recent Advances in Haematology*, ed. Brain, M. C. & Goldberg, A. London: Churchill.

Hunter, R. & Jones, D. M. (1967). Post-gastrectomy vitamin B_{12} deficiency in psychiatric practice. *Lancet*, **1**, 47.

Jensen, A. P. J. (1965). Myopati og andre neurologiske folgetilstande efter ventrikelresektion. *Ugeskrift for Laeger*, **127**, 823–829.

Johnson, H. D. & Hoffbrand, A. V. (1970). The influence of extent of resection, type of anastomosis, and of ulcer site on the haematological side effects of gastrectomy. *British Journal of Surgery*, **57**, 33–37.

Jones, C. T. & Williams, J. A. (1963). The effects of gastric operations on the gastric mucosa. In *Partial gastrectomy*, ed. Stammers, F. A. R. & Williams, J. A. pp. 122–149. London: Butterworth.

Jones, C. T., Williams, J. A., Cox, E. V., Meynell, M. J., Cooke, W. T. & Stammers, F. A. R. (1962). Peptic ulceration. Some haematological and metabolic consequences of gastric surgery. *Lancet*, **2**, 425–428.

Joske, R. A., Finckh, E. S. & Wood, I. J. (1955). Gastric biopsy: a study of 1000 consecutive successful gastric biopsies. *Quarterly Journal of Medicine*, **24**, 269–294.

Kniffen, J. C. & Quick, D. T. (1969). Neuromuscular disorder following gastric resection. *Archives of Internal Medicine*, **124**, 336–340.

Knox, J. D. E. & Delamore, I. W. (1960). Subacute combined degeneration of the cord after partial gastrectomy. *British Medical Journal*, **2**, 1494–1496.

Lous, P. & Schwartz, M. (1959). The absorption of vitamin B_{12} following partial gastrectomy. *Acta medica scandinavica*, **164**, 407–415.

Ogg, C. S. (1959). Intestinal diverticula. *British Medical Journal*, **2**, 888.

Olivarius, B. de F. & Roos, D. (1965). Responsibility after gastrectomy. *Lancet*, **2**, 1298.

Olivarius, B. de F. & Roos, D. (1968). Myelopathy following partial gastrectomy. *Acta neurologica scandinavica*, **44**, 347–362.

Ross, J. F., Belding, H. & Paegel, B. L. (1948). The development and progression of subacute combined degeneration of the spinal cord in patients with pernicious anaemia treated with synthetic pteroylglutamic (folic) acid. *Blood*, **3**, 68–90.

Rowlands, R. A. & Simpson, S. L. (1932). Addisonian anaemia following gastrectomy and gastrojejunostomy. *Lancet*, **2**, 1202–1209.

Salus, F. (1932). Zur Entstehung der funikulären Myelitis. *Klinische Wochenschrift*, **11**, 237–240.

Salus, F. & Reimann, F. (1934). Das Castlesche Ferment und die funikuläre Spinalerkrankung. Ein Beitrag zur Pathogenese des nervosen Krankheitssyndroms (VI. Untersuchungen zur Leberwirkung bei der Anaemia perniciosa). *Klinische Wochenschrift*, **13**, 986–990.
Schloesser, L. L., Deshpande, P. & Schilling, R. F. (1958). Biologic turnover rate of cyanocobalamin (vitamin B_{12}) in human liver. *Archives of Internal Medicine*, **101**, 306–309.
Schneider, J. P. & Carey, J. B. (1928). Clinical significance of primary achlorhydria. *Journal of the American Medical Association*, **91**, 1763–1768.
Tabaqchali, S., Okubadejo, O. A., Neale, G. & Booth, C. C. (1966). Influence of abnormal bacterial flora on small intestinal function. *Proceedings of the Royal Society of Medicine*, **59**, 1244–1246.
Temperley, I. J., Weir, D. G., Colliery, D. & Scott, J. M. (1969). Inhibition of free intrinsic factor activity by duodenal juice. *Gastroenterology*, **57**, 273–279.
Weir, D. G. & Gatenby, P. B. B. (1963). Subacute combined degeneration of the cord after partial gastrectomy. *British Medical Journal*, **2**, 1175–1176.
Wellbourn, R., Hughes, R. & Wells, C. (1951). Vitamin B deficiencies after gastric operations. *Lancet*, **1**, 939–945.
Wells, C. & MacPhee, I. W. (1954). Partial gastrectomy: ten years later. *British Medical Journal*, **2**, 1128–1132.
Williams, J. A. (1967). Postgastrectomy problems. *British Medical Journal*, **2**, 403–405, 467–469.
Williams, J. A., Hall, G. S., Thompson, A. G. & Cooke, W. T. (1969). Neurological disease after partial gastrectomy. *British Medical Journal*, **2**, 210–212.

Gastric lesions other than gastrectomy

Alsted, G. (1937). Pernicious anaemia after nitric acid corrosion of the stomach. *Lancet*, **1**, 76–79.
Ardeman, S. & Chanarin, I. (1963). A method for the assay of human gastric intrinsic factor and for the detection and titration of antibodies against intrinsic factor. *Lancet*, **2**, 1350–1354.
Ardeman, S. & Chanarin, I. (1965). Assay of intrinsic factor in the diagnosis of Addisonian pernicious anaemia. *British Journal of Haematology*, **11**, 305–314.
Ardeman, S. & Chanarin, I. (1966). Intrinsic factor secretion in gastric atrophy. *Gut*, **7**, 99–101.
Brandes, T. (1921). Uber die Beziehungen der perniziösen Anämie zum Magencarcinom. *MedizinischeKlinik*, **17**, 189–192.
Callender, S. T., Witts, L. J., Allison, P. R. & Gunning, A. (1961). Some metabolic and haematological effects of oesophago-jejunostomy with by-pass of the stomach. *Gut*, **2**, 150–157.
Chanarin, I. (1969). *The Megaloblastic Anaemias*. Oxford & Edinburgh: Blackwell.
Chanarin, I. (1970). Pernicious anaemia and other vitamin B_{12} deficiency states. *Abstracts of World Medicine*, **44**, 73–85.
Dreyfus, P. M. (1971). Nutritional disorders of the nervous system. In *Cecil–Loeb's Textbook of Medicine*, ed. Beeson, P. B. & McDermott, W., 13th edition. Philadelphia: Saunders.
Garvey, J. L. & Stern, L. D. (1924). Combined sclerosis of the spinal cord and carcinoma of the stomach. *American Journal of the Medical Sciences*, **168**, 847–852.
Grinker, R. R. (1926). Pernicious anemia, achylia gastrica and combined cord degeneration and their relationship. *Archives of Internal Medicine*, **38**, 292–302.
Hoffbrand, A. V. (1971). The megaloblastic anaemias. In *Recent Advances in Haematology*, ed. Brain, M. C. & Goldberg, A. London: Churchill.
Hurst, A. F. (1934). The clinical importance of achlorhydria. *British Medical Journal*, **2**, 665–669.
Jandl, J. H. (1971). Pernicious anaemia. In *Cecil–Loeb's Textbook of Medicine*, ed. Beeson, P. B. & McDermott, W. 13th edition, pp. 1466–1470. Philadelphia: Saunders.
Joske, R. A., Finckh, E. S. & Wood, I. J. (1955). Gastric biopsy: a study of 1000 consecutive successful gastric biopsies. *Quarterly Journal of Medicine*, **24**, 269–294.
Morson, B. C. (1966). The stomach. In *Systemic Pathology*, ed. Payling Wright, G. & Symmers, W. St. C., Vol. 1, pp. 481–514. London: Longmans.

Nonne, M. (1906). Ueber Myelitis intrafunicularis und über kombinierte Strangerkrankung bei Alcoholismus chronicus. *Monatsschrift für Psychiatrie und Neurologie*, **20**, 497–528.
Pearson, H. A., Vinson, R. & Smith, R. T. (1964). Pernicious anemia with neurologic involvement in childhood. *Journal of Pediatrics*, **65**, 334–339.
Porges, O. (1929). Magenkrankheiten, ihre Diagnose und Therapie. In *Zwölf klinischen Vorlesungen*, p. 63. Berlin: Urban & Schwarzenberg.
Reisner, E. H., Wolff, J. A., McKay, R. J. & Doyle, E. F. (1951). Juvenile pernicious anemia. *Pediatrics*, **8**, 88–106.
Simpson, C. K. (1931). A case of Addison's anaemia with subacute combined degeneration of the cord associated with carcinoma of the stomach. *Guy's Hospital Reports*, **11**, 392–406.
Waterfield, R. L. & Shackle, J. W. (1923). The diagnosis of Addison's (pernicious) anaemia: two cases of severe anaemia. *Guy's Hospital Reports*, **73**, 206–224.
Wood, I. J., Ralston, M., Ungar, B. & Cowling, D. C. (1964). Vitamin B_{12} deficiency in chronic gastritis. *Gut*, **5**, 27–37.

Structural lesions of the small bowel

Badenoch, J., Bedford, P. D. & Evans, J. R. (1955). Massive diverticulosis of the small intestine with steatorrhoea and megaloblastic anaemia. *Quarterly Journal of Medicine*, **N.S. 24**, 321–330.
Barker, W. H. & Hummel, L. E. (1939). Macrocytic anemia in association with intestinal strictures and anastomoses. *Bulletin of Johns Hopkins Hospital*, **64**, 215–254.
Blachford, R. D. & Dawson, D. W. (1956). Association of jejunal diverticulosis with macrocytic anaemia. *British Medical Journal*, **1**, 1407–1408.
Chanarin, I. (1969). *The Megaloblastic Anaemias*. Oxford & Edinburgh: Blackwell.
Chernov, A. J., Doe, W. F. & Gompertz, D. (1972). Intrajejunal volatile fatty acid in the stagnant loop syndrome. *Gut*, **13**, 103–106.
Cooke, W. T., Cox, E. V., Fone, D. J., Meynell, M. J. & Gaddie, R. (1963). The clinical and metabolic significance of jejunal diverticulosis. *Gut*, **4**, 115–131.
Dack, G. M. & Petran, E. (1934). Bacterial activity in different levels of intestine and in isolated segments of small and large bowel in monkeys and in dogs. *Journal of Infectious Diseases*, **54**, 204–220.
Dawson, A. M. & Isselbacher, K. J. (1960). Studies on lipid metabolism in the small intestine with observations on the role of bile salts. *Journal of Clinical Investigation*, **39**, 730–740.
Dubos, R. (1966). The microbiota of the gastrointestinal tract. *Gastroenterology*, **51**, 868–874.
Fairley, N. H. & Kilner, T. P. (1931). Gastro-jejuno-colic fistula, with megalocytic anemia simulating sprue. *Lancet*, **2**, 1335–1341.
Floch, M. H., Gershengoren, W., Diamond, S. & Hersh, T. (1970). Cholic acid inhibition of intestinal bacteria. *American Journal of Clinical Nutrition*, **23**, 8–10.
Gall, L. S. (1970). Normal fecal flora in man. *American Journal of Clinical Nutrition*, **23**, 1457–1465.
Gianella, R. A., Broitman, S. A. & Zamcheck, N. (1971). Vitamin B_{12} uptake by intestinal microorganisms: Mechanism and relevance to syndromes of intestinal bacterial overgrowth. *Journal of Clinical Investigation*, **50**, 1100–1107.
Glanvill, R. & Hurst, A. F. (1930). A case of Addison's anaemia with achlorhydria resulting from gastro-jejunostomy performed for gastric ulcer. *Guy's Hospital Reports*, **10**, 411–413.
Halsted, J. A., Lewis, P. M. & Gasster, M. (1956). Absorption of radioactive vitamin B_{12} in the syndrome of megaloblastic anemia associated with intestinal stricture or anastomosis. *American Journal of Medicine*, **20**, 42–52.
Harvey, E. A. & Murphy, W. P. (1933). Pernicious anemia without achlorhydria. *Annals of Internal Medicine*, **6**, 1393–1406.
Hersh, T., Floch, M. H., Binder, H. J., Conn, H. O., Prizont, R. & Spiro, H. M. (1970). Disturbance of the jejunal and colonic bacterial flora in immunoglobulin deficiencies. *American Journal of Clinical Nutrition*, **23**, 1595–1601.
Hill, M. J. & Drasar, B. S. (1968). Degradation of bile salts by human intestinal bacteria. *Gut*, **9**, 22–27.

Hurst, A. F. (1933). A case of Addison's anaemia with subacute combined degeneration of the spinal cord and normal gastric secretion following chronic obstruction of the ileum. *Guy's Hospital Reports*, **83**, 47–52.

Hurst, A. F. (1934). The clinical importance of achlorhydria. *British Medical Journal*, **2**, 665–669.

James, O. F. W., Agnew, J. E. & Bouchier, I. A. D. (1973). Assessment of the ^{14}C-glycocholic acid breath test. *British Medical Journal*, **2**, 191–195.

Krevans, J. R., Conley, C. L. & Sachs, M. (1954). Influence of certain diseases on the absorption of vitamin B_{12} from the gastrointestinal tract. *Journal of Clinical Investigation*, **33**, 949–950.

Lee, R. E. & Finby, N. (1958). Jejunal and ileal diverticulosis. *Archives of Internal Medicine*, **102**, 97–102.

Little, W. D., Zerfas, L. G. & Trusler, H. M. (1929). Chronic obstruction of the small bowel; result of 2 entero-enterostomies and apparently the cause of pernicious anemia. *Journal of the American Medical Association*, **93**, 1290–1291.

Midtvedt, T. & Norman, A. (1967). Bile acid transformations by microbial strains belonging to genera found in intestinal contents. *Acta pathologica et microbiologica scandinavica*, **71**, 629–638.

Mollin, D. L., Booth, C. C. & Baker, S. J. (1957). The absorption of vitamin B_{12} in control subjects, in Addisonian pernicious anaemia and in the malabsorption syndrome. *British Journal of Haematology*, **3**, 412–428.

Naish, J. & Capper, W. M. (1953). Intestinal cul-de-sac phenomena in man. *Lancet*, **2**, 597–600.

Neale, G., Gompertz, D., Schönsby, H., Tabaqchali, S. & Booth, C. C. (1972). The metabolic and nutritional consequences of bacterial overgrowth in the small intestine. *American Journal of Clinical Nutrition*, **25**, 1409–1417.

Neale, G., Lambert, R. A. & Gorbach, S. L. (1969). The production of indole by bacteria in vitro. *Gut*, **10**, 1056–1057.

Nicol, W. A. (1960). Non-Addisonian megaloblastic anaemia, complicated by subacute combined degeneration of the cord. *British Medical Journal*, **1**, 322–324.

Palmer, E. D. (1953). Further observations on post-operative gastritis: histopathologic aspects with a note on jejunitis. *Gastroenterology*, **25**, 405–415.

Ragins, H. & Oberhelman, H. A., Jr (1960). Anemia associated with a stagnant ('blind') jejunal loop. *Archives of Surgery*, **80**, 524–527.

Richmond, J. & Davidson, S. (1958). Subacute combined degeneration of the spinal cord in non-Addisonian megaloblastic anaemia. *Quarterly Journal of Medicine*, **N.S. 27**, 517–531.

Salus, F. (1932). Zur Entstehung der funikulären Myelitis. *Klinische Wochenschrift*, **11**, 237–240.

Scudamore, H. H., Hagedorn, A. B., Wollaenger, E. E. & Owen, C. A. (1958). Diverticulosis of the small intestine and macrocytic anemia with a report of 2 cases and studies on absorption of radioactive vitamin B_{12}. *Gastroenterology*, **34**, 66–82.

Starzl, T. E., Butz, G. W., Jr & Hartman, C. F. (1961). The blind-loop syndrome after gastric operations. *Surgery*, **50**, 849–858.

Tabaqchali, S. (1970). The pathophysiological role of small intestinal bacterial flora. *Scandinavian Journal of Gastroenterology*, Supplementum 6, 139–163.

Tabaqchali, S., Okubadejo, O. A., Neale, G. & Booth, C. C. (1966). Influence of abnormal bacterial flora on small intestinal function. *Proceedings of the Royal Society of Medicine*, **59**, 1244–1246.

Taylor, W. G. (1930). Intestinal diverticulosis, pernicious anemia, bilateral suprarenal apoplexy: report of a case. *New England Journal of Medicine*, **202**, 269–271.

Townsend, S. R. & Cameron, D. G. (1957). Megaloblastic anemia associated with diverticula of the small bowel. *American Journal of Medicine*, **23**, 668–670.

Wilkinson, R. W. (1955). Subacute combined degeneration of the spinal cord with megaloblastic anaemia due to spontaneous ileocolic fistula. *Lancet*, **1**, 74–85.

Woltman, H. W. & Heck, F. J. (1937). Funicular degeneration of the spinal cord without pernicious anemia. *Archives of Internal Medicine*, **60**, 272–300.

Regional enteritis, intestinal tuberculosis and gut resection

Allcock, E. (1961). Absorption of vitamin B_{12} in man following extensive resection of the jejunum, ileum and colon. *Gastroenterology*, **40**, 81–85.

Best, C. N. (1959). Subacute combined degeneration of spinal cord after extensive resection of ileum in Crohn's disease. *British Medical Journal*, **2**, 862–864.

Bitsch, V., Christiansen, P. M., Faber, V. & Rodbro, P. (1966). Gastric secretory patterns before and after vagotomy. *Lancet*, **1**, 1288–1291.

Booth, C. C. (1963). Absorption from the small intestine. *Scientific Basis of Medicine, Annual Reviews*, 171–196. London: Athlone Press.

Booth, C. C. & Mollin, D. L. (1957). Importance of ileum in the absorption of vitamin B_{12}. *Lancet*, **2**, 1007.

Booth, C. C. & Mollin, D. L. (1959). The site of absorption of vitamin B_{12} in man. *Lancet*, **1**, 18–21.

Chanarin, I. (1969). *The Megaloblastic Anaemias*. Oxford & Edinburgh: Blackwell.

Hoffbrand, A. V. (1971). The megaloblastic anaemias. In *Recent Advances in Haematology*, ed. Brain, M. C. & Goldberg, A. London: Churchill.

Hoffbrand, A. V., Stewart, J. S., Booth, C. C. & Mollin, D. L. (1968). Folate deficiency in Crohn's disease: incidence, pathogenesis and treatment. *British Medical Journal*, **2**, 71–75.

Kahn, I. J., Jeffries, G. H. & Sleisenger, M. H. (1966). Malabsorption in intestinal scleroderma. *New England Journal of Medicine*, **274**, 1339–1344.

McIntyre, P. A., Sachs, M. V., Krevans, J. R. & Conley, C. L. (1956). Symposium on hematology. Pathogenesis and treatment of macrocyte anemia; information obtained with radioactive vitamin B_{12}. *Archives of Internal Medicine*, **98**, 541–549.

Meynell, M. J., Cooke, W. T., Cox, E. V. & Gaddie, R. (1957). Serum-cyanocobalamin level in chronic intestinal disorders. *Lancet*, **1**, 901–904.

Plum, P. & Warburg, F. (1939). Haematological changes especially megaloblastic anaemia in regional ileitis. *Acta medica scandinavica*, **102**, 449–475.

Richmond, J. & Davidson, S. (1958). Subacute combined degeneration of the spinal cord in non-Addisonian megaloblastic anaemia. *Quarterly Journal of Medicine*, **N.S. 27**, 517–531.

Salen, G., Goldstein, I. & Wirts, C. W. (1966). Malabsorption in intestinal scleroderma, relation to bacterial flora and treatment with antibiotics. *Annals of Internal Medicine*, **64**, 834–841.

Tabaqchali, S. (1970). The pathophysiological role of small intestinal bacterial flora. *Scandinavian Journal of Gastroenterology*, Supplementum 6, 139–163.

Intestinal helminthiasis

Björkenheim, B. (1966). Optic neuropathy caused by vitamin B_{12} deficiency in carriers of the fish tapeworm Diphyllobothrium latum. *Lancet*, **1**, 688–690.

Björkenheim, G. (1951). Neurological changes in pernicious tapeworm anaemia. *Acta medica scandinavica*, **140**, Supplementum 260.

Bonsdorff, B. von (1956). Pathogenesis of vitamin B_{12} deficiency with special reference to tapeworm pernicious anaemia. In *Vitamin B_{12} und Intrinsic Factor. I. Europäisches Symposion Hamburg*, 1956, ed. Heinrich, H. C. p. 311. Stuttgart: Enke.

Faust, E. C. & Russell, P. R. (1964). *Craig and Faust's Clinical Parasitology*, 7th edition. London: Kimpton.

Minnich, W. (1892). Zur Kenntniss der im Verlauf der perniciösen Anämie beobachteten Spinalerkrankungen. *Zeitschrift für klinische Medizin*, **21**, 264–314.

Nyberg, W. (1958a). Absorption and excretion of vitamin B_{12} in subjects infected with Diphyllobothrium latum and in non-infected subjects following oral administration of radioactive vitamin B_{12}. *Acta haematologica*, **19**, 90–98.

Nyberg, W. (1958b). The uptake and distribution of Co^{60} labelled vitamin B_{12} by the fish tapeworm. *Experimental Parasitology*, **71**, 179–190.

Nyberg, W., Gräsbeck, R., Saarni, M. & von Bonsdorff, B. (1961). Serum vitamin B_{12} levels and incidence of tapeworm anaemia in a population heavily infected with Diphyllobothrium latum. *American Journal of Clinical Nutrition*, **9**, 606–612.

Nyberg, W., Gräsbeck, R. & Sippola, V. (1958). Urinary excretion of radiovitamin B_{12} in carriers of Diphyllobothrium latum. *New England Journal of Medicine*, **259**, 216–219.

Palva, I. (1962). Vitamin B_{12} deficiency in fish tapeworm carriers. A clinical and laboratory study. *Acta medica scandinavica*, **171**, Supplementum 374, 1–86.

Salokannel, J. (1970). Intrinsic factor in tapeworm anaemia. *Acta medica scandinavica*, supplementum 517, 1–51.

Woltman, H. W. & Heck, F. J. (1937). Funicular degeneration of the spinal cord without pernicious anemia. *Archives of Internal Medicine*, **60**, 272–300.

Other causes of malabsorption of vitamin B_{12}

Brizard, C. P. & Fraisse, H. (1973). Maladie d'Imerslund-Najman-Grasbeck avec syndrome neuro-anémique. *Lyon Médical*, **229**, 59–63.

Donaldson, R. M. & Katz, J. H. (1963). Exchange between free and gastric juice-bound cyanocobalamin. *Journal of Clinical Investigation*, **42**, 534–545.

François, P., Revol, L., Germain, D. & Bourlier, V. (1967). Le syndrome d'Imerslund. *Annales de Pédiatrie (Semaine des hôpitaux de Paris)*, **43**, 490–503.

Gräsbeck, R., Gordin, R., Kantero, I. & Kuhlback, B. (1960). Selective vitamin B_{12} malabsorption and proteinuria in young people: a syndrome. *Acta medica scandinavica*, **167**, 289–296.

Heinivaara, O. & Palva, I. P. (1964). Malabsorption of vitamin B_{12} during treatment with para-aminosalicylic acid. A preliminary report. *Acta medica scandinavica*, **175**, 469–471.

Imerslund, O. (1960). Idiopathic chronic megaloblastic anaemia in children. *Acta paediatrica scandinavica*, **49**, Supplementum 119, 1–115.

Jacobson, E. D., Chodos, R. B. & Faloon, W. W. (1960). An experimental malabsorption syndrome induced by neomycin. *American Journal of Medicine*, **28**, 524–533.

Katz, M., Sook, K. L. & Cooper, B. A. (1972). Vitamin B_{12} malabsorption due to a biologically inert intrinsic factor. *New England Journal of Medicine*, **287**, 425–429.

Latner, A. L., Hodson, A. W. & Smith P. A. (1962). Intestinal absorption of coenzyme B_{12} in the normal and fluoro-acetate poisoned rat. *Lancet*, **2**, 230.

Mackenzie, I. L. & Donaldson, R. M. (1969). Vitamin B_{12} absorption and the intestinal cell surface. *Federation Proceedings*, **28**, 41–45.

Mackenzie, I. L., Donaldson, R. M., Kopp, W. L. & Trier, J. S. (1968). Antibodies to intestinal microvillus membranes. II. Inhibition of intrinsic factor-mediated attachment of vitamin B_{12} to hamster brush borders. *Journal of Experimental Medicine*, **128**, 375–386.

Mackenzie, I. L., Donaldson, R. M., Trier, J. S. & Mathan, V. I. (1972). Ileal mucosa in familial selective vitamin B_{12} malabsorption. *New England Journal of Medicine*, **286**, 1021–1025.

Mohamed, S. D., McKay, E. & Galloway, W. H. (1966). Juvenile familial megaloblastic anaemia due to selective malabsorption of vitamin B_{12}. *Quarterly Journal of Medicine*, **35**, 433–453.

Perman, G., Gullberg, R., Reizenstein, P. G., Spellmann, B. & Allgen, L. G. (1960). A study of absorption patterns in malabsorption syndromes. *Acta medica scandinavica*, **168**, 117–125.

Peters, T. J. & Hoffbrand, A. V. (1970). Absorption of vitamin B_{12} by the guinea-pig. I. Subcellular localisation of vitamin B_{12} in the ileal enterocyte during absorption. *British Journal of Haematology*, **19**, 369–382.

Reynolds, E. H., Hallpike, J. F., Philips, B. M. & Mathews, D. M. (1965). Reversible absorptive defects in megaloblastic anaemia. *Journal of Clinical Pathology*, **18**, 593–598.

Rosenthal, H. L., Cutler, L. & Sobieszczanka, W. (1970). Uptake and transport of vitamin B_{12} in subcellular fractions of intestinal mucosa. *American Journal of Physiology*, 358–362.

Salokannel, S. J., Palva, I. P. & Takkunen, J. T. (1970). Malabsorption of vitamin B_{12} during treatment with slow release potassium chloride. *Acta medica scandinavica*, **187**, 431–432.

Shimoda, S. S., Saunders, D. R. & Rubin, C. E. (1968). The Zollinger–Ellison syndrome with steatorrhea. II. The mechanisms of fat and vitamin B_{12} malabsorption. *Gastroenterology*, **55**, 705–723.

Webb, D. I., Chodos, R. B., Mahar, C. Q. & Faloon, N. W. (1968). Mechanism of vitamin B_{12} malabsorption in patients receiving colchicine. *New England Journal of Medicine*, **279**, 845–850.

Practical problems and pitfalls

Chanarin, I. (1969). *The Megaloblastic Anaemias.* Oxford & Edinburgh: Blackwell.

Edwin, E., Holten, K., Norum, K. R., Schrumpf, A. & Skaug, O. E. (1966). Serum vitamin B_{12} and chlorpromazine. *Lancet*, **1**, 316–317.

Hakami, N., Neiman, P. E., Canellos, G. P. & Lazerson, J. (1971). Neonatal megaloblastic anaemia due to inherited transcobalamin II deficiency in two siblings. *New England Journal of Medicine*, **285**, 1163–1170.

Herbert, V. (1964). Studies of folate deficiency in man. *Proceedings of the Royal Society of Medicine*, **57**, 377.

Herbert, V., Gottlieb, C. W. & Altschule, M. D. (1965). Apparent low serum vitamin B_{12} levels associated with chlorpromazine: an artefact. *Lancet*, **2**, 1052–1053.

Lees, F. (1961). Radioactive vitamin B_{12} absorption in the megaloblastic anaemia caused by anticonvulsant drugs. *Quarterly Journal of Medicine*, **30**, 231–248.

Mollin, D. L. & Waters, A. H. (1968). Nutritional megaloblastic anaemia. *Symposium of the Swedish Nutritional Foundation*, **6**, 121–134.

Raven, J. L., Robson, M. B., Morgan, J. L. & Hoffbrand, A. V. (1972). Comparison of 3 methods for measuring vitamin B_{12} in serum. Radioisotopic, Euglena gracilis and Lactobacillus leichmannii. *British Journal of Haematology*, **22**, 21–31.

Scott, C. R., Hakami, N., Teng, C. C. & Sagerson, R. N. (1972). Hereditary transcobalamin II deficiency: the role of transcobalamin II in vitamin B_{12}-mediated reactions. *Journal of Pediatrics*, **81**, 1106–1110.

Scott, R. B., Kammer, R. B., Burgher, W. F. & Middleton, F. G. (1968). Reduced absorption of vitamin B_{12} in two patients with folic acid deficiency. *Annals of Internal Medicine*, **69**, 111-114.

CHAPTER SIX

Other Vitamin Deficiencies

THIAMINE DEFICIENCY

The minimum dietary requirement of thiamine in man is of the order of 0·4 mg/1000 kcal. Although bacteria in the gut may synthesise the vitamin there is no evidence that this represents an available source. Thiamine requirements are critically dependent on metabolic rate and on the proportion of carbohydrate calories in the total dietary intake. It should be remembered that patients with gastrointestinal disease who are maintained on parenteral feeding are likely to derive most of their calories from dextrose and therefore to need extra thiamine.

Absorption and storage

Thiamine is one of the very few water-soluble vitamins to be absorbed by active transport. In man the maximum daily absorption of orally administered thiamine ranges from 8 to 15 mg and can be achieved on an oral intake of 40 mg, given in divided doses with food. Larger doses saturate the absorption mechanism and are excreted in the faeces (Friedemann et al, 1948). Most of the absorption takes place from the proximal small intestine (Middleton and Grice, 1964). In several animal species low doses of thiamine seem to be absorbed both in vivo and in vitro by active transport—larger doses being absorbed by passive diffusion (Rindi and Ventura, 1972). Alcohol, whether in the blood or in the intestinal lumen, interferes with the absorption of thiamine (Thomson, Baker and Leevy, 1970) and this may contribute to the occurrence, in alcoholic patients, of thiamine deficiency syndromes despite ingestion of food containing established minimum daily requirements of the vitamin. There is also evidence that chronic malnutrition may itself interfere with thiamine absorption (Thomson et al, 1970).

Raw carp contains thiaminases and a diet in which such a delicacy figures prominently may contribute to the development of beri-beri in certain parts of the world. Certain bacteria (such as *Bacillus thiaminolyticus*) also contain enzymes capable of splitting the thiamine molecule into its pyrimidine and thiazole moieties. It has been claimed that some 3 per cent of people in Japan harbour this intestinal organism and show consequent thiamine deficiency (Marks, 1968).

Absorbed thiamine is not stored to any significant extent (Greengard, 1970). In fact, the body of a healthy human adult probably has a total thiamine content of less than 25 mg (Davidson and Passmore, 1965): the amount present in a few tablets. This accounts for the comparative speed with which signs and symptoms of thiamine deficiency may develop.

Malabsorption of thiamine

Dietary thiamine deficiency undoubtedly has profound clinical and neuropathological repercussions. The absorption of thiamine is probably impaired in some gastroenterological conditions (see below). It might therefore be thought that many conditions characterised by malabsorption would cause classical syndromes of thiamine deficiency. This, however, has seldom been reported. We suspect that the deficiency produced by malabsorption is rarely as severe as that occurring in patients with a defective intake. It should, moreover, be noted that whereas neurologists frequently assess—in the context of peripheral neuropathy—whether or not their patients are thiamine depleted, gastroenterologists do not seem to do so. It is therefore possible that neuropathy due to thiamine deficiency may be more common in cases of malabsorption than generally believed.

Welbourn, Hughes and Wells (1951) described the occurrence of various vitamin deficiency states following gastric operations. The clinical features suggested that vitamins other than vitamin B_{12} (to which we have already referred) were at times involved. Mild neuropathy was encountered in several cases. Some striking therapeutic responses to specific medication were reported, including a patient who developed encephalopathic symptoms which improved following the administration of thiamine. It was claimed that studies of blood pyruvate levels in these patients had shown that subclinical thiamine deficiency might be much commoner than established syndromes such as beri-beri or Wernicke's encephalopathy, but no data were given. Although minor alterations in food intake may have contributed, the authors felt that malabsorption was primarily responsible. They incriminated post-operative vomiting or anorexia, intestinal hurry, lack of acid secretion from the gastric remnant and 'diversion' of vitamins by intestinal bacteria. Girdwood (1956), on the other hand, could find no evidence of malabsorption of thiamine in 10 patients with tropical and 'non-tropical' sprue. The technique used was rather cumbersome and insensitive, however, consisting in microbiological assays of thiamine in the urine following both injection and oral administration of thiamine to both patients and controls.

That impaired absorption of thiamine may occur in patients with disease of the gastrointestinal tract was clearly established by Thomson (1966). Using ^{35}S-thiamine, he showed that in control subjects absorption of the vitamin occurred mainly within the first two hours and that practically all of the oral dose absorbed was excreted during the first 24 hours (a large parenteral 'flushing' dose of non-radioactive thiamine hydrochloride had been given concurrently with the oral dose). In eight patients with untreated coeliac disease proven by jejunal biopsy, similar tests showed a significant reduction in the excretion of labelled thiamine. Intravenously administered thiamine was excreted normally. In these cases there was no correlation between thiamine malabsorption and other absorptive defects or the severity of the changes shown by jejunal biopsy. Thirteen patients with coeliac disease, treated by a gluten-free diet, showed no significant difference from the control group in their ability to absorb thiamine. No evidence of thiamine malabsorption was found in eight patients with gastroenterostomies, in four patients with pernicious anaemia or in three patients with histamine-fast achlorhydria following gastric surgery.

Devastating thiamine deficiency (presenting as Wernicke's encephalopathy) may complicate any gastrointestinal disease producing severe vomiting and occur quite independently of any history of alcoholism. One of Wernicke's (1881) original patients was a young woman with an oesophageal stricture developing following the suicidal ingestion of sulphuric acid. Other cases of Wernicke's encephalopathy have occurred in the context of such disorders as

(a) carcinoma of stomach (Neubürger, 1936)
(b) carcinoma of head of pancreas (Neubürger, 1936)
(c) carcinoma of rectum (Neubürger, 1936)
(d) metastatic malignant melanoma in stomach (Neubürger, 1936)
(e) postoperative peritonitis (Neubürger, 1936)
(f) intestinal obstruction from other causes (Wagener and Weir, 1937)
(g) 'chronic gastritis' (Neubürger, 1937)
(h) ascending cholangitis, gastric ulceration and peritonitis (Edelmann and Leidler, 1938)

The common denominator of all these conditions is, of course, recurrent vomiting. Wernicke's encephalopathy is also well documented as a complication of hyperemesis gravidarum, where the vomiting is not due to primary gastroenterological disorder.

Clinical features of thiamine deficiency

The main neurological effects of thiamine deficiency consist of peripheral neuropathy (beri-beri), Wernicke's encephalopathy and Korsakoff's psychosis. These dramatic disorders are well described in a number of articles and monographs (Wernicke, 1881; Vedder, 1913; Campbell and Biggart, 1939; Campbell and Russell, 1941; Hibbs, 1946; de Wardener and Lennox, 1947; Cruickshank, 1950; Dreyfus and Herbert, 1961; Victor, Adams and Collins, 1971) and will not be reviewed here.

We would like to stress two clinical points which may be less well known. The first is that thiamine deficiency in infancy may present with unexpected features such as neck stiffness and spasticity of the limbs, punctuated at times by paroxysms of muscular rigidity. There may be aphonia due to laryngeal paresis or oedema of the vocal cords (Haridas, 1937). Anorexia and vomiting usually herald such attacks and it has been suggested that these symptoms may themselves be manifestations of thiamine deficiency. Although this and similar clinical pictures have usually been encountered in infants breast-fed by thiamine-depleted mothers (Tanaka, 1934) there is no reason to suppose that it might not complicate unrelieved infantile hypertrophic pyloric stenosis.

The second point is that 'beri-beri' (whether in its 'dry' or 'wet' forms) and Wernicke's encephalopathy are probably only the more striking manifestations of a more common deficiency state, the clinical features of which include anorexia, nausea, impaired gastrointestinal motility, vague muscle pains, paraesthesiae and heaviness of the legs, personality disturbance, altered behaviour and hypotension (Williams et al, 1940, 1942). Those with experience of thiamine deficiency in areas where it is endemic will certainly have seen many such cases, responding promptly to specific therapy. It is this sort of clinical presentation which should perhaps be expected and sought for in patients with malabsorption.

Laboratory diagnosis of thiamine deficiency

Thiamine may be assayed chemically (Haugen, 1960), chromatographically (Kingsley, 1961), and biochemically (Horwitt and Kreisler, 1949; Brin, 1962; Dreyfus, 1962). Microbiological methods, although more time-consuming, are, however, probably more sensitive and more specific, and can certainly be applied to very much smaller samples. Baker et al (1964) report a sensitive technique (using the protozoan flagellate *Ochromonas danica*) applicable to whole blood, serum, urine, cerebrospinal fluid, muscle and brain. The mean serum level was 21 ng/ml (range 18 to 62 ng/ml).

According to Marks (1968) the concentration of cocarboxylase in human erythrocytes is about 100 ng/ml. In plasma it is much lower (i.e. about 10 ng/ml) and in leucocytes higher (up to 1000 ng/ml). Fennelly et al (1964), also using a microbiological method of estimation, found the mean whole blood thiamine in their normal controls to be $43 \pm 17{\cdot}2$ ng/ml. Patients with Wernicke's encephalopathy had blood levels ranging from 2·5 to 10 ng/ml. The mean concentration of thiamine in human liver is 8 ng/ml (Baker et al, 1964). Patients with fatty liver lose over 50 per cent of their scanty hepatic stores.

Urinary thiamine excretion. In a normal adult, about 1 mg of thiamine is utilised daily. This is roughly equivalent to the minimum daily requirement. On low dietary intakes, a 24-hour sample of urine will therefore contain no thiamine. An increased thiamine intake will first saturate the tissue stores, then appear in the urine as pyrimidine and thiamine. These facts form the basis of certain simple, semi-quantitative tests of thiamine deficiency (Mason and Williams, 1942). The 24-hour excretion of urinary thiamine may be estimated before and after a 10 mg intramuscular injection of thiamine. Normal subjects will excrete between 60 and 80 per cent of the dose during this period, thiamine-depleted patients much less (Baker et al, 1964). Urinary thiamine excretion per gram of creatinine, in random urine samples, may also provide an index of thiamine saturation. Adults on an adequate thiamine intake should excrete between 66 and 130 μg of thiamine per gram of creatinine (*Manual for Nutrition Surveys*, 1963).

Serum pyruvate in thiamine deficiency. Although thiamine deficiency in man and in many animal species results in a rise of serum pyruvate, basal levels of serum pyruvate are of little value in early diagnosis. When depletion is severe, basal levels of pyruvic and lactic acid may be raised, but this is not constant (Horwitt, 1948). The determination of the serum levels of lactic and pyruvic acids following a glucose load was used for many years as an index of thiamine deficiency (Beuding, Stein and Wortis, 1940; Williams et al, 1943). Such data are only of diagnostic value if correlated with the blood sugar at any given time. Failure to appreciate this point resulted in the method falling into disrepute. Mild exercise (walking up and down steps for one minute) carried out 60 minutes after the ingestion of glucose further increases the metabolic load and makes it possible to demonstrate abnormalities in the metabolism of thiamine-depleted subjects at an early stage. Horwitt (1948) described an 'index of carbohydrate metabolism' relating glucose, pyruvate and lactate at any given time, which correlated well with thiamine deficiency.

Red cell transketolase. During the 1950s it was realised that these tests were not very specific and that abnormal results might be encountered in conditions other than thiamine deficiency (Earl et al, 1953). Attention began being focused on other more recently discovered functions of thiamine, namely its involvement in transketolase reactions (Horecker and Smyrniotis, 1953; Racker, de la Haba and Leder, 1953).

Brin, Shohet and Davidson (1956, 1958) showed that transketolase activity was markedly depressed in the erythrocytes of thiamine-deficient rats. Wolfe, Brin and Davidson (1958) then established that the same applied in human beings with Wernicke's encephalopathy. Because of the reduced transketolase activity, the erythrocyte pentose concentration increases in thiamine deficiency. Brin (1962) studied the relative rates of onset of the biochemical transketolase defect, the pyruvate decarboxylation defect and the appearance of clinical signs of thiamine deficiency in a group of healthy medical students maintained on a thiamine-deficient diet. The transketolase defect appeared early and fairly constantly.

Even greater specificity could be added to the estimation of red cell transketolase by adding thiamine pyrophosphate to the red cell haemolysates and observing the percentage increase in the formation of hexose. Dreyfus and Moniz (1962) describe a method applicable to very small samples. Haemolysed whole blood is incubated with an excess of ribose-5-phosphate. The result of the test is expressed both in absolute terms (micrograms of sedoheptulose-7-phosphate produced per millilitre of haemolysate per hour—in normal adult subjects values of sedoheptulose-7-phosphate range from 100 to 160 μg/ml/h) and as the amount, expressed as a percentage, by which the transketolase activity is enhanced when thiamine pyrophosphate is added to the system (the TPP effect).

RIBOFLAVINE DEFICIENCY

Minimum dietary requirements of riboflavine are of the order of 0·6 mg/1000 kcal. The vitamin is synthesised by intestinal microorganisms but faecal riboflavine appears to be within bacterial cells and there is no evidence that it can be absorbed (Greengard, 1970).

Absorption and storage

Dietary riboflavine is readily absorbed by passive diffusion and there is no evidence of saturation of the absorptive mechanism with oral doses of up to 20 mg (Matthews, 1967). The fact that peak urinary excretion occurs within two hours of an orally administered dose and that it is only possible to maintain sustained excretion of the vitamin for two hours after administration of the last dose suggests prompt absorption from the proximal small intestine (Morrison and Campbell, 1960; Campbell and Morrison, 1963).

Riboflavine is stored in liver, spleen, kidney and cardiac muscle. These stores are well maintained, even in the presence of severely restricted intake.

Malabsorption of riboflavine

Signs of ariboflavinosis were described in several patients following partial gastrectomy (Welbourn, Hughes and Wells, 1951) and attributed to malabsorption. Girdwood (1956), on the other hand, could find no evidence of impaired absorption of riboflavine in patients with coeliac disease.

Malabsorption of riboflavine was incriminated in one case of the 'burning feet' syndrome, well documented by Lai and Ransome (1970).

A 21-year-old Indian housewife, seen in Singapore, complained of intolerable nocturnal dysaesthesiae in the feet, of insidious onset and of about two weeks' duration. There had been five pregnancies but no glossitis or gastrointestinal symptoms. The dietary intake of riboflavine was inadequate. There were no abnormal neurological, ophthalmic or cutaneous signs, but she was apprehensive of bearing her weight on her feet. The serum B_{12} was 515 pg/ml and the folic acid 1·4 ng/ml. The serum pyruvate was 0·3 mg/100 ml. The marrow was normoblastic. There was impaired absorption of xylose, glucose and vitamin A. Jejunal biopsy showed partial villous atrophy. She was started on daily injections of 6 mg of riboflavine and within three days from being 'distraught with pain' had become symptom-free. The authors attribute the (unproven) ariboflavinosis to a combination of defective intake, enhanced utilisation by repeated pregnancies, and impaired absorption (the absorptive defect being, as it so often is in the tropics, of undetermined aetiology).

Clinical features of riboflavine deficiency

In man, the clinical effects of riboflavine deficiency are manifested mainly on *the eye* (corneal vascularisation which may be associated with a sense of 'grittiness', 'conjunctivitis', photophobia, lachrymation and blepharospasm), on *mucocutaneous junctions* (cheilosis, angular stomatitis), and on *the skin* (nasolabial seborrhoea, scrotal and vulval dermatitis). Neurological disorders are occasionally encountered in animals (Brozek and Grande, 1960) but their significance is controversial (Patek, Post and Victor, 1941; Follis, 1948). They must be very rare in man and some have denied their existence (Horwitt, 1954). The 'burning feet' syndrome has occasionally been attributed to riboflavine deficiency (Landor and Pallister, 1935; Peraita, 1946). Others have reported little success in the treatment of this condition with riboflavine (Gopalan, 1946; Cruickshank, 1952).

Laboratory diagnosis of riboflavine deficiency

Riboflavine can be estimated photometrically, fluorimetrically, polarographically, microbiologically, and by animal assay. These various methods are reviewed by Strohecker and Henning (1966). Microbiological techniques are probably the most accurate for concentrations occurring in biological fluids. Using a microbiological method involving *Tetrahymena pyriformis*, Fennelly et al (1964) reported normal serum levels varying from 100 to

500 ng/ml. According to Marks (1968) the normal red cell riboflavine concentration varies from 200 to 280 ng/ml.

The red cell riboflavine concentration correlates poorly with dietary intake and symptoms of frank deficiency may occur in the presence of normal blood levels (Marks, 1968). The urinary excretion of riboflavine (compared to that of creatinine) has been used as a test of deficiency. With adequate intake and absorption, urinary riboflavine excretion should range from 80 to 270 μg per gram of creatinine (*Manual for Nutrition Surveys*, 1963).

NICOTINIC ACID DEFICIENCY

The dietary requirements of nicotinic acid (niacin) can also be met by nicotinamide or tryptophan. The discovery, in 1945, by Krehl and his colleagues that tryptophan was transformed into nicotinic acid by mammalian tissues was an important event in vitamin research, for B vitamins cannot as a rule be synthesised by higher animals. It has been estimated that 60 mg of dietary tryptophan is equivalent to 1 mg of nicotinic acid (Greengard, 1970). The minimum daily requirement of nicotinic acid is about 6 mg/1000 kcal.

It was thought for a long time that diets based on maize actually contained a pellagra-producing factor. It is now known that such diets do not provide an adequate amount of tryptophan and that those consuming them need dietary nicotinic acid from other sources, which they usually cannot get.* It is perhaps a reflection of changing concepts in medical thought that maize was implicated as a poison long before it was considered an incomplete food.

At one time it was believed that nicotinic acid was involved in the metabolism of alcohol. 'Alcoholic pellagra' was the name given to a condition occurring in patients 'whose calories are derived largely from alcohol with a reduced intake of vitamin-rich foods needed to ensure its proper combustion' (Bean, Spies and Blankenhorn, 1944). There is no evidence that nicotinic acid has any such function and the undoubtedly increased occurrence of pellagra amongst alcoholics is probably related to other factors, such as reduced total nicotinic acid intake or possibly impaired absorption.

The amount of dietary tryptophan available for conversion into nicotinic acid seems to depend on the amount of certain other amino-acids available for making protein. A high dietary intake of these amino-acids spares tryptophan for nicotinamide synthesis. A high leucine intake, paradoxically, increases nicotinic acid requirements. Millet (ragi), widely consumed in certain parts of India is rich in leucine and it has been known for several years that the administration of leucine to pellagrins could precipitate mental symptoms (Gopalan and Srikantia, 1960) and cause a deterioration of the EEG. The in vitro synthesis of nicotinamide nucleotides by human erythrocytes is significantly reduced by leucine (Raghuramulu et al, 1965). The biochemical basis of the reaction is poorly understood.

---

* That pellagra is not more prevalent among the Arab nations, where maize is still often an important source of dietary protein, may possibly be due to the widespread consumption of coffee, which contains substantial amounts of the vitamin (McCance and Widdowson, 1960; Dreyfus, 1966).

Absorption and storage

Nicotinic acid and nicotinamide are very efficiently absorbed by passive diffusion from all portions of the gut. The absorption of tryptophan is by an active transport mechanism which is defective in Hartnup disease (p. 17). Little is known about the storage of nicotinic acid.

Malabsorption and 'secondary' pellagra

Pellagra has often been attributed to disorders of the gastrointestinal tract and there is a vast literature relating to 'secondary' pellagra, well reviewed by Eusterman and O'Leary (1931), Strauss (1934) and Bean, Spies and Blankenhorn (1944). A glance at this literature is fruitful, if only as a lesson as to how ideas have evolved on the subject of conditioned deficiency diseases. Moreover, it illustrates some general problems concerning the relationship of nutritional deficiency to malabsorption.

'Secondary' pellagra has been described as occurring in association with every conceivable disorder of the alimentary tract, from inadequate dentition (Killingworth, 1912; Smith and Moore, 1915) to fistula-in-ano (Turner, 1929; Bean et al, 1944). The list includes oral thrush (Shelley, 1927), pharyngitis (Bean et al, 1944), oesophageal carcinoma (Eusterman and O'Leary, 1931; Harris, 1941), oesophagitis due to the ingestion of corrosive agents (Bean et al, 1944), carcinoma of the stomach (Rolph, 1916; Sutton, 1926; O'Leary, 1928), gastric syphilis (Turner, 1929; Eusterman and O'Leary, 1931), partial gastrectomy (Levy-Simpson, 1935; Bean et al, 1944; Welbourn, Hughes and Wells, 1951), gastroenterostomy (Bender, 1925; O'Leary, 1928; Eusterman and O'Leary, 1931), 'gastric neurosis' (Bean et al, 1944), duodenal ulcer with pyloric obstruction (Eusterman and O'Leary, 1931; Levy-Simpson, 1935), stenosis of the jejunum (Turner, 1929), ileal disease (Nuzum, 1925), idiopathic steatorrhoea (Bennett, Hunter and Vaughan, 1932), coeliac disease (Lightwood and Smallpiece, 1937), regional enteritis (Golden, 1936), intestinal tuberculosis (Ellis, 1930; Langworthy, 1931; Bean and Spies, 1940), operations for appendicitis (Jelks, 1916), ulcerative colitis (Barnes, 1926; Bean and Spies, 1940; Harris, 1941), gastrocolic fistula (Mackie, Eddy and Mills, 1940; Bean and Spies, 1940), megacolon (Thaysen, 1932), Hirschsprung's disease (Bean et al, 1944), carcinoma of the colon (Eusterman and O'Leary, 1931; Harris, 1941), dysentery (Pasha, 1939; Bean and Spies, 1940), rectal stricture (Crutchfield, 1928; Bean et al, 1944), rectal abscess (Turner, 1929), recto-vaginal fistula (Scott, 1938), carcinoma of the rectum (Shattuck, 1923) and 'intemperate and repeated catharsis' (Stannus, 1937). Parasitic intestinal disease such as amoebiasis (Jelks, 1927; Fakhry, 1932), ankylostomiasis (Sambon, 1912; Parrish, 1917) and schistosomiasis (Fakhry, 1932; Biggam and Ghalioungui, 1933; Pasha, 1939) have also been incriminated with varying degrees of conviction. In many of these cases neurological complaints were prominent.

We have lengthily enumerated these alleged causes of 'secondary' pellagra not because we accept all of them as such, nor even to display a mass of esoteric and often irrelevant information, but because these 'causes' stress, in startling fashion, our changing concepts of the nature of pellagra, and because they provide an ever-constant reminder of the difficulty in differentiating between chance associations and causal relationships.

In some of the reports the association must have been fortuitous. Cases were often recorded from areas where pellagra was endemic. In other instances the reduced food intake associated with illness, pain, fever or surgery may have 'tipped the balance' in a subject already on the threshold of nicotinic acid deficiency of dietary origin. Vomiting obviously played a role in some patients.

Reviewing obstructive lesions of the gastrointestinal tract as a cause of pellagra, O'Leary (1928) claimed that the lesion 'played essentially a mechanical role, in that it prevented the ingestion or retention of sufficient food, or food containing enough vitamins. The influence of these obstructive lesions in producing symptoms of pellagra is evidenced by the rapid disappearance of the signs of the disease following surgical removal or relief of the obstruction'. He added, ominously, that 'as a rule the patients were so ill that operative interference was attended by a high mortality'.

Whether gastrointestinal disease ever actually impairs the absorption of ingested nicotinic acid once it has reached the intestine is more debatable. Current concepts of non-ionic diffusion, taking place throughout the small intestine, make it difficult to conceive of such an event. Yet it would be a bold clinician who could peremptorily dismiss all the previous literature on the subject. The very high incidence of achlorhydria in pellagrins, while possibly reflecting the impact of nicotinic acid deficiency on the stomach, might conceivably have an alternative significance, as might the undoubtedly increased occurrence of pellagra following partial gastrectomy. There is no firm evidence that the stomach produces a substance necessary for the absorption of dietary nicotinic acid although early reports of a beneficial effect of neutralised gastric juice in the treatment of human pellagra (Sydenstricker et al, 1936; Petri and Wanscher, 1937; Petri et al, 1937) do not seem to have been adequately followed up.

Acute nicotinamide deficiency encephalopathy (see p. 107) occurring in the context of known malabsorption due to jejunal diverticulosis was described by Tabaqchali and Pallis (1970). The patient, a 66-year-old woman, developed stupor, with bilateral severe cogwheel rigidity. There were marked grasping and pouting reflexes. Both the clinical state and EEG responded dramatically to an intravenous injection of nicotinamide. In this case, both protein malabsorption and bacterial colonisation of the small gut might have resulted in a proportion of the dietary tryptophan no longer being available for nicotinic acid synthesis. Other factors, such as elimination of nicotinic-acid-synthesising bacteria by a course of antibiotics given shortly before the patient lapsed into stupor may also have played a part.

Clinical features of nicotinic acid deficiency

The clinical features of nicotinic acid deficiency include *cutaneous lesions* (the classical pellagrous rash, resembling sunburn, appearing first on the back of the hands), *lesions of the gastrointestinal tract* (gingivitis, stomatitis, glossitis and enteritis, often associated with anorexia, gastric achylia, burning abdominal pain or diarrhoea), and *effects on the nervous system* (pellagrous 'psychoneurosis', pellagrous dementia and acute encephalopathy or Jolliffe's syndrome).

Various other neurological disturbances have been described in nicotinic acid-deficient patients (peripheral neuropathy, myelopathy, amblyopia) but it is difficult to determine whether these really belong to the neuropathology of pellagra or whether they are due to deficiency of other substances, known or unknown. Those interested in the alleged myelopathy of pellagra are referred to articles by Langworthy (1931), Greenfield and Holmes (1939), Hsü (1942) and Shulack and Peters (1945). Denny-Brown (1947) stated that it was highly doubtful whether any degenerative lesion of the nervous system could be attributed solely to nicotinic acid deficiency, the neuropathological features of human pellagra probably resulting from multiple deficiencies. Signs of peripheral neuropathy in pellagrins have been discussed by Biggam and Ghalioungui (1933) and by Lewy, Spies and Aring (1940) who felt that they were usually due to associated thiamine deficiency rather than to the nicotinic acid deficiency itself. The syndrome of 'burning feet' has been reported as improving following injection of the vitamin (Denny-Brown, 1947; Cruickshank, 1950).

Goldsmith et al (1952) produced a pure deficiency state in seven women, fed a diet low in nicotinic acid and with just enough tryptophan to maintain nitrogen balance. Pyridoxine and riboflavine supplements were given. The women were 'essentially free of organic disease' but had 'some type of psychoneurosis'. Frank neurological symptoms were not encountered, although apathy and depression were seen. Administration of the vitamin to pellagrins produces a striking and prompt improvement in the mental symptoms associated with the disease. These may include amnesia, hallucinations, delirium and mania, and be very prominent features of the condition. In patients with frank psychosis but questionable cutaneous or oral evidence of pellagra, nicotinic acid may produce dramatic improvement (Greengard, 1970), establishing a link between specific vitamin deficiency and the mental disorder. The administration of nicotinic acid does not, however, benefit the peripheral nervous symptoms commonly encountered in pellagrins (Lewy et al, 1940; Grande and Peraita, 1941) and may, in fact, exacerbate them.

Jolliffe's syndrome (acute nicotinic acid deficiency encephalopathy) is encountered in states of severe deficiency of abrupt onset. It is characterised by clouding of consciousness, marked sucking and grasping reflexes and rigidity of extrapyramidal type. Classical stigmata of pellagra may be absent. Cleckley, Sydenstricker and Geeslin (1939) pointed out that cerebral manifestations might be the first evidence of severe or complete depletion of nicotinic acid. 'Hebetude grading into profound stupor' might occur even when the usual clinical features of pellagra were absent. The authors described 19 stuporous patients showing remarkable improvement after intravenous nicotinic acid therapy. They stressed that such patients fell into a high mortality group, 'usually inadequately diagnosed as cerebromalacia, hospitalised as a gesture and perfunctorily treated until death from broncho-pneumonia'. Jolliffe et al (1940) stressed that whereas nicotinic acid deficiency encephalopathy might occasionally be seen in endemic pellagrins, it was in fact more often encountered in chronic alcoholics or other malnourished individuals, particularly when they developed acute intercurrent illnesses such as pneumonia, lung abscess, perforated ulcer, or subarachnoid haemorrhage. In such patients there may be none of the usual tell-tale signs of pellagra. Spillane (1947) points out that in localities where pellagra is not endemic the true nature of such nervous disturbances may pass unrecognised in the absence of the cutaneous signs of this disease. According to Jolliffe and his colleagues (1940) 'the encephalopathic syndrome represents a partial deficiency. Patients showing the encephalopathic syndrome without signs of pellagra would represent a complete nicotinic acid deficiency which develops so rapidly that the structural changes in the mouth and skin characteristic of pellagra do not have time to occur'.

Laboratory diagnosis of nicotinic acid deficiency

Baker and Sobotka (1962) describe a microbiological assay involving *Tetrahymena pyriformis*. Nicotinic acid concentration in whole blood, in 28 normal subjects, ranged from 3·9 to 9·6 μg/ml. Less than 1 per cent of this quantity was present in serum. Fennelly et al (1964) report that chronic alcoholics showing features of pellagra had a mean blood nicotinic acid level of 2·6 μg/ml, but blood level determinations do not usually give accurate indications of deficiency.

Loading tests have been widely used but the excretion of *N'*-methylnicotinamide and its 6-pyridone derivative in the urine seem to depend on the methylating ability of the patient as well as on his intake of nicotinic acid. For field surveys the estimation of methyl nicotinic derivatives per gram of creatinine in random urine samples is probably the most reliable simple test. Excretion of less than 0·5 mg of *N'*-methylnicotinamide per gram of creatinine suggests deficiency (*Manual for Nutrition Surveys*, 1963).

PYRIDOXINE DEFICIENCY

Pyridoxine, pyridoxal and pyridoxamine are three closely related naturally occurring compounds, any of which may be designed vitamin B_6. The physiologically active forms of vitamin B_6 are pyridoxal phosphate and pyridoxamine phosphate.

Isonicotinic acid hydrazide (INAH), a drug used in the treatment of pulmonary tuberculosis, may impair the synthesis of pyridoxal phosphate. It reacts with pyridoxal to form a hydrazone which is excreted in the urine. In much higher concentrations INAH also inhibits reactions in which pyridoxal phosphate participates as a coenzyme. Penicillamine may also act as an antagonist to pyridoxine (Jaffe, Altman and Merryman, 1964).

Absorption and storage

The adult minimum daily dietary requirement is of the order of 2 mg. Absorption is thought to be by passive diffusion. Brain, Stewart and Booth (1963) showed that peak urinary excretion occurred within two hours of an oral dose. Brain and Booth (1964) later demonstrated that absorption was predominantly proximal. Using tritium-labelled pyridoxine, they showed that patients with extensive resections of distal small intestine still absorbed appreciable amounts of an orally administered test dose. In one instance normal absorption was achieved in a patient with only four feet of residual proximal small intestine. It is not known whether vitamin B_6 is ever stored as such.

Malabsorption of pyridoxine

Using rather a crude technique (microbiological urinary assay of pyridoxine following oral ingestion of a test dose), Girdwood (1956) could find no evidence of malabsorption of pyridoxine in 10 patients with coeliac disease and tropical sprue. Such malabsorption was, however, later demonstrated in patients suffering from these conditions (Kowlessar et al, 1961; Sigler et al, 1962). Baker and Sobotka (1962) demonstrated subnormal levels of serum pyridoxine in patients with 'non-tropical sprue'.

Brain and Booth (1964) studied the absorption of tritium-labelled pyridoxine hydrochloride (a method which circumvents many of the shortcomings of microbiological assays) in normal controls, in patients with coeliac disease (in whom the diagnosis had been confirmed by jejunal biopsy), and in patients with steatorrhoea due to other causes. Abnormalities were only found in six of the 13 patients with coeliac disease. The severity of the malabsorption did not correlate well with other parameters of small bowel disease such as impaired folate or xylose absorption, degree of steatorrhoea or severity of changes in the jejunal mucosa.

Morris, Ajdukiewicz and Read (1970) showed that some 50 per cent of patients with coeliac disease (proven by jejunal biopsy) had low serum levels of pyridoxal. Neuropathy was very rare. Nerve conduction velocities in coeliac patients with a low serum pyridoxal level were not significantly different from those in coeliac patients with normal levels. The significance of this study will be referred to later, in our discussion of the neuropathy of coeliac disease.

Clinical features of pyridoxine deficiency

Nasolabial seborrhoea, glossitis and stomatitis have been reported. *Epileptic seizures* occur in animals maintained on pyridoxine-deficient diet and there is evidence that pyridoxine deficiency may cause seizures in human beings, especially in infancy (Snyderman et al, 1953; Coursin, 1954; May, 1954; Hunt et al, 1954). Seizures may also be a feature of INAH-induced pyridoxine deficiency in adults (Reilly et al, 1953).

Neurological manifestations of pyridoxine deficiency may be induced by the administration of pyridoxine antagonists such as 4-deoxypyridoxine, which has been administered experimentally to human beings. These manifestations are said to include *polyneuritis* (Vilter et al, 1953). A peripheral neuropathy with features of the 'burning feet' syndrome is encountered in patients receiving INAH (Biehl and Vilter, 1954). Pyridoxine deficiency has been suggested as yet another cause of the 'burning feet' syndrome in patients not receiving such drugs (Denny-Brown, 1947). Patients with acute porphyria are thought to have a consumptive pyridoxal phosphate deficiency (Cavanagh and Ridley, 1967), though there is no evidence that such deficiency is responsible for any of the neurological manifestations.

Laboratory diagnosis of pyridoxine deficiency

Pyridoxal may be estimated in plasma directly (Toepfer, Polansky and Hewston, 1961) or by a tyrosine decarboxylase method described by Hamfelt (1962). Normal values according to Hamfelt (1964) vary with age in a highly significant manner, from a mean of 16·3 ng/ml for children under the age of one year to 3·4 ng/ml for patients over the age of 60. The cause of the reduced level of serum pyridoxal-5-phosphate in elderly people is not known. It did not seem to be of dietary origin. Malabsorption was considered but not specifically tested for. Hagberg, Hamfelt and Hansson (1966) describe estimations of serum pyridoxal in 18 children between the ages of seven months and 14 years, used as normal controls. The mean level was 11·2 ng/ml (SEM $\pm$ 9·6).

Baker et al (1966) describe a microbiological assay using *Tetrahymena pyriformis*. Using this technique the mean concentrations of vitamin B_6 in whole blood, serum and erythrocytes, in normal subjects, were found to be 37, 44 and 20 ng/ml, respectively.

The estimation of red cell glutamic transaminases may provide some indication of pyridoxine deficiency but the reduction is non-specific and more reliable tests are available for detecting the deficiency.

Xanthurenic acid excretion after tryptophan load

Greenberg et al (1949) showed that xanthurenic acid could be found in the urine of human beings deficient in pyridoxine, especially if the diet had a high tryptophan content. Pyridoxal phosphate catalyses important enzymic reactions along the pathway from tryptophan to nicotinic acid. In pyridoxine deficiency various intermediate products of tryptophan metabolism (kynurenine, hydroxykynurenine) and their degradation products (kynurenic acid and xanthurenic acid) appear in the urine, sometimes in considerable amounts (Dalgleish, 1952). The abnormality is particularly striking after a tryptophan load and appears to be one of the earliest manifestations of vitamin B_6 deficiency in man (Baker et al, 1964; Sauberlich, 1964).

The administration of desoxypyridoxine to human beings (to induce a pyridoxine deficiency state) may result in an 8 to 10-fold increase in the amount of xanthurenic acid excreted in the urine following a test dose of tryptophan (Glazer et al, 1951). A correlation appears to exist between the amount of xanthurenic acid excreted in the urine and the severity of the pyridoxine deficiency (Baker et al, 1964; Sauberlich, 1964). These observations form the basis of useful diagnostic tests of pyridoxine deficiency.

The tests, unfortunately, have not been standardised. Hughes et al (1966) review various procedures. A useful technique is to keep the patient on a diet devoid of bananas or liver for three days and then to administer an oral dose of 100 mg/kg body weight of L-tryptophan (or 200 mg/kg of DL-tryptophan) dissolved in fruit juice. The urine is collected over the next 24 hours. Xanthurenic acid may be estimated in the urine by the methods of Satoh and Price (1958) modified by Cohen, Fishman and Jenkins (1966), or by the method of Weller and Fichtenbaum (1961).

Normal individuals will excrete less than 50 mg (and usually less than 25 mg) of xanthurenic acid in the 24 hours following such a test dose of tryptophan. ('Control' 24-hour urine collections, in normal adults, seldom contain more than 15 mg of apparent xanthurenic acid.) In the presence of pyridoxine deficiency the excretion of xanthurenic acid following a tryptophan load may reach 100 to 500 mg in the first 24 hours (Sauberlich, 1967). Hagberg et al (1966) define as abnormal a xanthurenic acid excretion above 3·8 μmol/kg body weight/24 h (or of more than 0·78 per cent of the ingested dose of L-tryptophan). When interpreting the results of a tryptophan load test, it is important to keep in mind that the amount of xanthurenic acid excreted (related to body weight) increases with age (Meuwisse, Gamstorp and Tryding, 1968). Normal children on a normal diet do not excrete more than 3 mg/day of xanthurenic acid (Hughes et al, 1966). Many of the elderly patients with low serum pyridoxal levels reported by Hamfelt (1964) had abnormal xanthurenic acid excretion which returned to normal following the administration of pyridoxine.

PANTOTHENIC ACID DEFICIENCY

Absorption and storage

The minimum required daily intake of pantothenic acid is about 10 mg. Absorption is thought to be by passive diffusion, throughout the gastro-intestinal tract. Intake and excretion are approximately equal, suggesting that the vitamin is not appreciably destroyed or stored in the body. Of an administered dose, 70 per cent will appear in the urine and 30 per cent in the faeces (Oldham, Davis and Roberts, 1946).

Malabsorption of pantothenic acid

This has not been documented, to our knowledge.

Clinical features of pantothenic acid deficiency

The neurological features of pantothenic acid deficiency are far from clear. The syndrome of 'burning feet', as encountered in malnourished populations, is of course believed by some to arise on the basis of pantothenic acid deficiency. Gopalan (1946) reported that the condition responded well to treatment with pantothenic acid, but this has not been confirmed by other investigators (Bibile et al, 1957).

Pantothenic acid deficiency is difficult to reproduce experimentally and is seldom seen in peacetime because of the ubiquitous occurrence of the vitamin. In fact, experimental deficiency can only be produced with any certainty by the concurrent use of a semi-synthetic diet and the oral administration of a pantothenic acid antagonist (omega-methylpantothenic acid). Bean and Hodges (1954) showed, perhaps inevitably, that the syndrome of 'burning feet' could be produced by this regime. Hodges et al (1959) later reported that in healthy human volunteers this regime produced a more generalised syndrome characterised by fatigue, headache, weakness, emotional lability, incoordination, paraesthesiae, muscle cramps and gastrointestinal disturbances such as nausea and vomiting.

Laboratory diagnosis of pantothenic acid deficiency

This cannot be established with certainty. A microbiological assay, using *Lactobacillus plantarum* (formerly *L. arabinosus*) is described by Baker and Sobotka (1962). Estimations in 367 normal subjects revealed a mean whole blood level of 0·56 μg/ml (range 0·22 to 1·9 μg/ml). The serum level of pantothenic acid may be increased in patients with liver disease (Fennelly et al, 1964).

VITAMIN A DEFICIENCY

Vitamin A (vitamin A alcohol or retinol) is only found in foods of animal origin. Milk and eggs, and the liver of cattle and fish, contain substantial amounts of preformed vitamin A. A chemically distinct form (vitamin A_2) occurs in certain fish liver oils. The plant pigment β-carotene (provitamin A) is widely distributed, and is rather wastefully converted to physiologically active vitamin A in the mucosa of the small intestine. In man the main intake of vitamin A is in the form of esters such as retinyl palmitate. Synthetic preparations of retinol and β-carotene are today widely used to 'reinforce' the natural content of certain foodstuffs. One international unit (IU) of vitamin A is equivalent to 0·344 μg of synthetic vitamin A acetate, or to 0·3 μg of crystalline 'all-trans' vitamin A alcohol.

Vitamin A plays important roles in retinal physiology and in the maintenance of the integrity of certain epithelial surfaces, particularly those of the conjunctiva and cornea, but also those of the respiratory, urinary and alimentary tracts. The vitamin is also involved in sterol metabolism. It is needed for the normal growth and health of tissues, probably being involved—in a manner as yet not clearly understood—in the metabolism of glycoproteins.

Absorption and storage

It has been claimed that the absorption of vitamin A is by a process of active transport (Loran et al, 1961; Skala and Hruba, 1964), but it seems more likely that entry into the cell is through the micellar phase which seems obligatory for the uptake, by the intestinal mucosa, of various non-polar solutes. Other stages preceding the appearance of vitamin A in the lymph may be energy-dependent (see p. 7–8). The complexities of the process are fully discussed by Roels (1967). Absorption is accelerated in the presence of emulsifying agents such as bile salts but is not critically dependent on their presence. It is markedly reduced in the presence of low dietary fat (Roels, Trout and Dujacquier, 1958) or of impaired fat absorption, of which impairment vitamin A absorption is itself a useful measure.

The absorption of vitamin A is also impaired in the presence of a reduced dietary intake of protein and in liver disease. Popper, Steigmann and Zevin (1943) showed that flat vitamin A tolerance curves in patients with liver disease were not due to depletion of liver stores of vitamin A (i.e. the curves obtained were not saturation curves) but were genuinely due to malabsorption. The mechanism remains obscure but does not seem to be related to an insufficiency of bile salts (Mandel, 1970). Carotene absorption is less efficient than that of preformed vitamin A. It is dependent on bile salts and is greatly decreased in all patients with steatorrhoea. Retinol, conjugated to form a β-glucuronide, undergoes enterohepatic circulation and oxidation to retinoic acid, which has powerful growth-promoting properties but no effect on the retina.

Vitamin A is stored mainly in the liver. The liver of a healthy individual on a Western diet contains between 300 000 and 500 000 IU of vitamin A (Moore, 1957). Hepatic stores are capable of maintaining a normal plasma level, possibly for up to a year, even in the presence of grossly reduced intake or absorption. In the blood, retinol is bound to retinol-binding protein (RBP), a simple polypeptide with a molecular weight of about 21 000. RBP, present in plasma at a concentration of 40 to 50 μg/ml, itself forms a protein–protein complex with prealbumin. Deficiencies of the prealbumin carrier-protein may account for low blood vitamin A levels in cases of kwashiorkor (Scrimshaw and Behar, 1961). Patients with liver disease also show a low level of prealbumin. There is some evidence that retinol deficiency itself may interfere with the release (but not with the formation) of RBP.

Malabsorption of vitamin A

In a comprehensive review of night blindness as a criterion of vitamin A deficiency, Jeghers (1937) showed that in the absence of eye disease night blindness was the earliest and most constant manifestation of vitamin A deficiency. The usual cause was defective intake but the condition could also arise as a result of impaired absorption or interference with the conversion of carotene to vitamin A. Other causes were disturbances of vitamin A storage in the liver or release from the liver. Vomiting, various types of gastrointestinal and gastrocolic fistulae, changes in the gastrointestinal mucosa, pancreatic insufficiency and chronic diarrhoeas could all hinder the proper absorption of vitamin A.

Vitamin A deficiency and impaired dark adaptation is common with every variety of liver disease (Jeghers, 1937). Haig, Hecht and Patek (1938) found impaired dark adaptation in 13 out of 14 patients with alcoholic cirrhosis, none of whom were jaundiced. The cone threshold was impaired as well as the rod threshold and the authors commented prophetically that vitamin A might have 'a chemical relation to visual violet resembling the one it has to visual purple'. Harris and Moore (1947) investigated 30 patients with infective hepatitis. Reduced plasma vitamin A and carotene levels were common, as were failure of the plasma level to rise and the excretion of large amounts of vitamin A in the faeces after massive oral dosage. The authors comment that the disturbances were of complex nature, involving failure of absorption of vitamin A, and failures of both deposition and release of vitamin A from the liver. Low levels (often as low as 30 IU/100 ml plasma) were found in the early stages of the disease, whereas it might take months to reach such low levels on the basis of defective intake. Studying dark adaptation in patients with infective hepatitis, Craik, MacPherson and Harris (1947) found a significant reduction in mean final rod threshold in 37 patients examined early in the course of the disease, compared with age-matched controls.

There are few studies relating dark adaptation to the more common malabsorption syndromes such as sprue and coeliac disease. Chesney and McCoord (1934) and May, McCreary and Blackfan (1942) describe 'secondary' vitamin A deficiency in various types of malabsorption.

Clinical features of vitamin A deficiency

When people eat little food of animal origin they are critically dependent on carotene as a source of vitamin A. When, in addition, their diet contains no green vegetables—either through ignorance or, as in certain tropical areas, because they are not available—when, for instance, the diet consists mainly of rice (which contains no carotene), the scene is set for the tragedy of childhood blindness.

Vitamin A deficiency is widespread in many parts of the world. On the Indian subcontinent, in South-East Asia, and in Central and South America whole communities may be affected. The keratinising effects of vitamin A deficiency on the conjunctiva and cornea (*xerophthalmia*) may, unless treated, proceed to *keratomalacia* and *blindness*. This may occur fairly abruptly, following attacks of diarrhoea, measles, febrile tuberculosis or meningococcal meningitis, all of which seem abruptly to enhance vitamin A requirements.

The earliest repercussion of vitamin A deficiency is, however, far less dramatic and consists of *impaired adaptation to vision in the dark* (Hume and Krebs, 1949; McLaren, 1967). The association of night blindness (nyctalopia) with vitamin A deficiency has been known for many years. Facts and figures concerning the prevalence of nyctalopia are, however, hard to come by. The disorder can be documented by rod scotometry (Livingston, 1944) or dark adaptometry (Jayle and Ourgand, 1950). If the dark-adapted subject is asked to look into a black sphere it can be noted at what stage he first perceives a point source of light, gradually increasing in brightness. The lowest perceptible intensity of light (the bleaching of the smallest quantity of rhodopsin that gives rise to a subjectively perceptible nerve impulse) is a measure of rhodopsin concentration in the rods. These techniques require cooperative subjects and trained personnel, although the equipment itself is not very expensive. More objective procedures such as electroretinography (Jacobson, 1961; Dhanda, 1955) require more complex equipment. An impairment of dark adaptation is said to be detectable when the plasma level of vitamin A falls below 50 IU (15 μg)/100 ml (Hume and Krebs, 1949).

While the effects of hypovitaminosis A on the cornea and on dark adaptation will be familiar to most neurologists and gastroenterologists, the effects on the fundus (*Uyemura's syndrome*) are less well known. Numerous white spots appear, which lie along the course of the vessels, their diameter less than that of the vessel itself. Unlike the spots of retinitis punctata albescens, the spots due to hypovitaminosis A disappear following appropriate therapy (Uyemura, 1928; Fuchs, 1959; Teng, 1965).

Obstructive hydrocephalus has been reported in puppies whose mothers were fed insufficient vitamin A during pregnancy (Millen, Woollam and Lamming, 1953). There is no evidence to date that this occurs in human subjects. Malformations of the skull have also been reported in puppies brought up on vitamin A-deficient diets and may affect the nervous system by mechanical compression. Mellanby (1947) dramatically described these blind, deaf and anosmic animals, in whom 'the skull and vertebrae had lost their primary function of protecting the nervous system and had become destructive agents'. Raised intracranial pressure has been reported as a manifestation of vitamin A deficiency in man on a few occasions (Cornfeld and Cooke, 1952; Bass and Caplan, 1955). Such an occurrence must be very rare, however, the usual relationship between vitamin A and raised intracranial pressure in man being the very opposite. Iatrogenic or accidental hypervitaminosis A is a well-known cause of symptoms resembling intracranial tumour.* It should be noted that both hydrocephalus and cranial deformities may also occur after excessive amounts of the vitamin have been given to animals (Calhoun et al, 1965).

Laboratory diagnosis of vitamin A deficiency

The most commonly applied tests have been the estimation of vitamin A and carotenoid concentrations in serum. The estimation of retinol in biological fluids was for a long time a tedious procedure, depending on the vitamin's growth-promoting effect on vitamin A-depleted rats (Harris, 1960). A chemical technique adaptable to very small samples was reported by Neeld and Pearson (1963). Photometric and spectrophotometric methods of assay are reviewed by Strohecker and Henning (1966). They are not very accurate at low concentrations. The biological assay techniques for vitamin A are reviewed by Roels and Mahadevan (1967).

Plasma vitamin A levels are not an accurate index of tissue depletion. In healthy individuals, in Great Britain, they were found to range between 50 and 300 IU (15 to 90 μg)/100 ml (Leitner, Moore and Sharman, 1952). In a study in South India the *mean* serum vitamin A in apparently healthy children was 80 IU (24 μg)/100 ml (Chandra et al, 1960). Dowling and Wald (1958) have shown that in vitamin A-depleted rats, the liver stores have to be totally depleted before there is a fall in serum levels. The concentration of retinal rhodopsin only decreased at a still later stage. McLaren (1966) has shown that, in man, *liver concentrations of vitamin A* could be estimated in biopsy samples, providing a better indication of hypovitaminosis than concentrations in plasma (the normal liver concentration is above 45 μg/g fresh liver). In states of protein malnutrition, as has been mentioned, serum levels may be very low without this necessarily implying a depletion of tissue stores (Arroyave et al, 1961). Serum carotenoid levels closely reflect recent dietary intake and are no index of hepatic stores of vitamin A. In healthy individuals they may vary from 15 to 370 μg/100 ml (Leitner et al, 1952).

References

Thiamine deficiency

Baker, H., Frank, O., Fennelly, J. J. & Leevy, C. M. (1964). A method for assaying thiamine status in man and animals. *American Journal of Clinical Nutrition*, **14**, 197–201.

* As is well known the syndrome may be encountered in Eskimos or polar explorers who have partaken of polar bear liver. The liver of the polar bear (*Thalarctos maritimus*) contains about 10 000 μg/g (or about 33 000 IU/g) of vitamin A (Russell, 1967).

Beuding, E., Stein, M. H. & Wortis, H. (1940). Blood pyruvate curves following glucose ingestion in normal and thiamine deficient subjects. *Journal of Biological Chemistry*, **140,** 697–703.

Brin, M. (1962). Erythrocyte transketolase in early thiamine deficiency. *Annals of the New York Academy of Sciences*, **98,** 528–541.

Brin, M., Shohet, S. S. & Davidson, C. S. (1956). Effect of thiamine deficiency on mammalian erythrocyte metabolism. *Federation Proceedings*, **15,** 224.

Brin, M., Shohet, S. S. & Davidson, C. S. (1958). The effect of thiamine deficiency on the glucose oxidative pathway of rat erythrocytes. *Journal of Biological Chemistry*, **230,** 319–326.

Campbell, A. C. P. & Biggart, J. H. (1939). Wernicke's encephalopathy (polioencephalitis haemorrhagica superior): its alcoholic and non-alcoholic incidence. *Journal of Pathology and Bacteriology*, **48,** 245–262.

Campbell, A. C. P. & Russell, W. R. (1941). Wernicke's encephalopathy: the clinical features and their probable relationship to vitamin B deficiency. *Quarterly Journal of Medicine*, **N.S. 10,** 41–64.

Cruickshank, E. K. (1950). Wernicke's encephalopathy. *Quarterly Journal of Medicine*, **19,** 327–338.

Davidson, S. & Passmore, R. (1965). *Human Nutrition and Dietetics*. Edinburgh & London: Livingstone.

de Wardener, H. E. & Lennox, B. (1947). Cerebral beri-beri (Wernicke's encephalopathy). Review of 52 cases in Singapore P.o.W. hospital. *Lancet*, **1,** 11–17.

Dreyfus, P. M. (1962). Clinical application of blood transketolase determinations. *New England Journal of Medicine*, **267,** 596–598.

Dreyfus, P. M. & Herbert, V. (1961). Effects of thiamine deficiency on the central nervous system. *American Journal of Clinical Nutrition*, **9,** 414–425.

Dreyfus, P. M. & Moniz, R. (1962). The quantitative histochemical estimation of transketolase in the nervous system of the rat. *Biochimica et biophysica acta*, **65,** 181–189.

Earl, C. J., El Hawary, M. F. S., Thompson, R. H. S. & Webster, G. R. (1953). Blood-pyruvate levels in subacute combined degeneration of cord. *Lancet*, **1,** 115–116.

Edelmann, A. & Leidler, R. (1938). Ein Fall von pankreohepatischem Syndrom mit toxisch-enzephalitischen Herden in beiden hinteren Längsbündeln und im periaquäduktiellen Grau der hinteren Vierhügel. *Confinia neurologica*, **1,** 202–216.

Fennelly, J., Frank, O., Baker, H. & Leevy, C. M. (1964). Peripheral neuropathy of the Alcoholic. I. Aetiological role of aneurin and other B-complex vitamins. *British Medical Journal*, **2,** 1290–1292.

Friedemann, T. E., Kmieciak, T. C., Keegan, P. K. & Sheft, B. B. (1948). Absorption, destruction and excretion of orally administered thiamin by human subjects. *Gastroenterology*, **11,** 100–114.

Girdwood, R. H. (1956). Absorption in sprue of vitamins of the B complex. *Lancet*, **2,** 700–701.

Greengard, P. (1970). Water soluble vitamins. I. The vitamin B complex. In *The Pharmacological Basis of Therapeutics*, ed. Goodman, L. S. & Gilman, A. 4th edition, Ch. 73. New York: Macmillan.

Haridas, G. (1937). Infantile beri-beri. *Journal of the Malaya Branch, British Medical Association*, **1,** 26–37.

Haugen, H. N. (1960). The determination of thiamine in urine by the thiochrome method. *Scandinavian Journal of Clinical and Laboratory Investigation*, **12,** 253–260.

Hibbs, R. E. (1946). Beri-beri in Japanese prison camp. *Annals of Internal Medicine*, **25,** 270–282.

Horecker, B. L. & Smyrniotis, P. Z. (1953). The coenzyme function of thiamine pyrosphosphate in pentose metabolism. *Journal of the American Chemical Society*, **75,** 1009–1010.

Horwitt, M. K. (1948). Biochemical observations (Section II). In Investigations of Human Requirements for B-Complex Vitamins. *Bulletin of the National Research Council (U.S.A.)*, **116,** 12–46.

Horwitt, M. K. & Kreisler, O. (1949). The determination of early thiamine deficient status by estimation of blood lactic and pyruvic acids after glucose administration and exercise. *Journal of Nutrition*, **37,** 411–427.

Kingsley, G. R. (1961). Clinical chemistry. *Analytical Chemistry*, **33**, 13–32.
Marks, J. (1968). *The Vitamins in Health and Disease*. London: Churchill.
Manual for Nutrition Surveys (1963) 2nd edition, pp. 244–249. Interdepartmental Committee on Nutrition for National Defense, National Institutes of Health, Bethesda, Maryland.
Mason, H. L. & Williams, R. D. (1942). The urinary excretion of thiamine as an index of the nutritional level: assessment of the value of a test dose. *Journal of Clinical Investigation*, **21**, 247–255.
Middleton, E. J. & Grice, H. C. (1964). Vitamin absorption studies. IV. Site of absorption of C14-riboflavin and S35-thiamine in the rat. *Canadian Journal of Biochemistry*, **42**, 353–358.
Neubürger, K. (1936). Über die nichtalkoholische Wernickesche Krankheit, insbesondere über ihr Vorkommen beim Krebsleiden. *Virchows Archiv für pathologische Anatomie und Physiologie und für klinische Medizin*, **298**, 68–86.
Neubürger, K. (1937). Wernickesche Krankheit bei chronischer Gastritis. Ein Beitrag zu den Beziehungen zwischen Magen und Gehirn. *Zeitschrift für die gesamte Neurologie und Psychiatrie*, **160**, 208–225.
Racker, E., de la Haba, G. & Leder, I. G. (1953). Thiamine pyrophosphate, a coenzyme of transketolase. *Journal of the American Chemical Society*, **75**, 1010–1011.
Rindi, G. & Ventura, U. (1972). Thiamine intestinal transport. *Physiological Reviews*, **52**, 821–827.
Tanaka, T. (1934). So-called breast milk intoxication. *American Journal of Diseases of Childhood*, **47**, 1286–1298.
Thomson, A. D. (1966). The absorption of radioactive sulphur-labelled thiamine hydrochloride in control subjects and in patients with intestinal malabsorption. *Clinical Science*, **31**, 167–179.
Thomson, A. D., Baker, H. & Leevy, C. M. (1970). Patterns of ^{35}S-thiamine hydrochloride absorption in the malnourished alcoholic patient. *Journal of Laboratory and Clinical Medicine*, **76**, 34–45.
Vedder, E. B. (1913). *Beri-beri*. New York: Wood.
Victor, M., Adams, R. D. & Collins, G. H. (1971). *The Wernicke-Korsakoff Syndrome*. Philadelphia: Davis.
Wagener, H. P. & Weir, J. F. (1937). Ocular lesions associated with postoperative and gestational nutritional deficiency. *American Journal of Ophthalmology*, **20**, 253–259.
Welbourn, R., Hughes, R. & Wells, C. (1951). Vitamin B deficiencies after gastric operations. *Lancet*, **1**, 939–945.
Wernicke, C. (1881). *Lehrbuch der Gehirnkrankheiten fur Aerzte und Studirende*. Kassel: Fischer.
Williams, R. D., Mason, H. L., Power, M. H. & Wilder, R. M. (1943). Induced thiamine (vitamin B_1) deficiency in man. *Archives of Internal Medicine*, **71**, 38–52.
Williams, R. D., Mason, H. L. Smith, B. F. & Wilder, R. M. (1942). Induced thiamine (vitamin B_1) deficiency and the thiamine requirement of man: further observations. *Archives of Internal Medicine*, **69**, 721–738.
Williams, R. D., Mason, H. L., Wilder, R. M. & Smith, B. F. (1940). Observations on induced thiamine (vitamin B_1) deficiency in man. *Archives of Internal Medicine*, **66**, 785–799.
Wolfe, S. J., Brin, M. & Davidson, C. S. (1958). The effect of thiamine deficiency on human erythrocyte metabolism. *Journal of Clinical Investigation*, **37**, 1476–1484.

Riboflavine deficiency

Brozek, J. & Grande, F. (1960). Abnormalities of neural function in the presence of inadequate nutrition. In *Handbook of Physiology* (*Section 1: Neurophysiology*), Vol. III, Ch. 79. Washington: American Physiological Society.
Campbell, J. A. & Morrison, A. B. (1963). Some factors affecting the absorption of vitamins. *American Journal of Clinical Nutrition*, **12**, 162–169.
Cruickshank, E. K. (1952). Dietary neuropathies. *Vitamins and Hormones*, **10**, 1–45.
Fennelly, J., Frank, O., Baker, H. & Leevy, C. M. (1964). Peripheral neuropathy of the alcoholic. I. Aetiological role of aneurin and other B-complex vitamins. *British Medical Journal*, **2**, 1290–1292.

Follis, R. H. (1948). *The Pathology of Nutritional Diseases*. Springfield: Thomas.
Girdwood, R. H. (1956). Absorption in sprue of vitamins of the B complex. *Lancet*, **2**, 700–701.
Gopalan, C. (1946). 'Burning-feet' syndrome. *Indian Medical Gazette*, **81**, 22–26.
Greengard, P. (1970). Water soluble vitamins. I. The vitamin B complex. In *The Pharmacological Basis of Therapeutics*, ed. Goodman, L. S. & Gilman, A. 4th edition, Ch. 73. New York: Macmillan.
Horwitt, M. K. (1954). In *Vitamins III*, ed. Sebrell, W. H. & Harris, R. S. p. 387. New York: Academy Press.
Lai, C. S. & Ransome, G. A. (1970). Burning feet syndrome. Case due to malabsorption and responding to riboflavine. *British Medical Journal*, **1**, 151–152.
Landor, J. V. & Pallister, R. A. (1935). Avitaminosis B_2. *Transactions of the Royal Society of Tropical Medicine and Hygiene*, **29**, 121–134.
Manual for Nutrition Surveys (1963), 2nd edition, pp. 244–249. Interdepartmental Committee on Nutrition for National Defense, National Institutes of Health, Bethesda, Maryland.
Marks, J. (1968). *The Vitamins in Health and Disease*. London: Churchill.
Matthews, D. M. (1967). Absorption of water soluble vitamins. *British Medical Bulletin*, **23**, 258–262.
Morrison, A. B. & Campbell, J. A. (1960). Vitamin absorption studies. 1. Factors influencing the excretion of oral test doses of thiamine and riboflavin by human subjects. *Journal of Nutrition*, **72**, 435–440.
Patek, A. J., Post, J. & Victor, J. (1941). Riboflavin deficiency in the pig. *American Journal of Physiology*, **133**, 47–55.
Peraita, M. (1946). Deficiency neuropathies observed in Madrid during the Civil War (1936–1939). *British Medical Journal*, **2**, 784.
Strohecker, R. & Henning, H. M. (1966). *Vitamin Assay: Tested Methods*. Berlin: Springer-Verlag.
Welbourn, R., Hughes, R. & Wells, C. (1951). Vitamin B deficiencies after gastric operations. *Lancet*, **1**, 939–945.

Nicotinic acid deficiency

Baker, H. & Sobotka, H. (1962). Microbiological assay methods for vitamins. *Advances in Clinical Chemistry*, **5**, 173–235.
Barnes, J. M. (1926). Typical pellagra syndrome developing in a patient with chronic ulcerative colitis while under hospital treatment. *Annals of Clinical Medicine*, **4**, 552.
Bean, W. B. & Spies, T. D. (1940). Vitamin deficiencies in diarrheal states. *Journal of the American Medical Association*, **115**, 1078–1081.
Bean, W. B., Spies, T. D. & Blankenhorn, M. A. (1944). Secondary pellagra. *Medicine (Baltimore)*, **23**, 1–77.
Bender, W. L. (1925). Pellagra secondary to lesions of the stomach interfering with nutrition. *Journal of the American Medical Association*, **84**, 1250–1253.
Bennett, T. I., Hunter, D. & Vaughan, J. M. (1932). Idiopathic steatorrhoea (Gee's disease). *Quarterly Journal of Medicine*, **1**, 603–677.
Biggam, A. G. & Ghalioungui, P. (1933). Pellagra: its clinical features and pathology, *Lancet*, **2**, 1198–1203.
Cleckley, H. M., Sydenstricker, V. P. & Geeslin, L. E. (1939). Nicotinic acid in the treatment of atypical psychotic states associated with malnutrition. *Journal of the American Medical Association*, **112**, 2107–2110.
Cruickshank, E. K. (1950). Wernicke's encephalopathy. *Quarterly Journal of Medicine*, **19**, 327–338.
Crutchfield, E. D. (1928). Pellagra. *Archives of Dermatology and Syphilology*, **17**, 650.
Denny-Brown, D. (1947). Neurological conditions resulting from prolonged and severe dietary restriction. *Medicine (Baltimore)*, **26**, 41–113.
Dreyfus, P. M. (1966). Nutritional disorders of the nervous system. I. Specific vitamin deficiencies. *Medical Science*, **17**, 44–50 (March), 44–48 (April).
Ellis, R. W. B. (1930). Pellagra secondary to gastrointestinal disease. *American Journal of Diseases of Children*, **39**, 1036–1044.

Eusterman, G. B. & O'Leary, P. A. (1931). Pellagra secondary to benign and carcinomatous lesions and dysfunction of gastrointestinal tract (13 cases). *Archives of Internal Medicine*, **47**, 633–649.

Fakhry, A. (1932). Incidence, parasitological findings and treatment of pellagra in Kafr-El-Zayat Ankylostoma Hospital. *Journal of the Egyptian Medical Association*, **15**, 53–64.

Fennelly, J., Frank, O., Baker, H. & Leevy, C. M. (1964). Peripheral neuropathy of the alcoholic. I. Aetiological role of aneurin and other B-complex vitamins. *British Medical Journal*, **2**, 1290–1292.

Golden, R. (1936). The small intestine and diarrhea. *American Journal of Roentgenology, Radium Therapy and Nuclear Medicine*, **36**, 892–901.

Goldsmith, G. A., Sarrett, H. P., Register, U. D. & Gibbens, J. (1952). Studies of niacin requirement in man. I. Experimental pellagra in subjects on corn diets low in niacin and tryptophan. *Journal of Clinical Investigation*, **31**, 533–542.

Gopalan, C. & Srikantia, S. G. (1960). Leucine and pellagra. *Lancet*, **1**, 954–957.

Grande, F. & Peraita, M. (1941). *Avitaminosis y sistema nervioso.* Barcelona: Miguel Servet.

Greenfield, J. G. & Holmes, J. MacD. (1939). A case of pellagra—the pathological changes in the spinal cord. *British Medical Journal*, **1**, 815–819.

Greengard, P. (1970). Water soluble vitamins. I. The vitamin B complex. In *The Pharmacological Basis of Therapeutics*, ed. Goodman, L. S. & Gilman, A., 4th edition, Ch. 73. New York: Macmillan.

Harris, S. (1941). *Clinical Pellagra.* St. Louis: Mosby.

Hsü, Y. K. (1942). Pathologic anatomy of human nervous system in avitaminosis. *Archives of Neurology and Psychiatry*, **48**, 271–319.

Jelks, J. L. (1916). Discussion symposium on pellagra. *Southern Medical Journal*, **9**, 36–37.

Jelks, J. L. (1927). Pellagra: is pellagra an infection; or is pellagra due solely to an unbalanced or insufficient diet? *Journal of Tennessee State Medical Association*, **20**, 233–239.

Jolliffe, N., Bowman, K. M., Rosenblum, L. A. & Fein, H. D. (1940). Nicotinic acid deficiency encephalopathy. *Journal of the American Medical Association*, **114**, 307–312.

Killingworth, S. A. (1912). Dental findings in insane pellagrins. *Transactions of the National Association for the Study of Pellagra*, **2**, 405.

Krehl, W. A., Teply, L. J., Sarma, P. S. & Elvehjem, C. A. (1945). Growth-retarding effect of corn in nicotinic acid-low rations and its counteraction by tryptophane. *Science*, **101**, 489–490.

Langworthy, O. R. (1931). Lesions of the central nervous system characteristic of pellagra. *Brain*, **54**, 291–302.

Levy-Simpson, S. (1935). Secondary pellagra. *Quarterly Journal of Medicine*, **N.S. 4**, 191–201.

Lewy, F. H., Spies, T. D. & Aring, C. D. (1940). The incidence of neuropathy in pellagra: the effect of cocarboxylase upon its neurological signs. *American Journal of Medical Sciences*, **199**, 840–849.

Lightwood, R. & Smallpiece, V. (1937). Coeliac disease with a conditioned vitamin deficiency resembling but not typical of pellagra. *Proceedings of the Royal Society of Medicine*, **31**, 71–73.

McCance, R. A. & Widdowson, E. M. (1960). The composition of foods. *M.R.C. Special Report Series No.* 297, p. 180. London: H.M.S.O.

MacKie, T. T., Eddy, W. H. & Mills, M. A. (1940). Vitamin deficiencies in gastrointestinal disease. *Annals of Internal Medicine*, **14**, 28–41.

Manual for Nutrition Surveys (1963), 2nd edition, pp. 244–249. Interdepartmental Commission on Nutrition for National Defense, National Institutes of Health, Bethesda, Maryland.

Nuzum, F. R. (1925). Pellagra associated with annular carcinoma of the terminal portion of the ileum. *Journal of the American Medical Association*, **85**, 1861–1862.

O'Leary, P. A. (1928). Pellagra: a study of 34 cases in localities where pellagra is not endemic. *Northwest Medicine*, **27**, 319–323.

Parrish, E. M. (1917). Discussion symposium on pellagra. *Southern Medical Journal*, **10**, 388.

Pasha, S. A. (1939). Observations on the effects of various modes of treatment on pellagrous patients. *Journal of Tropical Medicine and Hygiene*, **42**, 329–333.

Petri, S. & Wanscher, O. (1937). Some cases of pellagra and polyneuritis treated with stomach preparations. *Acta medica scandinavica*, **91**, 370–377.

Petri, S., Wanscher, O., Stubbe Teglbjaerg, E. & Stubbe Teglbjaerg, H. P. (1937) Über die Behandlung der Pellagra mit Ventrikelprepäraten. *Acta medica scandinavica*, **93**, 450–486.

Raghuramulu, N., Srikantia, S. G., Rao, B. S. N. & Gopalan, C. (1965). Nicotinamide nucleotides in the erythrocytes of patients suffering from pellagra. *Biochemical Journal*, **96**, 837–838.

Rolph, F. W. (1916). Cancer of the stomach and pellagra in the same patient. *Canadian Medical Association Journal*, **N.S. 6**, 323–324.

Sambon, L. W. (1912). Special points of epidemological interest in pellagra. *Transactions of the National Association of the Study of Pellagra*, **2**, 81.

Scott, W. M. (1938). Pellagra secondary to lesions of the gastrointestinal tract. *New Orleans Medical and Surgical Journal*, **90**, 403.

Shattuck, G. C. (1923). Factors apparently influencing the development of pellagra in Massachusetts. *Boston Medical and Surgical Journal*, **188**, 889.

Shelley, H. M. (1927). Observations of pellagra in Nyasaland. *Lancet*, **1**, 74–75.

Shulack, N. R. & Peters, M. (1945). Spinal cord changes with avitaminosis. *Journal of Nervous and Mental Diseases*, **102**, 359–366.

Smith, D. L. & Moore, G. Y. (1915). Pyorrhoea alveolaris as cause of pellagra. *Southern Medical Journal*, **8**, 692.

Spillane, J. D. (1947). *Nutritional Disorders of the Nervous System*, pp. 103–114. Edinburgh: Livingstone.

Stannus, H. S. (1937). Pellagra: Theories of causation. *Tropical Diseases Bulletin*, **34**, 183–204.

Strauss, M. B. (1934). The role of the gastrointestinal tract in conditioning deficiency disease. *Journal of the American Medical Association*, **103**, 1–4.

Sutton, I. C. (1926). Pellagra. *American Journal of Medical Sciences*, **172**, 374–382.

Sydenstricker, V. P., Armstrong, E. S., Derrick, C. J. & Kemp, P. S. (1936). Intrinsic deficiency in pellagra. *American Journal of Medical Sciences*, **192**, 1–9.

Tabaqchali, S. & Pallis, C. (1970). Reversible nicotinamide-deficiency encephalopathy in a patient with jejunal diverticulosis. *Gut*, **11**, 1024–1028.

Thaysen, T. E. H. (1932). Secondary pellagra with report of 4 cases. *Verhandlung der Deutschen Gesellschaft für innere Medizin*, **44**, 429–439.

Turner, R. H. (1929). Pellagra associated with organic disease of the gastrointestinal tract. *American Journal of Tropical Medicine and Hygiene*, **9**, 129–137.

Welbourn, R., Hughes, R. & Wells, C. (1951). Vitamin B deficiencies after gastric operations. *Lancet*, **1**, 939–945.

Pyridoxine deficiency

Baker, E. M., Canham, J. E., Nunes, W. T., Sauberlich, H. E. & McDowell, M. E. (1964). Vitamin B_6 requirement for adult men. *American Journal of Clinical Nutrition*, **15**, 59–66.

Baker, H., Frank, O., Ning, M., Gellene, R. A., Hutner, S. H. & Leevy, C. M. (1966). A protozoological method for detecting clinical vitamin B_6 deficiency. *American Journal of Clinical Nutrition*, **18**, 123–133.

Baker, H. & Sobotka, H. (1962). Microbiological assay methods for vitamins. *Advances in Clinical Chemistry*, **5**, 173–235.

Biehl, J. P. & Vilter, R. W. (1954). Effect of isoniazid on vitamin B_6 metabolism: its possible significance in producing isoniazid neuritis. *Proceedings of the Society for Experimental Biology and Medicine*, **85**, 389–392.

Brain, M. C. & Booth, C. C. (1964). The absorption of tritium-labelled pyridoxine HCl in control subjects and in patients with intestinal malabsorption. *Gut*, **5**, 241–247.

Brain, M. C., Stewart, J. S. & Booth, C. C. (1963). The absorption of tritiated pyridoxine in the rat and in man. In *Radioaktive Isotope in Klinik und Forschung*, ed. Fellinger, K., & Hofer, R. Band **V**, 475. Munich: Urban & Schwarzenberg.

Cavanagh, J. B. & Ridley, A. R. (1967). The nature of the neuropathy complicating acute intermittent porphyria. *Lancet*, **2**, 1023–1024.

Cohen, G., Fishman, R. A. & Jenkins, A. L. (1966). A fluorometric method for the determination of xanthurenic acid in urine. *Journal of Laboratory and Clinical Medicine*, **67**, 520–527.

Coursin, D. B. (1954). Convulsive seizures in infants with pyridoxine-deficient diet. *Journal of the American Medical Association*, **154**, 406–408.

Dalgleish, C. E. (1952). The relation between pyridoxin and tryptophan metabolism studied in the rat. *Biochemical Journal*, **52**, 3–14.

Denny-Brown, D. (1947). Neurological conditions resulting from prolonged and severe dietary restriction. *Medicine*, **26**, 41–113.

Girdwood, R. H. (1956). Absorption in sprue of vitamins of the B complex. *Lancet*, **2**, 700–701.

Glazer, H. S., Mueller, J. F., Thompson, C., Hawkins, V. R. & Vilter, R. W. (1951). A study of urinary excretion of xanthurenic acid and other tryptophan metabolites in human beings with pyridoxine deficiency induced by deoxypyridoxine. *Archives of Biochemistry and Biophysics*, **33**, 243–251.

Greenberg, L. D., Bohr, D. F., McGrath, H. & Rinehart, J. F. (1949). Xanthurenic acid excretion in the human subject on a pyridoxine deficient diet. *Archives of Biochemistry*, **21**, 237–239.

Hagberg, B., Hamfelt, A. & Hansson, O. (1966). Tryptophan load tests and pyridoxal-5-phosphate levels in epileptic children. *Acta paediatrica scandinavica*, **55**, 363–370.

Hamfelt, A. (1962). A method of determining pyridoxal phosphate in blood by decarboxylation of L-tyrosine ^{14}C (U). *Clinica chimica acta*, **7**, 746.

Hamfelt, A. (1964). Age variation of vitamin B_6 metabolism in man. *Clinica chimica acta*, **10**, 48–54.

Hughes, P. A. M., Bower, B. D., Raine, D. N. & Syed, N. (1966). Metabolism of tryptophan in childhood epilepsy. *Archives of Disease in Childhood*, **41**, 642–651.

Hunt, A. D., Stokes, J., McCrory, W. W. & Stroud, H. H. (1954). Pyridoxine dependency: report of case of intractable convulsions in an infant controlled by pyridoxine. *Pediatrics*, **13**, 140–145.

Jaffe, I. A., Altman, K. & Merryman, P. (1964). Antipyridoxine effect of penicillamine in man. *Journal of Clinical Investigation*, **43**, 1869–1873.

Kowlessar, O. D., Haeffner, L. J., Benson, G. & Sleisenger, M. H. (1961). Evidence of deficiency of vitamin B_6 in non-tropical sprue. *Journal of Clinical Investigation*, **40**, 1055.

May, C. D. (1954). Vitamin B_6 in human nutrition: a critique and an object lesson. *Pediatrics*, **14**, 269–279.

Meuwisse, G., Gamstorp, I. & Tryding, N. (1968). Effect of phenytoin on the tryptophan load test. *Acta paediatrica scandinavica*, **57**, 115–120.

Morris, J. S., Ajdukiewicz, A. B. & Read, A. E. (1970). Neurological disorders in adult coeliac disease. *Gut*, **11**, 549–554.

Reilly, R. H., Killam, K. F., Jenney, E. H., Marshall, W. H., Tausig, T., Apter, N. S. & Pfeiffer, C. C. (1953). Convulsant effects of isoniazid. *Journal of American Medical Association*, **152**, 1317–1321.

Satoh, K. & Price, J. M. (1958). Fluorometric determination of kynurenic acid and xanthurenic acid in human urine. *Journal of Biological Chemistry*, **230**, 781–789.

Sauberlich, H. E. (1964). Human requirements for vitamin B_6. *Vitamins and Hormones*, **22**, 807–823.

Sauberlich, H. E. (1967). Pyridoxine. In *The Vitamins* (*Chemistry, Physiology, Pathology, Methods*), ed. György, P. & Pearson, W. N., Vol. II, Ch. 6. New York: Academic Press.

Sigler, M. H., Sheehy, T. W., Santini, R. & Rubini, M. E. (1962). Xanthurenic aciduria in tropical sprue. *American Journal of the Medical Sciences*, **244**, 197–201.

Snyderman, S. E., Holt, L. E., Carretero, R. & Jacobs, K. (1953). Pyridoxine deficiency in human infant. *Journal of Clinical Nutrition*, **1**, 200–207.

Toepfer, E. W., Polansky, M. M. & Hewston, E. M. (1961). Fluorometric determination of pyridoxamine by conversion to pyridoxal cyanide compound. *Analytical Biochemistry*, **2**, 463–469.

Vilter, R. W., Mueller, J. F., Glazer, H. S., Jarrold, T., Abraham, J., Thompson, C. & Hawkins, V. R. (1953). The effect of vitamin B_6 deficiency induced by desoxypyridoxine in human beings. *Journal of Laboratory and Clinical Medicine*, **42**, 335–357.

Weller, H. & Fichtenbaum, M. (1961). Der Tryptophanbelastungstest als Nachweis eines vitamin B_6—Mangels bei Arteriosclerose. *Klinische Wochenschrift*, **39**, 1275–1280.

Pantothenic acid deficiency

Baker, H. & Sobotka, H. (1962). Microbiological assay methods for vitamins. *Advances in Clinical Chemistry*, **5**, 173–235.

Bean, W. B. & Hodges, R. E. (1954). Pantothenic acid deficiency induced in human subjects. *Proceedings of the Society for Experimental Biology and Medicine*, **86**, 693–698.

Bibile, S. W., Lionel, N. D. W., Dunuwille, R. & Perera, G. (1957). Pantothenol and the burning feet syndrome. *British Journal of Nutrition*, **11**, 434–439.

Fennelly, J., Frank, O., Baker, H. & Leevy, C. M. (1964). Peripheral neuropathy of the alcoholic. I. Aetiological role of aneurin and other B-complex vitamins. *British Medical Journal*, **2**, 1290–1292.

Gopalan, C. (1946). 'Burning-feet' syndrome. *Indian Medical Gazette*, **81**, 22–26.

Hodges, R. E., Bean, W. B., Ohlson, M. A. & Bleiler, R. (1959). Human pantothenic acid deficiency produced by omega-methyl pantothenic acid. *Journal of Clinical Investigation*, **38**, 1421–1425.

Oldham, H. G., Davis, M. V. & Roberts, L. J. (1946). Thiamine excretion and blood levels of young women on diets containing varying levels of the B vitamins with some observations on niacin and pantothenic acid. *Journal of Nutrition*, **32**, 163–180.

Vitamin A deficiency

Arroyave, G., Wilson, D., Mendez, J., Behar, M. & Scrimshaw, N. S. (1961). Serum and liver vitamin A and lipids in children with severe protein malnutrition. *American Journal of Clinical Nutrition*, **9**, 180–185.

Bass, M. H. & Caplan, J. (1955). Vitamin A deficiency in infancy. *Journal of Pediatrics*, **47**, 690–695.

Calhoun, M. C., Rousseau, J. E. Jr., Hall, R. C. Jr, Eaton, H. D., Nelson, S. W. & Lucas, J. J. (1965). Cisternal cerebrospinal fluid pressure during development of chronic bovine hypervitaminosis A. *Journal of Dairy Science*, **48**, 729–732.

Chandra, H., Venkatachalam, P. S., Belavadi, B., Reddy, V. & Gopalan, C. (1960). Some observations on vitamin A deficiency in Indian children. *Indian Journal of Child Health*, **9**, 589–595.

Chesney, J. & McCoord, A. B. (1934). Vitamin A of serum following administration of haliver oil in normal children and in chronic steatorrhea. *Proceedings of the Society for Experimental Biology and Medicine*, **31**, 887.

Cornfeld, D. & Cooke, R. F. (1952). Vitamin A deficiency: case report. *Pediatrics*, **10**, 33–39.

Craik, K. J. W., MacPherson, S. J. & Harris, A. D. (1947). Vitamin A in infective hepatitis. Addendum on dark-adaptation. *British Medical Journal*, **1**, 558–559.

Dhanda, R. P. (1955). Electroretinography in night blindness and other vitamin A deficiencies. *Archives of Ophthalmology*, **54**, 841–849.

Dowling, J. E. & Wald, G. (1958). Nutritional night blindness. *Annals of the New York Academy of Sciences*, **74**, 256–265.

Fuchs, A. (1959). White spots of the fundus combined with night blindness and xerosis (Uyemura's syndrome). *American Journal of Ophthalmology*, **48**, 101–103.

Haig, C., Hecht, S. & Patek, A. J. (1938). Vitamin A and rod-cone dark adaptation in cirrhosis of the liver. *Science*, **87**, 534–536.

Harris, A. D. & Moore, T. (1947). Vitamin A in infective hepatitis. *British Medical Journal*, **1**, 553–557.

Harris, P. L. (1960). Bio-assay of vitamin A compounds. *Vitamins and Hormones*, **18**, 341–370.

Hume, E. M. & Krebs, H. A. (1949). Vitamin A requirements of human adults. *Medical Research Council Special Report Series* No. 264. London: H.M.S.O.

Jacobson, J. H. (1961). *Clinical Electroretinography*, ed. Lyle, D. J. Springfield, Illinois: Thomas.

Jayle, G. E. & Ourgand, A. G. (1950). *La vision nocturne et ses troubles*. Paris: Masson.
Jeghers, H. (1937). Night blindness as a criterion of vitamin A deficiency: Review of the literature with preliminary observations of the degree and prevalence of vitamin A deficiency among adults in both health and disease. *Annals of Internal Medicine*, **10**, 1304–1334.
Leitner, Z. A., Moore, T. & Sharman, I. M. (1952). Vitamin A carotenoids and tocopherol levels in the blood of two different classes of patient. *British Journal of Nutrition*, **6**, x-xi.
Livingston, P. C. (1944). Visual problems of aerial warfare; 'night' studies in dark-adapted eye. *Lancet*, **2**, 33–38.
Loran, M. R., Althausen, T. L., Spicer, F. W. & Goldstein, W. I. (1961). Transport of vitamin A across human intestine in vitro. *Journal of Laboratory and Clinical Medicine*, **58**, 622–626.
McLaren, D. (1967). Vitamins A and carotene: effects of vitamin A deficiency in man. In *The Vitamins: Chemistry, Physiology, Pathology, Methods*, ed. Sebrell, W. H. & Harris, R. S., Vol. I, Ch. I. New York & London: Academic Press.
McLaren, D. S. (1966). Present knowledge of the role of vitamin A in health and disease. *Transactions of the Royal Society of Tropical Medicine and Hygiene*, **60**, 436–462.
Mandel, H. G. (1970). Fat soluble vitamins. In *Pharmacological Basis of Therapeutics*, ed. Goodman, L. S. & Gillman, A., Ch. 75. New York: Macmillan.
May, C. D., McCreary, J. F. & Blackfan, K. D. (1942). Notes concerning the cause and treatment of coeliac disease. *Journal of Pediatrics*, **21**, 289–305.
Mellanby, E. (1947). Vitamin A and bone growth: the reversibility of vitamin A deficiency changes. *Journal of Physiology*, **105**, 382–399.
Millen, J. W., Woollam, D. H. M. & Lamming, G. E. (1953). Hydrocephalus associated with deficiency of vitamin A. *Lancet*, **2**, 1234–1237.
Moore, T. (1957). *Vitamin A*. London & New York: Elsevier.
Neeld, J. B. & Pearson, W. N. (1963). Macro and micro methods for the determination of serum vitamin A using trifluoracetic acid. *Journal of Nutrition*, **79**, 454–462.
Popper, H., Steigmann, F. & Zevin, S. (1943). On the variations of plasma vitamin A level after the administration of large doses of vitamin A in liver disease. *Journal of Clinical Investigation*, **22**, 775–783.
Roels, O. A. (1967). Vitamins A and carotene: biochemical systems. In *The Vitamins: Chemistry, Physiology, Pathology, Methods*, ed. Sebrell, W. H. & Harris, R. S., Vol. I, Ch. I. New York & London: Academic Press.
Roels, O. A. & Mahadevan, S. (1967). Vitamin A. In *The Vitamins: Chemistry, Physiology, Pathology, Methods*, ed. György, P. & Pearson, W. N., Vol. VI, Ch. 3. New York: Academic Press.
Roels, O. A., Trout, M. & Dujacquier, R. (1958). Carotene balance in boys in Ruanda where vitamin A deficiency is prevalent. *Journal of Nutrition*, **65**, 115–127.
Russell, F. E. (1967). Vitamin A content of polar bear liver. *Toxicon*, **5**, 61–62.
Scrimshaw, N. S. & Behar, M. (1961). Protein malnutrition in young children. *Science*, **133**, 2039–2047.
Skala, I. & Hruba, F. (1964). Accumulation of vitamin A by small intestine of the rat in vitro. *American Journal of Physiology*, **206**, 458–460.
Strohecker, R. & Henning, H. M. (1966). *Vitamin Assay: Tested Methods*. Berlin: Springer-Verlag.
Teng, K. H. (1965). Further contributions to the fundus—xerophthalmicus. *Ophthalmologica*, **150**, 219–238.
Uyemura, M. (1928). Ueber eine merkwürdige Augenhintergrundveränderung bei zwei Fällen von idiopathischer Hemeralopie. *Klinische Monatsblätter für Augenheilkunde*, **81**, 471–473.

CHAPTER SEVEN

Folate Deficiency

Whether folate deficiency per se is ever a cause of neurological symptoms and signs is controversial. Some of the relevant facts are briefly reviewed here. This is an area in which further developments may be anticipated.

Folates are widely distributed in plant and animal tissues, particularly high concentrations being found in liver, greens and yeast. In an average western diet three-quarters of the daily folate intake of about 700 μg will be in the form of pteroylpolyglutamates (Chanarin et al, 1968; Hurdle, Barton and Searles, 1968). Polyglutamates with more than three glutamic acid residues are not biologically active. They can only be assayed with *L. casei* after hydrolysis to 'free' folate (i.e. to the simpler tri-, di-, or mono-glutamate forms).

Folates are easily destroyed by cooking and thus the exact amount available will depend on both the type of food eaten and on the method of its preparation. Folic (pteroylglutamic) acid itself often constitutes less than 1 per cent of the folate content of an average western diet.

Folic acid is, however, both stable and readily available commercially in pure form (and as a tritiated variant). This is why most studies of folate absorption have been carried out with this substance, despite the fact that what happens during the absorption of natural folates probably differs from what happens during the absorption of folic acid itself.

Absorption and storage

Folic acid itself is rapidly absorbed from the duodenum and jejunum, up to 80 per cent of a dose as large as 15 mg being absorbable by this route (Hoffbrand, 1971). It is poorly absorbed from the ileum and hardly absorbed at all from the large intestine. There is controversy as to whether folic acid is absorbed unchanged or whether it is reduced and methylated in its passage through the intestinal cell, as first suggested by Baker et al (1965). Perhaps both processes occur according to the dose administered (Olinger, Bertino and Binder, 1973). In normal plasma, folate is present as 5-methyltetrahydrofolate.

Hepner et al (1968) have shown that folic acid may be absorbed against a concentration gradient in man. Further evidence that an active process is involved is provided by the existence of a genetically determined disorder in which there is specific malabsorption of folate. The condition, recently reviewed by Lanzkowsky (1970), will be referred to further on, as it has important neurological associations.

Dietary folate, biliary folate (Baker, Kumar and Swaminathan, 1965) and folate from desquamated intestinal cells are the three main sources of folate presented to the human intestine. Dietary folates are hydrolysed to pteroylmonoglutamate by an enzyme named folate conjugase or pteroylpolyglutamate hydrolase (or PPH) by Hoffbrand and Peters (1969). This probably takes place mainly in the jejunal mucosa. Natural folates differ from folic acid in that they are usually already reduced to the di- or tetra-hydrofolate form at positions 5, 6, 7 and 8 of their pteroyl portions. Natural folates that are not already fully reduced are probably converted to the tetra-hydro form in the enterocytes. Dietary folates also differ from folic acid in that they usually contain a methyl or formyl group at position 5 (or a formyl group at position 10) in the pteroyl portion. Methylation probably takes place during absorption of those folates not already containing a methyl group at this site (Perry and Chanarin, 1970).

The net result is that the major compound entering portal blood after ingestion of a wide variety of dietary folates is 5-methyltetrahydropteroylmonoglutamate. Hydrolysis of polyglutamates to monoglutamates occurs rapidly and proceeds optimally at a pH of between 4·0 and 5·0, possibly within the mucosal cell into which polyglutamate may have entered by a process of pinocytosis (Hoffbrand and Peters, 1970). The absorption of polyglutamates is rapidly saturated.

Malabsorption of folate

The commonest cause of folate deficiency is inadequate dietary intake. Folate deficiency may, however, also result from malabsorption. Such malabsorption has been well documented in untreated coeliac disease and in untreated tropical sprue. Croft, Loehry and Creamer (1968) have suggested that folate loss from sloughed intestinal cells may be considerable in these conditions and contribute to the deficiency. The malabsorption affects dietary folate more severely than folic acid itself but searches for a PPH-inhibiting substance or agent in these diseases have so far been inconclusive.

Malabsorption of pteroylglutamates may occur in dermatitis herpetiformis (Hoffbrand et al, 1970), following jejunal resection (Pavesio and Bosio, 1965; Baker, Thompson and Feingold, 1969), following partial gastrectomy (Markkanen, 1968; Chanarin, 1969), and in patients with Crohn's disease (Hoffbrand et al, 1968). In the last two conditions an inadequate diet is, however, the major contributory cause of the folate deficiency. Bacterial contamination of 'stagnant' intestinal loops (see p. 70) usually results in a raised serum folate (Hoffbrand, Tabaqchali and Mollin, 1966) although malabsorption of folic acid has also been reported in some such cases (Cooke et al, 1963).

Of particular interest to neurologists will be folate deficiency encountered in patients receiving such anticonvulsants as phenytoin or primidone. Various suggested mechanisms are reviewed by Hoffbrand (1971) but none has been proved conclusively. Possible mechanisms include (a) inhibition of PPH, with selective malabsorption of pteroylpolyglutamates (Hoffbrand and Necheles, 1968), and (b) malabsorption of folic acid itself, due either to inhibition of Na–K ATPase (Hepner et al, 1970) or the result of an increase in duodenal and jejunal pH (brought about by phenytoin) to a point where folic acid absorption is reduced (Benn et al, 1971).

Folate malabsorption in patients on the contraceptive pill has been reported by Shojania, Hornady and Barnes (1968) and it has been claimed (Streiff and Greene, 1970) that this occurs as a result of an inhibition of intestinal PPH but this has not been confirmed (Stephens et al, 1972).

Specific malabsorption of folate. The most cogent evidence that folate deficiency may have an effect upon the nervous system is derived from the study of a condition named *congenital specific folate malabsorption*. In 1961, Luhby et al described an infant with relapsing megaloblastic anaemia due to folate deficiency who could not be maintained in haematological remission on a normal diet, but only after massive and very unphysiological folic acid supplements had been added. Follow-up reports in 1965 (Luhby, Cooperman and Pesci-Bourel) and in 1967 (Luhby and Cooperman) mentioned that a female sibling was also affected. Both children absorbed fat, glucose and vitamin A normally, and neither had any radiologically demonstrable abnormality of the gastrointestinal tract. Both had developed a neurological disorder characterised by moderate mental and physical retardation, ataxia and seizures, the frequency of the latter being reduced by the administration of folic acid. The neurological condition seemed to be slowly progressive despite daily oral intake of folic acid of 60 mg. Neither child was able to transport folate normally from plasma to CSF. The authors attributed the severe isolated defect in folic acid transport across both the intestinal mucosa and the blood–CSF barrier to a new inborn error of metabolism.

In 1969, Lanzkowsky, Erlandson and Bezan reported in detail on a similar case, with a follow-up a year later (Lanzkowsky, 1970). A 20-year-old girl had suffered from recurrent megaloblastic anaemia since early childhood. She required a daily oral intake of at least 40 mg of folic acid to maintain her in haematological remission. Any attempt to reduce the oral folic acid resulted in stomatitis, anorexia, weight loss and anaemia. At the age of 9 she had developed epileptic seizures. Examination at the age of 19 showed profound mental retardation (but normal physical development, including sexual characteristics), dysarthria, 'an athetotic movement disorder of the upper limbs resembling extrapyramidal disease without tremor, ataxia or cerebellar signs', and punctate calcification of the basal ganglia, particularly of the caudate nuclei. Barium meal and jejunal biopsy were normal. She had a normal Schilling test and fat, glucose and vitamin A were normally absorbed. Following daily intramuscular injections of folic acid, plasma and erythrocyte folate levels rose but the CSF level remained unrecordably low despite the fact that the CSF folate concentration is normally three times that of plasma (Herbert and Zalusky, 1961; Herbert, 1964). The patient was shown to have a specific defect in the absorption of folic acid. Absorption was not enhanced when the folic acid was given in conjunction with lyophilised calf jejunum or pancreas, or in the form of pteroyldiglutamic acid, pteroyltriglutamic acid, formyltetrahydrofolic acid or methyltetrahydrofolic acid. Folate withdrawal resulted in a diminution in the number of seizures. Resumption of folate therapy increased the number of seizures. In contrast to the findings in the sibship described by Luhby, the neurological disorder, although profound, did not appear to be progressive.

This discussion of congenital folate deficiency associated with neurological signs would be incomplete without reference to the fact that within the last decade Japanese workers (Arakawa et al, 1963, 1966, 1967) have described three separate inborn errors of folate metabolism associated with mental retardation and abnormally *high* levels of folate activity in the serum. These patients seem to have had defects of folate metabolism, rather than of folate absorption. The determination of serum folate levels should clearly form part of the investigation of cases of mental retardation of uncertain cause. The finding of abnormally low (or abnormally high) levels should lead to a search for an inborn error of folate absorption (or metabolism).

Clinical features of folate deficiency

The *haematological repercussions* of folate deficiency are beyond the scope of this monograph. Other effects are less well documented. *Cutaneous pigmentation* may occur. Reporting on seven patients with nutritional megaloblastic anaemia due to folic acid deficiency, Gough et al (1963) stressed that in addition to pallor the patients all presented a greyish-brown pigmentation, particularly of exposed parts. In the absence of prematurely grey hair, this colour often suggested the true aetiological diagnosis before folic acid deficiency was confirmed.

The possible *neurological repercussions* of folate deficiency have been the subject of much controversy. Studies in this field are beset with problems. Many of the patients alleged to show involvement of the nervous system from this cause also suffer from conditions themselves likely to produce neurological signs. For instance, a low serum folate (which does not necessarily imply severe folate deficiency) is not uncommon in elderly patients (Hurdle and Picton-Williams, 1966; Batata et al, 1967) in whom neurological signs, sometimes unrelated to recognised clinical entities, are commonly present. Epileptics maintained on long-term anticonvulsant therapy present a similar problem. It is known that such therapy may result in low serum folate levels (Klipstein, 1964; Reynolds et al, 1966; Reynolds, 1972) and possibly also in peripheral neuropathy (Lovelace and Horwitz, 1968). In neither group of patients should it be inferred that folate deficiency is *responsible* for neurological abnormalities. Patients with organic dementia and folate deficiency are particularly difficult to assess. Dementia is not infrequently associated with lack of interest in food and this may lead to a folate deficiency (Batata et al, 1967) of nutritional origin. Considerable improvement in dementia or other organic psychiatric syndromes following the administration of folate, although suggestive of a causal relationship, must be interpreted cautiously. Dementia in the elderly often runs an episodic course and may appear spontaneously to improve for short periods. Moreover, the improved appetite induced by folate therapy in folate-deficient patients may result in the ingestion of other vitamins, deficiency of which may have been contributing to the clinical picture. A further difficulty is that several of the reported cases of alleged folate-responsive dementia received vitamin B_{12} (usually during the performance of a Schilling test) in the course of the investigation of their megaloblastic anaemia.

Herbert (1962) reported that four and a half months of self-imposed folate deprivation only produced insomnia, forgetfulness and irritability but no neurological signs. *Long, Childress and Bond (1963)* reported the case of a 47-year-old man who developed a megaloblastic anaemia after receiving phenytoin for three years in a dose of 400 mg daily. During this period he had on one occasion suffered from phenytoin intoxication. At the time he developed anaemia he had no neurological symptoms. Neurological examination was 'essentially within normal limits except for a "stocking-type" of hypalgesia in both legs, beginning just above the knees'. The sensory level was sharply demarcated. Other types of sensation were not impaired. No comment was made concerning the ankle jerks. Serum folate and B_{12} levels were not reported and the presence of neuropathy was not documented by electrophysiological means. The sensory findings promptly disappeared following the administration of oral folic acid in a dose of 10 mg b.d., which induced an adequate haematological response. 'Hysterical' sensory loss seems to us at least as plausible an interpretation of the findings as folate-induced neuropathy.

Anand (1964) described a man aged 60 with epilepsy due to cerebral cysticercosis. Following the administration of phenytoin for nine years, during the latter part of which period he also received phenobarbitone and primidone, the patient developed a megaloblastic anaemia, signs and symptoms suggestive of a severe peripheral neuropathy and an organic dementia. There was free acid in the gastric juice and the barium meal was normal. Serum folate and B_{12} levels were not reported. There was no response to cyanocobalamin (administered by an unspecified route) but prompt improvement following the oral administration of folic acid in a dose of 5 mg twice daily. Within six weeks the mental confusion had cleared, the patient was no longer incontinent of urine, and joint position sense had returned to the feet although the patient was reported as still ataxic. No comment is made concerning the knee and ankle jerks (originally absent) or concerning the plantar responses (originally extensor).

Hansen, Nordquist and Sourander (1964) described an epileptic aged 60 who had been receiving anticonvulsants for over 50 years, when he more or less synchronously developed signs and sympoms of megaloblastic anaemia and of a severe peripheral neuropathy, confirmed electrically. There were no clinical features suggestive of nicotinic acid or thiamine deficiency. The serum folic acid was markedly reduced at 0·7 ng/ml and the serum B_{12} was normal (350 pg/ml). Malnutrition was established by dietary history and malabsorption of folic acid by special tests. The patient fell, broke several ribs and died of bronchopneumonia. Necropsy revealed convolutional atrophy, with frontal and temporal loss of neurones, Ammon's horn sclerosis, Purkinje cell loss, and pallor of myelin staining in dorsal columns. Lumbar and sacral roots appeared fibrotic, but peroneal nerves were histologically normal. The authors suggested that 'the lesions of the cerebellum, spinal cord and root pouches might be connected with severe folic acid deficiency'. While admitting this to be possible, we feel this interpretation to be simplistic, ignoring as it does the effects of age, severe and longstanding epilepsy and possibly earlier phenytoin intoxication.

We have quoted these cases at some length as they illustrate the somewhat shaky foundations on which the concept of neuropathy due to folate deficiency was based. Misrepresentation of the original facts at times compounds the difficulties. For instance, Strachan and Henderson (1967) even claimed that there were confirmatory neuropathological findings of peripheral neuropathy and myelopathy in the prementioned patient of Long et al (1963)—in whom no necropsy had been performed—and in the case of Hansen et al (1964), in whose peripheral nerves the authors reported no abnormalities of either axons or myelin.

In a much-quoted paper published in 1965, Grant, Hoffbrand and Wells reported seven patients with folate deficiency of nutritional origin and chronic neurological disease. Serum folate levels ranged from 1·8 to 4·2 ng/ml, the serum B_{12} levels being normal in each case. Four patients had chronic spastic paraplegia without evidence of peripheral neuropathy and failed to show any neurological improvement following folate therapy. Of the remaining three patients one, a woman aged 39 described as having peripheral neuropathy (but also as having hyperaesthesiae over the lower *dorsal* dermatomes and a positive Lhermitte sign), improved dramatically after the administration of folic acid. Both neurological signs and symptoms disappeared. Another patient, a woman aged 43, was also alleged to have peripheral neuropathy (although the table shows her to have had brisk knee jerks, wasting of one thigh, loss of vibration sense confined to one leg, and incontinence of urine). She lost her sensory signs and symptoms after a few weeks of therapy with folic acid. The third patient to have shown improvement was a woman aged 47, deemed to have hereditary cerebellar ataxia of 10 years' duration and a superadded peripheral neuropathy. The sensory symptoms subsided following specific therapy. No comment is made about any change in the physical signs following treatment.

These three clinically very heterogeneous cases have been repeatedly referred to in the literature as providing evidence for the existence of a neuropathy due to folate deficiency (Strachan and Henderson, 1967; Brain, 1969; Ahmed, 1972). Grant et al (1965), it should be stressed, claimed that it was 'unjustifiable to conclude that the neurological syndromes (they were describing) . . . were the direct result of folate deficiency'. They believed a more plausible explanation to be that in some of their patients neurological disease had caused folate deficiency by interfering with appetite, and improved appetite following folate therapy had possibly resulted in increased intake of other essential dietary factors.

Some recently reported cases illustrate other diagnostic difficulties, in particular the association with alcoholism.

Dérot et al (1967) described a young woman aged 25 who after several months of anorexia and of excessive alcohol intake developed mental changes, melaena and oliguria. Her confusional state improved following haemodialysis but within a few days—and while receiving both thiamine and pyridoxine—she developed a neurological disturbance combining features of severe motor neuropathy in the lower limbs with bilateral cerebellar signs. The knee jerks were depressed and the ankle jerks absent. Sensation was normal. Treatment with a high calorie, high protein diet and iron supplements gradually improved her general condition and her macrocytic anaemia, but the neurological disturbance remained unaltered. The formiminoglutamic acid (FIGLU) test was then found to be strongly positive. The neurological signs improved rapidly following treatment with oral folic acid, in a daily dose of 20 mg. In our opinion the folate deficiency here was probably due to the combined effects of defective intake, alcoholism and excessive folate loss, such as is known to occur following dialysis (Whitehead et al, 1968; Sevitt and Hoffbrand, 1969). The onset of neuropathy in the wake of dialysis suggests that deficiency of other factors may also have been involved.

Ahmed (1972) reported a woman aged 63 who had been depressed and anxious for four years. No comment was made as to whether she had received any medication. She gradually developed weakness and numbness of the legs. On examination she was found to have a megaloblastic anaemia, exaggeration of all the tendon reflexes (including the ankle jerks), extensor plantar responses, impaired vibration sense in the legs and a positive Romberg sign. She had a serum folate of 0·6 ng/ml and a serum B_{12} of 300 pg/ml. The cause of the folate deficiency was not pursued. There was a haematological response to folic acid (10 mg thrice daily). The legs became stronger, and the sensory signs and symptoms subsided. The tendon reflexes remained brisk and the plantar responses extensor. There is no mention of the cervical spine having been x-rayed.

Pincus, Reynolds and Glaser (1972) gave perhaps the best-documented case of myelopathy associated with folate deficiency. A 69-year-old woman, who admitted to consuming 2 oz of whisky a day, developed pallor, fatigue and forgetfulness over a period of two months and more recent disorientation and diffuse weakness, maximal in the legs. She was found to have a megaloblastic anaemia and grossly abnormal liver function tests, with a serum B_{12} of over 2000 pg/ml, suggesting hepatic cirrhosis. The limbs were weak, the tendon reflexes being depressed in the arms and absent in the legs. The plantar responses were both extensor. Vibration sense was absent below the iliac crests, position sense depressed in the toes and there was hypalgesia over the feet. She was moderately demented, the EEG being abnormal. There was free acid in the gastric juice and a Schilling test showed that vitamin B_{12} could be absorbed normally. No reticulocyte response followed daily injections of vitamin B_{12} (1000 μg/day) for eight days, but a moderately good haematological response occurred after oral folic acid (10 mg/daily). Neurological improvement was slow but six months later the patient was alert and orientated with an intact memory. The tendon reflexes had returned in the lower limbs and the plantar responses were now flexor. Vibration sense was back to normal, although there were mild residual deficits of postural sensibility and of pain sense in the feet. The EEG had also improved. The authors commented that 'a clinical picture identical to that of subacute combined system degeneration can be associated with folate deficiency and responds to administration of folate'. Whether the alcoholic background played any contributory role in this case, as in the above-mentioned one, must be left a matter of conjecture.

The evidence for an encephalopathy due to folate deficiency rests on no firmer foundations.

Spillane (1959) mentioned the case of a middle-aged woman with an alleged folate-responsive encephalopathy. As far as is known, full details of this case remain unpublished.

Strachan and Henderson (1967) described two elderly women with nutritional folate deficiency and megaloblastic anaemia, moderate in the one case, severe in the other. Each patient presented with moderate dementia and had an abnormal EEG. In one case there were no abnormal neurological signs, in the other 'apparent impairment of vibratory sensibility in the legs'. The serum folate levels were 2·7 ng/ml and 0·6 ng/ml respectively. The initial serum vitamin B_{12} levels were 323 and 300 pg/ml. Both patients were given oral folic acid over a prolonged period. Their abnormal mental states improved strikingly but rather slowly, over a period of several months. Their EEGs became normal. Other measures aimed at improving the nutrition of the patients had also been resorted to, the second patient in particular receiving a transfusion of packed red cells. In view of the tendency of mild dementing processes in the elderly to be markedly aggravated by intercurrent illness (and of the fact that a wide variety of illnesses in this age group may present with 'reversible' organic dementia) we feel these two cases to constitute but slender evidence for the existence of a specific encephalopathy *due to* folate deficiency.

More recently Reynolds, Rothfeld and Pincus (1973) have attempted to assess the comparative prevalence of neurological signs in two groups of age and sex-matched hospital patients, the one comprising cases with severe folate deficiency (serum folate <3 ng/ml), the other cases with normal serum folate levels ($>6·9$ ng/ml). 'A significant increase of organic brain syndrome and pyramidal tract damage' and 'a higher prevalence of neuropathy' were found in the former group. The groups were small (24 and 21 patients), however, and both comprised a large number of alcoholics (12 and 8 cases respectively). The groups also contained diabetics, patients with malignant disease, patients who had undergone partial gastrectomy, malnourished patients with chronic renal disease and patients with malabsorption. Although these cases were fairly evenly distributed between the two groups, the presence of a majority of such cases in each group lessens the validity of the study. If all patients with such conditions (each of which may be associated with neurological complications) were eliminated, a comparison became possible between six patients in group A and six patients in group B. Of six (folate deficient) patients in group A, five had neurological abnormalities, whereas of six 'comparable' patients in group B all were neurologically normal except for one patient who was retarded and depressed.

A somewhat different, if equally tenuous, strand of evidence seeks to incriminate folate deficiency as a cause of chronic encephalopathy on the grounds that both are common in epileptics treated with anticonvulsants. Reynolds (1967) found that folic acid partially reversed the 'retarding' effect of anticonvulsants such as phenytoin, primidone, and phenobarbitone. As it also reversed the therapeutic (anti-epileptic) effects of these drugs, it was suggested that these drugs might act by inducing alterations of folate metabolism. Chanarin et al (1960) had earlier described the aggravation of seizures in a patient with drug-induced folate deficiency on administration of folic acid, although earlier still Hawkins and Meynell (1958) had claimed that the administration of folate lessened seizure frequency in epileptics with anticonvulsant-induced megaloblastic anaemia. Reynolds (1968) has even suggested that anticonvulsant-induced folate deficiency probably contributes to many of the psychiatric illnesses and other neurological abnormalities encountered in epileptics of long standing.

Folate and the nervous system

In 1961, Herbert and Zalusky had reported that the average concentration of folic acid was three times higher in the CSF than it was in blood. (Folic acid was assessed in terms of its growth-promoting action for *L. casei*.) None of the 16 patients studied by these authors had a ratio of less than 1·5 : 1. This was in striking contrast to their finding concerning protein-bound vitamin B_{12} (*E. gracilis* assay) where the mean CSF value was 22 pg/ml, the mean serum value being 546 pg/ml. Reynolds et al (1972) have recently confirmed that CSF folate levels are always higher than serum levels and have shown that there is a striking correlation between serum and CSF folate in normal controls, in psychiatric patients (before the administration of psychotropic drugs) and in epileptics receiving a wide variety of medication. Folate concentrations in both blood and CSF are significantly reduced in the latter group, as reported earlier by Wells and Casey (1967) and by Weckman and Lehtovaara (1969).

No other substance appears to be concentrated in the CSF to this degree (Davson, 1967). The significance of this is unclear; it might even mean that folate is selectively secreted by the choroid plexus and then *not* utilised by the brain (a teleological oxymoron). However, it seems that folate may have a physiological role in the central nervous system, for 5-methyltetrahydrofolic acid has been shown to be present in certain areas of the rat brain, and may be involved in the inactivation by transmethylation of serotonin (Korevaar et al, 1973). The selective concentration of folate in the CSF seems to operate even during the development of folate deficiency. Herbert (1964) showed that of 11 subjects with serum folate levels between 4·2 and 6·3 ng/ml all had normal CSF folates (19 to 39 ng/ml). Three patients with low serum folate levels of 2·2, 1·9 and <1·0 ng/ml respectively, had CSF folate levels of 7, 13 and 7·9 ng/ml.

As will have become apparent, it remains uncertain whether or not folate deficiency induces neurological disorder. *How* any such disorder might be induced is also unknown. The vague suggestion has been made that RNA synthesis might be impaired. Haltia (1970) fed newborn chicks for one month on a ration deficient in folic acid. The animals all developed low serum folate levels and clinical signs of folate deficiency characteristic for chicks (retarded growth, poor feathering and macrocytic anaemia). RNA content of Purkinje cells was significantly lower than that of control chicks, but this could well have been a non-specific effect of generalised nutritional deficiency. Body weight was severely reduced in the folate-depleted chicks, and in the early postnatal period Purkinje cell dendritic arborisation might have been impaired in the same way as occurs in protein–calorie malnourished mammals.

Laboratory diagnosis of folate deficiency

Folate deficiency should be suspected in any patient with megaloblastic anaemia or—in the absence of anaemia—in any patient with macrocytosis of the erythrocytes and hypersegmentation of polymorphs in the peripheral blood, and with megaloblasts and giant metamyelocytes in the marrow. Folate deficiency is likely if such changes are associated with a normal serum vitamin B_{12}, or if changes in the blood are gross while the serum vitamin B_{12} level is only slightly reduced (Mollin, Waters and Harris, 1962). Unlike what is sometimes seen in vitamin B_{12} deficiency, there is usually a good correlation between the severity of folate deficiency and the severity of its haematological repercussions. The diagnosis of folate deficiency is confirmed if the haematological abnormalities are corrected by physiological doses of folic acid (i.e. 200 μg/day).

In the complicated situations encountered in clinical practice, where several disease processes may be contributing to anaemia and where multiple deficiencies of haemopoietic factors may be present, it will be quicker to resort to biochemical tests to establish the presence of folate deficiency.

Serum folate level. This is estimated microbiologically using *L. casei* as the test organism. The test is extremely sensitive and considerable variations may occur when single samples are estimated several times in different laboratories, or even in the same laboratory. Mollin and Hoffbrand (1965) discuss some of the explanations for these variations. Most laboratories consider a serum folate below 3 ng/ml as definitely abnormal, levels between 3 and 5 ng/ml as equivocal and levels above 5 ng/ml as definitely normal (Hoffbrand, 1971).

Many antibiotics and folate antagonists will inhibit the growth of the test organism and give rise to 'false' low readings. Unless serum proteins are extracted before assay such readings may also be encountered in many patients with untreated coeliac disease and tropical sprue, whose serum may contain an agglutinating antibody (an IgG globulin) directed against an antigen on the body of *L. casei* (Cowan, 1969).

Serum folate has been tentatively identified as 5-methyltetrahydrofolate (5-methyl-THF) (Herbert, Larrabee and Buchanan, 1962). It is probably derived from liver and other tissue stores by a displacement mechanism, absorbed folic acid entering these tissues and displacing 5-methyl-THF from their cells (Whitehead and Cooper, 1967; Chanarin and McLean, 1967).

The serum folate falls fairly rapidly in a normal subject on a folate-deficient diet, presumably as a result of reduction of this displacement phenomenon. The fall will occur long before there is any reduction of tissue stores. In the presence of grossly reduced intake the tissue stores will probably last for about four months.

Red cell folate. There is 30 to 40 times more folate in red cells than in serum and the assessment of red cell folate provides a useful measure of tissue folate stores. A fall in red cell folate implies a fairly severe folate deficiency (Hoffbrand, Newcombe and Mollin, 1966).

Misleadingly high red cell folate levels are encountered in patients with a raised reticulocyte count. Misleadingly low levels are seen in some patients with megaloblastic anaemia due to B_{12} deficiency (Cooper and Lowenstein, 1964). As the serum folate levels may rise in such cases the ratio of red cell folate concentration to serum folate concentration (normally 30–40 : 1) will be markedly altered and may fall to about 10 : 1 in patients with severe B_{12} deficiency (Hoffbrand, Newcombe and Mollin, 1966).

FIGLU Excretion. Dietary histidine is broken down to glutamic acid, a process which involves the successive formation of urocanic acid, imidazole-propionic acid and formiminoglutamic acid (FIGLU). Folate is needed as a coenzyme in the last step of this metabolic sequence: the breakdown of FIGLU to glutamic acid. In folate deficiency FIGLU excretion is increased particularly after a loading dose of histidine.

The test is fully reviewed by Luhby and Cooperman (1964). FIGLU excretion may be measured by cellulose acetate electrophoresis (Kohn, Mollin and Rosenbach, 1961) or, more reliably, by spectrophotometry (Chanarin and Bennett, 1962). If urine is collected for eight hours following a loading dose of 15 g of L-histidine, normal subjects will excrete up to 17 mg of FIGLU. Results correlate well with those of the red cell folate assay (Hoffbrand, Newcombe and Mollin, 1966) and with estimations of liver folate stores (Chanarin et al, 1966).

FIGLU excretion may be increased, in the absence of folate deficiency, in some patients with uncomplicated vitamin B_{12} deficiency, as well as in patients with liver disease, carcinoma, Hodgkin's disease and myelosclerosis. False negative results may occur during pregnancy and in severe protein malnutrition. In view of these facts the estimation of FIGLU excretion is gradually falling out of favour, as a test of folate deficiency.

References

Ahmed, M. (1972). Neurological disease and folate deficiency. *British Medical Journal*, **1**, 181.

Anand, M. P. (1964). Iatrogenic megaloblastic anaemia with neurological complications. *Scottish Medical Journal*, **9**, 388–390.

Arakawa, T., Ohara, K., Kudo, Z., Tada, K., Hayashi, T. & Mizuno, T. (1963). 'Hyperfolic acidemia with formiminoglutamic aciduria following histidine loading' suggested for a case of congenital deficiency in formimino transferase. *Tohoku Journal of Experimental Medicine*, **80**, 370–382.

Arakawa, T., Fujii, M., Ohara, K., Watanabe, S., Karahashi, M., Kobayashi, M. & Hirono, H. (1966). Mental retardation with hyperfolic acidemia not associated with formiminoglutamic aciduria; cyclohydrolase deficiency syndrome. *Tohoku Journal of Experimental Medicine*, **88**, 341–352.

Arakawa, T., Narisawa, K., Tanno, K., Ohara, K., Higashi, O., Honda, Y., Tamura, T., Wada, Y., Mizuno, T., Hayashi, T., Hirooka, Y., Ohno, T. & Ikeda, M. (1967). Megaloblastic anemia and mental retardation associated with hyperfolic-acidemia: probably due to N^5 methyl-tetrahydrofolate transferase deficiency. *Tohoku Journal of Experimental Medicine*, **93**, 1–22.

Baker, H., Frank, O., Feingold, S., Ziffer, H., Gellene, R. A., Leevy, C. M. & Sobotka, H. (1965). The fate of orally and parenterally administered folates. *American Journal of Clinical Nutrition*, **17**, 88–95.

Baker, H., Thomson, A. D. & Feingold, S. (1969). Role of the jejunum in the absorption of folic acid and its polyglutamates. *American Journal of Clinical Nutrition*, **22**, 124–132.

Baker, S. J., Kumar, S. & Swaminathan, S. P. (1965). Excretion of folic acid in bile. *Lancet*, **1**, 685.

Batata, M., Spray, G. H., Bolton, F. G., Higgins, G., Wollner, L. (1967). Blood and bone marrow changes in elderly patients with special reference to folic acid, vitamin B_{12}, iron and ascorbic acid. *British Medical Journal*, **2**, 667–669.

Benn, A., Swan, C. H. J., Cooke, W. T., Blair, J. A., Matty, A. J. & Smith, M. E. (1971). Effect of intraluminal pH on the absorption of pteroylglutamic acid. *British Medical Journal*, **1**, 148–150.

Brain, M. C. (1969). The neurological manifestations of folate deficiency. In *Recent Advances in Neurology and Psychiatry*, ed. Brain, W. R. & Wilkinson, M., 8th edition. London: Churchill.

Chanarin, I. (1969). *The Megaloblastic Anaemias*. Oxford: Blackwell.

Chanarin, I. & Bennett, M. C. (1962). A spectrophotometric method for estimating formimino-glutamic acid and urocanic acid. *British Medical Journal*, **1**, 27–29.

Chanarin, I., Hutchinson, M., McLean, A. & Moule, M. (1966). Hepatic folate in man. *British Medical Journal*, **1**, 396–399.

Chanarin, I., Laidlaw, J., Loughridge, L. W. & Mollin, D. L. (1960). Megaloblastic anaemia due to phenobarbitone. The convulsant action of therapeutic doses of folic acid. *British Medical Journal*, **1**, 1099–1102.

Chanarin, I. & McLean, A. (1967). Origin of serum and urinary methyl tetra-hydrofolate in man. *Clinical Science*, **32**, 57–67.

Chanarin, I., Rothman, D., Perry, J. & Stratfull, D. (1968). Normal dietary folate, iron and protein intake with special reference to pregnancy. *British Medical Journal*, **2**, 394–397.

Cooke, W. T., Cox, E. V., Fone, D. J., Meynell, M. J. & Gaddie, R. (1963). The clinical and metabolic significance of jejunal diverticulosis. *Gut*, **4**, 115–135.

Cooper, B. A. & Lowenstein, L. (1964). Relative folate deficiency of erythrocytes in pernicious anemia and its correction with cyanocobalamin. *Blood*, **24**, 502–521.

Cowan, J. D. (1969). An investigation into factors affecting the Lactobacillus casei assay of folate in serum. Ph.D. thesis, London.

Croft, D. N., Loehry, C. A. & Creamer, B. (1968). Small-bowel cell-loss and weight-loss in the coeliac syndrome. *Lancet*, **2**, 68–70.

Dérot, M., Castaigne, P., Morel-Maroger, A. & Leclercq, A. (1967). Syndrome neurologique nutritionel complexe réversible par administration d'acide folique. *Bulletins et Mémoires de la Société Médicale des Hôpitaux de Paris*, **118**, 867–874.

Davson, H. (1967). *Physiology of the Cerebrospinal Fluid.* London: Churchill.

Gough, K. R., Read, A. E., McCarthy, C. F. & Waters, A. H. (1963). Megaloblastic anaemia due to nutritional deficiency of folic acid. *Quarterly Journal of Medicine*, **32,** 243–256.

Grant, H. C., Hoffbrand, A. V. & Wells, D. G. (1965). Folate deficiency and neurological disease. *Lancet*, **2,** 763–767.

Haltia, M. (1970). The effect of folate deficiency on neuronal RNA content. A quantitative cytochemical study. *British Journal of Experimental Pathology*, **51,** 191–196.

Hansen, H. A., Nordquist, P. & Sourander, P. (1964). Megaloblastic anaemia and neurological disturbances combined with folic acid deficiency; observations on an epileptic patient treated with anticonvulsants. *Acta medica scandinavica*, **176,** 243–251.

Hawkins, C. F. & Meynell, M. K. (1958). Macrocytosis and macrocytic anaemia caused by anticonvulsant drugs. *Quarterly Journal of Medicine*, **27,** 45–63.

Hepner, G. W., Aledort, L. M., Gerson, C. D., Cohen, N., Herbert, V. & Janowitz, H. D. (1970). Inhibition of intestinal ATPase by diphenylhydantoin and acetazolamide. *Clinical Research*, **18,** 382.

Hepner, G. W., Booth, C. C., Cowan, J., Hoffbrand, A. V. & Mollin, D. L. (1968). Absorption of crystalline folic acid in man. *Lancet*, **2,** 302–306.

Herbert, V. (1962). Experimental nutritional folate deficiency in man. *Transactions of the Association of American Physicians*, **75,** 307–320.

Herbert, V. (1964). Studies of folate deficiency in man. *Proceedings of the Royal Society of Medicine*, **57,** 377–384.

Herbert, V., Larrabee, A. R. & Buchanan, J. M. (1962). Studies on the identification of folate compound of human serum. *Journal of Clinical Investigation*, **41,** 1134–1138.

Herbert, V. & Zalusky, R. (1961). Selective concentration of folic acid activity in cerebrospinal fluid. *Federation Proceedings*, **20,** 453.

Hoffbrand, A. V. (1971). Folate absorption. *Journal of Clinical Pathology*, **24,** *Supplement 5*, 66–76.

Hoffbrand, A. V., Douglas, A. P., Fry, L. & Stewart, J. S. (1970). Malabsorption of dietary folate (pteroylpolyglutamates) in adult coeliac disease and dermatitis herpetiformis. *British Medical Journal*, **4,** 85–89.

Hoffbrand, A. V. & Necheles, T. F. (1968). Mechanism of folate deficiency in patients receiving phenytoin. *Lancet*, **2,** 528–530.

Hoffbrand, A. V., Newcombe, B. F. A. & Mollin, D. L. (1966). Method of assay of red cell folate and the value of the assay as a test for folate deficiency. *Journal of Clinical Pathology*, **19,** 17–28.

Hoffbrand, A.V. & Peters, T. J. (1969). The subcellular localization of pteroylpolyglutamate hydrolase and folate in guinea-pig intestinal mucosa. *Biochima et biophysica acta*, **192,** 479–485.

Hoffbrand, A. V. & Peters, T. J. (1970). Recent advances in clinical and biochemical aspects of folate. *Schweizerische Medizinische Wochenschrift*, **100,** 1954–1960.

Hoffbrand, A. V., Stewart, J. S., Booth, C. C. & Mollin, D. L. (1968). Folate deficiency in Crohn's disease: incidence, pathogenesis, and treatment. *British Medical Journal*, **2,** 71–75.

Hoffbrand, A. V., Tabaqchali, S. & Mollin, D. L. (1966). High serum folate levels in intestinal blind-loop syndrome. *Lancet*, **1,** 1339–1342.

Hurdle, A. D. F., Barton, D. & Searles, I. H. (1968). A method for measuring folate in food and its application to a hospital diet. *American Journal of Clinical Nutrition*, **21,** 1202–1207.

Hurdle, A. D. F. & Picton-Williams, T. C. (1966). Folic acid deficiency in elderly patients admitted to hospital. *British Medical Journal*, **2,** 202–205.

Klipstein, F. A. (1964). Subnormal serum folate and macrocytosis associated with anticonvulsant drug therapy. *Blood*, **23,** 68–86.

Kohn, J., Mollin, D. L. & Rosenbach, L. M. (1961). Conventional voltage electrophoresis for formimino-glutamic acid determination in folic acid deficiency. *Journal of Clinical Pathology*, **14,** 345–350.

Korevaar, W. C., Geyer, M. A., Knapp, S., Hsu, L. L. & Mandell, A. J. (1973). Regional distribution of 5-methyltetrahydrofolic acid in brain. *Nature New Biology*, **245,** 244–245.

Lanzkowsky, P. (1970). Congenital malabsorption of folate. *American Journal of Medicine*, **48**, 580–583.

Lanzkowsky, P., Erlandson, M. E. & Bezan, A. I. (1969). Isolated defect of folic acid absorption associated with mental retardation and cerebral calcification. *Blood*, **34**, 452–465.

Long, M. T., Childress, R. H. & Bond, W. H. (1963). Megaloblastic anemia associated with the use of anticonvulsant drugs. *Neurology*, **13**, 697–702.

Lovelace, R. E. & Horwitz, S. J. (1968). Peripheral neuropathy in long-term diphenylhydantoin therapy. *Archives of Neurology*, **18**, 69–77.

Luhby, A. L. & Cooperman, J. M. (1964). Folic acid deficiency in man and its interrelationship with vitamin B_{12} metabolism. *Advances in Metabolic Disorders*, **1**, 263–334.

Luhby, A. L. & Cooperman, J. M. (1967). Congenital megaloblastic anemia and progressive central nervous system degeneration. Further clinical and physiological characterization and therapy of syndrome due to inborn error of folate transport. *American Pediatric Society Inc. Annual meeting, Atlantic City, April, 1967.*

Luhby, A. L., Cooperman, J. M. & Pesci-Bourel, A. (1965). A new inborn error of metabolism: folic acid responsive megaloblastic anemia, ataxia, mental retardation and convulsions. *American Pediatric Society Inc. Annual Meeting, Philadelphia, May, 1965.*

Luhby, A. L., Eagle, F. J., Roth, E. & Cooperman, J. M. (1961). Relapsing megaloblastic anemia in an infant due to a specific defect in gastrointestinal absorption of folic acid. *American Journal of Diseases of Children*, **102**, 482–483.

Markkanen, T. (1968). Absorption tests with natural folate material in controls and in gastrectomized patients. *American Journal of Clinical Nutrition*, **21**, 473–481.

Mollin, D. L. & Hoffbrand, A. V. (1965). The diagnosis of folate deficiency. *Series Haematologica*, **3**, 1–18.

Mollin, D. L., Waters, A. H. & Harris, S. E. B. (1962). Clinical aspects of the metabolic interrelationships between folic acid and vitamin B_{12}. *In Vitamin B_{12} and Intrinsic Factor. 2 Europäisches Symposion Hamburg, 1961*, pp. 737–755. Stuttgart: Enke.

Olinger, E. J., Bertino, J. R. & Binder, H. J. (1973). Intestinal folate absorption. II. Conversion and retention of pteroylmonoglutamate by jejunum. *Journal of Clinical Investigation*, **52**, 2138–2145.

Pavesio, D. & Bosio, U. (1965). Il test di assorbimento dell'acido folico in alcune malattie intestinali infantili. *Minerva Pediatrica*, **17**, 1488–1491.

Perry, J. & Chanarin, I. (1970). Intestinal absorption of reduced folate compounds in man. *British Journal of Haematology*, **18**, 329–339.

Pincus, J. H., Reynolds, E. H. & Glaser, G. H. (1972). Subacute combined system degeneration with folate deficiency. *Journal of the American Medical Association*, **221**, 496–497.

Reynolds, E. H. (1967). Effects of folic acid on the mental state and fit frequency of drug-treated epileptic patients. *Lancet*, **1**, 1086–1088.

Reynolds, E. H. (1968). Mental effects of anticonvulsants and folic acid metabolism. *Brain*, **91**, 197–214.

Reynolds, E. H. (1972). Diphenylhydantoin: hematologic aspects of toxicity. In *Antiepileptic Drugs*, ed. Woodbury, D. M., Penry, J. K. & Schmidt, R. P. New York: Raven Press.

Reynolds, E. H., Gallacher, B. B., Mattson, R. H., Bowers, M. & Johnson, A. L. (1972). Relationship between serum and cerebrospinal fluid folate. *Nature*, **240**, 155–157.

Reynolds, E. H., Milner, D., Matthews, D. M. & Chanarin, I. (1966). Anticonvulsant therapy, megaloblastic haemopoiesis and folic acid metabolism. *Quarterly Journal of Medicine*, **35**, 521–537.

Reynolds, E. H., Rothfeld, P. & Pincus, J. H. (1973). Neurological disease associated with folate deficiency. *British Medical Journal*, **2**, 398–400.

Sevitt, L. H. & Hoffbrand, A. V. (1969). Serum folate and vitamin B_{12} levels in acute and chronic renal disease. Effect of peritoneal dialysis. *British Medical Journal*, **2**, 18–21.

Shojania, A. M., Hornady, G. & Barnes, P. H. (1968). Oral contraceptives and serum-folate levels. *Lancet*, **1**, 1376–1377.

Spillane, J. D. (1959). Clinical aspects of vitamin-B group disorders of the nervous system. In *Biochemical Aspects of Neurological Disorders*, ed. by Cumings, J. N. & Kremer, M., pp. 10–34. Oxford: Blackwell.

Stephens, M. E. M., Craft, I., Peters, T. J. & Hoffbrand, A. V. (1972). Oral contraceptives and folate metabolism. *Clinical Science*, **42**, 405–414.

Strachan, R. W. & Henderson, J. G. (1967). Dementia and folate deficiency. *Quarterly Journal of Medicine*, **36**, 189–204.

Streiff, R. R. & Greene, B. (1970). Drug inhibition of folate conjugase. In *Proceedings XIIIth International Congress of Haematology, Munich*, p. 377.

Weckman, N. & Lehtovaara, R. (1969). Folic acid and anticonvulsants. *Lancet*, **1**, 207–208.

Wells, D. G. & Casey, H. J. (1967). Lactobacillus casei CSF folate activity. *British Medical Journal*, **3**, 834–836.

Whitehead, V. M., Comty, C. H., Posen, G. A. & Kaye, M. (1968). Homeostasis of folic acid in patients undergoing maintenance hemodialysis. *New England Journal of Medicine*, **279**, 970–974.

Whitehead, V. M. & Cooper, B. A. (1967). Absorption of unaltered folic acid from the gastrointestinal tract in man. *British Journal of Haematology*, **13**, 679–686.

CHAPTER EIGHT

Neurological Complications of Coeliac Disease and Tropical Sprue

DEFINITIONS

There can be few fields of modern medicine where terminological and conceptual chaos is more prevalent than in the broad area covered by such terms as sprue (Manson, 1880), parasprue (Napier, 1943), idiopathic tropical steatorrhoea (Baker, 1957), idiopathic tropical diarrhoea with or without steatorrhoea (Jeejeebhoy et al, 1966), and tropical malabsorption syndrome (Jeejeebhoy et al, 1968). Similar but less florid confusion pervades the field of 'non-tropical sprue', and of its sundry synonyms and subdivisions such as idiopathic steatorrhoea, coeliac disease, adult coeliac disease, and gluten-sensitive enteropathy.

The chaos itself has interesting causes. New techniques, such as peroral jejunal biopsy and the study of absorption of particular substances (fat, xylose, folate, vitamin B_{12}), have yielded a vast harvest of fact which has not been associated with a commensurate harvest in understanding. Modern travel brought patients with certain types of malabsorption to laboratories equipped with dissecting microscopes and facilities for the microbiological assay and isotopic study of vitamin B_{12} long before these technical developments were available in those parts of the world where the diseases themselves were widespread. Conflicting reports appeared from different geographical areas concerning the prevalence there of particular syndromes. These contradictory data reflected both the very different criteria used in the diagnosis of sprue, and the wide variations in the local availability and reliability of certain investigative prodecures. Studies of 'normal' or 'control' populations, using some of the new techniques, yielded a surprising number of abnormal results, suggesting either that common local dietary ingredients or other environmental hazards may have hitherto unsuspected effects on gut morphology and absorptive physiology, or that a 'normal' population (or person) is merely one that has not been adequately investigated.

The current chaos is perhaps best epitomised in the following observations:

(a) A quarter of a century after the recognition of the role of wheat gluten in precipitating steatorrhoea in predisposed individuals, most textbooks still use the term 'idiopathic steatorrhoea' to refer to a condition the aetiology of which is at least partially understood. This devalues the use ot the word 'idiopathic' and may detract attention from other mechanisms of steatorrhoea. Strictly speaking—and if mere neurologists may be pardoned the heresy—'tropical sprue' is today probably the major 'idiopathic' steatorrhoea.

(b) It is now known that a substantial minority of patients with both 'tropical sprue' (Klipstein, 1968; Wellcome Trust, 1972) and 'coeliac disease' (Stewart et al, 1967; Gent and Creamer, 1968; Truelove and Reynell, 1972) need not have steatorrhoea at all (and may in fact have no abdominal symptoms whatsoever). To call coeliac disease 'idiopathic steatorrhoea' therefore also devalues the use of the word 'steatorrhoea', conceptually overemphasising one aspect of the total absorptive defect. Moreover, malabsorption in these diseases usually involves—and may even predominantly affect—substances other than fat. The persistence of the name 'idiopathic steatorrhoea' as a synonym for coeliac disease illustrates the tendency for names to linger on, long after the reality they refer to has altered: the condition usually referred to by these terms is neither 'idiopathic' nor necessarily associated with steatorrhoea.

(c) The jejunal mucosa in patients with tropical sprue may not differ from that of control subjects from the same region, who do not exhibit malabsorption (Tandon et al, 1966; Baker and Mathan, 1968; Klipstein et al, 1968; Jeejeebhoy et al, 1968). Similar structural changes in the bowel may also be found in clinically asymptomatic patients who show evidence of malabsorption on formal testing. This raises doubts about the allegedly central significance of changes in gut morphology in the diagnosis of certain types of malabsorption, as well as interesting philosophical (or even philological) problems as to what constitutes a disease.

(d) Finally, jejunal biopsies from patients with tropical sprue may, during the early phase of their illness, show a normal architecture (England, 1968). This again raises questions (but this time of a different order) concerning the relation of structural changes to disordered absorptive function.

In an excellent editorial devoted to the definition of tropical sprue, Klipstein and Baker (1970) conclude that 'no single clinical manifestation or laboratory abnormality can be construed as diagnostic of tropical sprue in persons who present with symptomatic malabsorption'. Response to therapy with folic acid or antibiotics cannot be deemed a diagnostic criterion either (Wellcome Trust, 1972). Neither, unfortunately, can 'gluten-sensitive enteropathy' be defined in terms of its response to a gluten-free diet, for some patients with this condition will initially respond to such a diet but fail to do so after a relapse. One is irresistibly reminded of certain paragraphs of Lewis Carroll (1865).*

* 'I said pig' replied Alice 'and I wish you wouldn't keep appearing and vanishing so suddenly: you make one quite giddy.'

'All right', said the Cat; and this time it vanished quite slowly, beginning with the end of the tail, and ending with the grin, which remained some time after the rest of it had gone.

"Well! I've often seen a cat without a grin' thought Alice, 'but a grin without a cat! It's the most curious thing I ever saw in all my life!'

It is perhaps best to avoid using the words 'idiopathic steatorrhoea' altogether. In the course of the last 50 years an increasing number of conditions occurring either in the tropics or in temperate climates (or in both) have been recognised as causing malabsorption (with or without steatorrhoea) and assigned specific names. The words 'idiopathic steatorrhoea' should certainly not be used when malabsorption is due to an identifiable cause—or where such a cause can be incriminated with at least reasonable certainty.

'Tropical sprue' and 'coeliac disease' should probably be thought of as syndromes, rather than as disease entities. The cause of tropical sprue is unknown. The commonest cause of coeliac disease is gluten-sensitive enteropathy but there may be others. It is difficult relevantly to discuss the neurological complications of these conditions when the conditions themselves are so difficult to define. The task can only be attempted at the cost of a certain 'tidying up' of reality and by conforming, at least to some extent, with current practice.

For the purpose of this review we shall therefore refer to 'tropical sprue' and to 'coeliac disease' as if they were distinct nosological conditions (which is almost certainly true), and as if each were a single disease entity (which is almost certainly untrue). We will use the words 'coeliac disease' as synonymous with 'gluten-sensitive enteropathy', while fully aware of the occasional inadequacy of this identification.

Tropical sprue and coeliac disease can therefore be thought of as two diseases of the small bowel characterised by striking changes in gut morphology, widespread malabsorption and a rather similar symptomatology. The two conditions have very different epidemiological characteristics and almost certainly different aetiologies. Both may be complicated by a variety of neurological symptoms and signs.

The main feature of each of these diseases will first be summarised. We will then deal with certain common neurological symptoms encountered in both conditions, before turning to the rarer, more serious, and possibly more specific complications of each.

COELIAC DISEASE: GENERAL ASPECTS

In coeliac disease, gluten derived from wheat and rye exerts a deleterious effect on the villi of the small intestine. Before this fact was discovered coeliac disease was indeed an 'idiopathic steatorrhoea'. The pathological alterations in the intestinal mucosa, when fully developed, produce the picture of subtotal villous atrophy. The changes are more marked in the upper jejunum than in more distal parts of the small intestine, and are rapidly reversible on withdrawal of gluten from the diet. First described by Paulley (1954) the appearances are not pathognomonic of coeliac disease, and even in this condition their degree may vary. The characteristic histological lesion is, however, produced rapidly following the local instillation of gluten into either jejunum or ileum. It only affects areas distal to the site of instillation (Rubin et al, 1962). This probably explains the predominantly proximal distribution of the changes in gut morphology in patients with coeliac disease.

The precise aetiology of coeliac disease remains unknown. The intestinal mucosa from untreated coeliac patients certainly liberates less amino-acids from dipeptides and from the more complex peptides of gluten than does the mucosa of normal subjects but these abnormalities return to normal when the coeliac patient is treated (Douglas et al, 1970) suggesting that the abnormality in the untreated patient is secondary to the mucosal damage. There is no evidence for the hypothesis that coeliac disease is due to a primary enzyme deficiency. Readers interested in the immunological aspects of the problem are referred to articles by Crabbé, Douglas and Hobbs (1970), Asquith, Housley and Cooke (1970) and Asquith, Thompson and Cooke (1970).

Clinical features

Various absorptive defects may occur. Failure to recognise the nature of biochemically restricted forms of malabsorption may lead to serious diagnostic errors.

Steatorrhoea is usually present but its occurrence will depend on fat intake and it may be absent in up to 25 per cent of cases (Gent and Creamer, 1968). Steatorrhoea is partly a direct result of jejunal involvement, and partly related to an excess of unconjugated bile salts in the gut, resulting from bacterial overactivity in stagnant, atonic loops of bowel (Spiro, 1970). The general malnutrition of these patients may result in secondary pancreatic insufficiency, which may further contribute to steatorrhoea. To these disturbances may be added a functional pancreatic insufficiency, from failure of the secretin–pancreozymin mechanism, itself a consequence of the mucosal atrophy. Diarrhoea is usual, although some 20 per cent of patients may not complain of this symptom (Cooke, Peeney and Hawkins, 1953).

Hypoproteinaemia is not uncommon in patients with coeliac disease. It may be due to protein loss from the gut, but it is also in part a result of anorexia and of the general malnutrition resulting from malabsorption. *Abdominal distension* may result from the action of colonic bacteria on unabsorbed carbohydrate. Malabsorption of iron leads to hypochromic *anaemia*, while folate malabsorption may produce megaloblastic changes in the marrow and peripheral blood.

Hypomagnesaemia may be responsible for 'calcium-resistant tetany', although *tetany* and *fits* are generally a consequence of impaired vitamin D absorption and of hypocalcaemia, which also produce *osteomalacia*, pseudofractures and bone pain. Vitamin K deficiency may result in hypoprothrombinaemia and *spontaneous haemorrhages*, which may be cutaneous or take the form of haemarthrosis or melaena.

Total body potassium is often grossly reduced, as faecal losses may attain 100 mEq/day during acute phases of the disease. Hypokalaemia, however, is rare. *Intestinal atony* and *general muscular weakness* have been attributed to this depletion of body potassium.

Even the absorption of water is impaired.

Other clinical features of the disease (possibly related to malabsorption of water-soluble vitamins) include *glossitis* and occasionally *stomatitis*. There may be *hyperpigmentation of the skin*, pigmentation of the oral mucosa, *hypotension*, *clubbing* of the nails and *splenic atrophy*. Gastric secretion is usually normal. Patients may simply show mild *chronic ill-health*, many cases probably going undiagnosed because of the alliterative stress, in undergraduate teaching, on the 'foul, frothy, fatty, floating faeces'. The condition should be considered in any patient with refractory iron deficiency anaemia, megaloblastic anaemia due to folate deficiency, unexplained oedema or bone pain, haemorrhagic tendency due to hypoprothrombinaemia, mild tetany, or loss of weight, particularly if associated with a change in bowel habit. The presentation may be purely neurological and coeliac disease should also be thought of, as we shall stress, in any patient with unexplained myopathy or peripheral neuropathy.

TROPICAL SPRUE: GENERAL ASPECTS

This disease of unknown aetiology (Klipstein, 1968) differs from coeliac disease in several respects. It is found in certain parts of the world (South India, Ceylon, South-East Asia, Hong Kong and the Caribbean Islands) but not in others (such as Africa or South America). Within endemic areas its prevalence again varies widely. Its occasional occurrence in epidemic form (Mathan and Baker, 1968), clinically rapid rate of onset, and often excellent response to antibiotics suggest that infection plays some role in aetiology, although what this role is and what agents might be responsible are still unsettled questions. The disease affects the well-nourished and under-nourished with complete impartiality.

Tropical sprue is often defined by exclusion, for instance as a malabsorption syndrome occurring in people resident in (or who have resided in) certain parts of the tropics, known aetiological factors such as pancreatic insufficiency, intestinal tuberculosis, certain types of parasitic infestation of the bowel and gluten-sensitive enteropathy having been excluded.

Tropical sprue, like coeliac disease, is characterised by widespread malabsorption, again related to changes in structure of the mucous membrane of the small intestine. The whole of the small bowel is affected, the most persistently involved area being the distal ileum. Jejunal biopsy reveals partial villous atrophy, the changes in structure being generally less severe than those encountered in coeliac disease. The exact significance of these changes is the subject of much controversy. In some parts of the world such as South India (Baker, Mathan and Joseph, 1962), Haiti (Klipstein, Samloff and Schenk, 1966), Puerto Rico (Swanson and Thomassen, 1965) and Thailand (Sprinz et al, 1962) similar changes have been described in large numbers of asymptomatic individuals. Whether this represents a subclinical form of the disease or a response of the bowel to some dietary ingredient or other environmental hazard remains undetermined.

The main difference between tropical sprue and coeliac disease (apart from the interesting epidemiological characteristics and the fact that the former responds to certain antibiotics while the latter responds to the withdrawal of gluten from the diet) seems to be the differing frequency with which certain symptoms and signs are encountered in the two conditions.

Megaloblastic anaemia, in early tropical sprue, is often due to folate deficiency. In the more chronic cases it is almost always due, in part at least, to malabsorption of vitamin B_{12}. Osteomalacia and tetany are rare in tropical sprue (Rodriguez-Molina, 1954), common in coeliac disease (Sencer, 1957; Green and Wollaeger, 1960). The areas in which tropical sprue is endemic are often also areas in which malnutrition is widespread: this may account for the more frequent occurrence of obvious vitamin deficiency syndromes in tropical sprue, such as glossitis, angulostomatitis and rashes of pellagrous type.

NEUROLOGICAL FEATURES OF COELIAC DISEASE AND TROPICAL SPRUE: GENERAL ASPECTS

Paraesthesiae in the limbs, in both diseases, may be due to latent tetany, pain to osteomalacia, faintness to hypotension and weakness to hypokalaemia or to the non-specific effects of gross wasting. Occasional patients are encountered, however, in whom paraesthesiae are associated with abnormal neurological signs. When such a neuropathy complicates a condition characterised by widespread malabsorption it is difficult and usually pointless to seek to incriminate one particular factor. Some factors have to be specifically considered, however, in view of the known or claimed association of their deficiency with lesions of the central and peripheral nervous system.

Vitamin B_{12} and coeliac disease

In coeliac disease the most profound structural alterations are found in the proximal gut (duodenum and jejunum). The changes become less severe, or may be absent altogether, as the distal ileum is approached (Rubin et al, 1962; McCarthy et al, 1964). The absorption of vitamin B_{12} might therefore be expected to be normal in most cases. Most patients with coeliac disease, although exhibiting malabsorption of fat, xylose and folate, in fact absorb vitamin B_{12} normally (Chanarin, 1969). However, a substantial minority—97 out of 231 patients (42 per cent) reviewed by Chanarin—had reduced serum vitamin B_{12} levels, while impaired vitamin B_{12} absorption was present in a similar proportion of patients. Stewart et al (1967) showed that there was some correlation between vitamin B_{12} malabsorption, fat absorption and the extent of the ileal lesion. Previously impaired vitamin B_{12} absorption returns to normal after these patients have been put on a gluten-free diet (Benson, Kowlessar and Sleisenger, 1964)

Most patients with coeliac disease and a low serum vitamin B_{12} have malabsorption of vitamin B_{12} (Mollin, Booth and Baker, 1957), suggesting that their low B_{12} levels are not the result of primary folate deficiency. Very low levels of serum B_{12} such as may be found in untreated pernicious anaemia or in patients with distal ileal lesions, are only exceptionally encountered.

Vitamin B_{12} and tropical sprue

Severe neurological complications are *less* common in tropical sprue than in coeliac disease. Malabsorption of vitamin B_{12} is, however, more frequently encountered in tropical sprue than in coeliac disease and, in chronic cases, proves more difficult to reverse.

Tropical sprue affects the whole of the small intestine. The maximal changes are in the ileum. The vast majority of patients have low serum levels of vitamin B_{12} and nearly 100 per cent will show impaired vitamin B_{12} absorption (Chanarin, 1969). Really low serum levels (below 60 pg/ml) may be encountered in chronic cases. It should be remembered in this context that tropical sprue tends to occur in areas where the mean serum B_{12} level may, for dietary reasons alone, be lower than that encountered in the West.

It will be realised from these observations that vitamin B_{12} deficiency, although common in coeliac disease and very common in tropical sprue, is unlikely to be the sole cause—or even the main cause—of the neurological complications of these diseases. Not only are the clinical and pathological features of these complications not consonant with the known syndromes of vitamin B_{12} deficiency, as will be discussed, but they occur most frequently in the condition least often associated with severe B_{12} deficiency. What some of these neurological complications resemble most are some of the syndromes, discussed elsewhere in this monograph, that may follow partial gastrectomy (Williams et al, 1969), or be associated with diverticulosis of the small bowel (Cooke et al, 1963). These syndromes are often unrelated to vitamin B_{12} deficiency.

Folate status in coeliac disease and in tropical sprue

As discussed in Chapter 7, it is not yet established whether folate deficiency may cause neurological signs. Our own opinion is that there is probably no neurology of folate deficiency. As the matter is not finally settled, however —and as unexplained neurological signs and symptoms are not uncommon in coeliac disease and in tropical sprue—the main facts concerning the folate status of such patients are worth brief mention.

Impaired folate absorption is present in 90 per cent of patients with coeliac disease (Chanarin, 1969). These patients have low serum folate levels (Waters, 1963; Klipstein, 1966), low red cell folate levels (Hoffbrand, Newcombe and Mollin, 1966), and increased urinary excretion of formiminoglutamic acid (Chanarin, Bennett and Berry, 1962; Chanarin, 1963) whether or not they are previously given an oral L-histidine load. Megaloblastic anaemia in the great majority of patients with coeliac disease is due to folate deficiency.

The serum folate was low in 131 out of 150 patients (87 per cent) with tropical sprue reviewed by Chanarin (1969). There is conflicting information concerning folate absorption in tropical sprue (Butterworth et al, 1957; Jeejeebhoy et al, 1966). Both megaloblastic anaemia and other non-neurological features of acute tropical sprue respond to folate therapy (O'Brien and England, 1964, 1966).

NEUROLOGICAL COMPLICATIONS OF TROPICAL SPRUE

Neurological signs are not very uncommon in tropical sprue. In a well-documented study of malabsorption in Singapore, Wye and Khoo (1969) described 20 patients with tropical sprue. Weakness and muscle wasting were present in 65 per cent of the patients; 40 per cent of the cases had evidence of peripheral neuropathy. The authors make the interesting comment that at the time of writing no case of adult coeliac disease had been documented in an Asian in Singapore. All the patients in whom jejunal biopsy had been performed had shown an abnormal mucosa (usually partial villous atrophy). Megaloblastic anaemia was the commonest presentation, at times severe enough to cause congestive cardiac failure. Only about half the patients showed steatorrhoea. Folate levels were low in all cases. Vitamin B_{12} levels were below 150 pg/ml in 25 per cent of cases and serum calcium levels below 8·5 mg/100 ml in 37·5 per cent of cases. There was no correlation between the degree of malabsorption—as represented by the severity of steatorrhoea—and the extent and severity of the villous atrophy, lending weight to the view put forward by Jeejeebhoy et al (1966) that malabsorption in tropical sprue is not directly related to the gross mucosal lesion.

Writing from an endemic sprue area in South India, Iyer et al (1973) describe a detailed neurological, electromyographic and electroencephalographic study of 24 unselected cases of tropical sprue. Patients were defined as suffering from this condition if they showed malabsorption (as evidenced by two or more of the triad steatorrhoea, xylose malabsorption, vitamin B_{12} malabsorption) in the absence of gluten-sensitive enteropathy, tuberculous enteritis, postgastrectomy syndrome or other known cause. In this series fatigue and weakness were very frequent complaints. In addition, 15 patients had proximal weakness in the lower limbs and, to a lesser extent, in the upper limbs. Eight of these 15 patients also had obvious proximal wasting and 10 exhibited a myopathic EMG pattern. Of the patients with a myopathic EMG, six showed pseudomyotonia (rapid repetitive discharges resembling myotonia but lacking a decremental character) in both proximal and distal muscle groups. Six patients complained of paraesthesiae in the limbs. Objective distal tactile loss with hypalgesia and loss of ankle jerks was only detected in one patient, who also showed loss of vibration sense up to the iliac crests, impaired postural sense in the toes and bilateral extensor plantar responses. Eight patients, however, showed definite evidence of peripheral neuropathy on electrodiagnostic testing, either in the form of reduced conduction velocity in peripheral nerves (motor, sensory, or both), and/or in the form of diminished amplitude of the sensory evoked potentials. Tetany was detected in only one case. No correlation between peripheral 'neuropathy' and serum folate levels could be detected. Of the eight patients with peripheral neuropathy, five had a megaloblastic marrow, of whom four had low serum B_{12} levels (80, 64, 149 and 120 pg/ml, respectively). Five patients complained of night blindness, presumably due to the combined effects of a defective vitamin A intake and impaired absorption. Three patients showed slow cerebration, defective recent memory and emotional lability, either singly or in combination, and five had an abnormal EEG characterised by slow, bilateral, predominantly frontotemporal dysrhythmias.

Myopathy

The myopathy of tropical sprue recalls the myopathy that may follow partial gastrectomy (Ekbom et al, 1964; Jensen, 1965), the myopathy associated with osteomalacia (Prineas, Mason and Henson, 1965; Smith and Stern, 1967) and the myopathies reported in protein–calorie malnutrition (Sachdev, Taori and Pereira, 1971) and in various conditions characterised by general wasting (Adams, Denny-Brown and Pearson, 1962; Harriman,

1966; Tomlinson, Walton and Rebeiz, 1969). Proximal muscle wasting may also be encountered in patients with coeliac disease (Hall, 1968), but in these cases the wasting seemed to have at least a neurogenic component.

The pseudomyotonia associated with sprue myopathy reported by Iyer et al (1973) apparently subsided within two to three weeks of hospitalisation, a feature which suggested to the authors that it might be due to the effects of electrolyte imbalance on the stability of the muscle membrane. Two of the six patients exhibiting this phenomenon had hypokalaemia and another two low serum calcium levels.

Histological studies have not to date been reported in the myopathy complicating tropical sprue.

Peripheral neuropathy

Patients with tropical sprue often experience paraesthesiae. Stefanini (1948), reporting his experiences among over a thousand Italian prisoners of war in India suffering from tropical sprue, described paraesthesiae as occurring in just over 17 per cent. Writing from Puerto Rico, another endemic area for tropical sprue, Rodriguez-Molina (1954) described a prevalence of paraesthesiae of 14 per cent (although this report is vitiated, for our immediate purpose, by the statement that tropical sprue and idiopathic steatorrhoea 'are manifestations or phases of one disease entity').

As previously mentioned, paraesthesiae in patients with malabsorption are often attributed to hypocalcaemia or to anaemia. Abnormal physical signs suggestive of a peripheral neuropathy are, however, at times encountered in tropical sprue (Mackie and Fairley, 1929; Rodriguez-Molina, 1954; Jeejeebhoy et al, 1968; Wye and Khoo, 1969). The detailed electrodiagnostic studies reported by Iyer et al (1973) suggest that subclinical peripheral neuropathy may in fact be quite common. In their cases there was a definite correlation between the presence of neuropathy and a megaloblastic bone marrow, although no correlation with folate levels. Half their patients with neuropathy had serum B_{12} levels below 140 pg/ml. Unfortunately no tests were carried out in the remaining patients to exclude other vitamin deficiencies.

No pathological studies have been reported, to our knowledge, to determine the nature of the peripheral neuropathy complicating tropical sprue.

Myelopathy

Although there is malabsorption of vitamin B_{12} in nearly every case of tropical sprue, and although low serum levels are very common, subacute combined degeneration of the spinal cord (SCD) is usually stated to be a very rare complication or not to occur at all (Stefanini, 1948; Green and Wollaeger, 1960; Sheehy, Perez-Santiago and Rubini, 1961), and this despite the fact that many of these patients have received treatment with folic acid. Fairley (1934), who had a vast experience of the condition, wrote 'I have never observed subacute combined degeneration in sprue, though neuritic manifestations are common enough'. Well-documented accounts of myelopathy complicating tropical sprue are as difficult to discover as in other patients with non-Addisonian megaloblastic anaemia.

Hotz and Lüthy (1939) described in a single case necropsy findings which were compatible with a diagnosis of SCD. Mollin and Booth (1972), in their comprehensive review of chronic tropical sprue in London, also reported a single instance of myelopathy (Case 11) associated with a serum B_{12} level of 10 pg/ml. Iyer et al (1973) likewise described a single case.

In certain parts of the world both tropical sprue and unexplained myelopathy are relatively common. Jeejeebhoy, Wadia and Desai (1967) discussed the possible significance of this association. They reported 12 patients seen in Bombay who presented with neuropathy and myelopathy of obscure origin. Clinically, the dominant feature was a sensory ataxia associated in some patients with spastic paraparesis. Peripheral nerve involvement was confined to a mild sensory neuropathy. Mental changes and optic atrophy were also seen. Gastrointestinal symptoms were either slight or absent. Eight of the patients were shown to have vitamin B_{12} deficiency associated with malabsorption of vitamin B_{12}. In these cases considerable neurological improvement followed the administration of vitamin B_{12}. Four patients, clinically indistinguishable from the first eight, did not have vitamin B_{12} deficiency and did not improve following the administration of this vitamin. In six of the patients with malabsorption of vitamin B_{12} this did not improve following the administration of intrinsic factor, the patients also exhibiting malabsorption of fat, D-xylose and folic acid. The authors concluded that vitamin B_{12} deficiency appeared to be an important cause of obscure so-called 'nutritional myelopathy' in India, and that it was often based on malabsorption, itself due to clinically latent tropical sprue. In two patients the absorption of vitamin B_{12} improved with IF. The authors argued that these were also instances of tropical sprue, associated with the gastric atrophy now known to be an occasional feature of the disease (Floch et al, 1963). Of the patients with myelopathy presumed due to vitamin B_{12} deficiency, four showed partial villous atrophy on jejunal biopsy. Six of 11 patients studied showed steatorrhoea.

NEUROLOGICAL COMPLICATIONS OF COELIAC DISEASE

These follow the same general pattern as in tropical sprue, the main difference being perhaps the occurrence in coeliac disease of a severe encephalo-myelo-radiculo-neuropathy, of unknown aetiology, and the relative rarity with which myopathic complications have so far been reported.

Some of the early reports of neurological complications in patients with coeliac disease are difficult to categorise, because of inadequate data. Thaysen (1932) described three patients with non-tropical sprue who had shown transient extensor plantar responses. Cooke, Peeney and Hawkins (1953), in a review of 100 patients with 'idiopathic steatorrhoea', reported two cases with 'symptoms simulating subacute combined degeneration of the cord'. Both had absent reflexes, extensor plantar responses, and absent vibration sense; they were bedridden 'but after a short period of treatment became fully ambulant'.

In 1957 Sencer described the neurological symptoms and signs encountered in 94 patients with malabsorption, presumed due to coeliac disease. Forty-nine patients (52 per cent) had features suggesting involvement of the nervous system. Twenty patients had evidence of tetany but no objective reflex or sensory changes. Ten patients had experienced paraesthesiae and were found to be anaemic but had no abnormal neurological signs. A further 12 patients had reflex or sensory abnormalities on examination. There were two cases of severe myeloradiculopathy (referred to by the authors as 'pseudo-tabes'). In a review of 124 patients with 'non-tropical sprue' Green and Wollaeger (1960) encountered six patients with neurological signs. Abnormalities included peripheral neuropathy, areflexia and (in one case) 'subacute combined sclerosis'.

Myopathy

A 'regressive vacuolar myopathy' was reported by Coërs, Telerman-Toppet and Cremer (1971, 1972) in a patient with chronic diarrhoea associated with steatorrhoea, impaired absorption of xylose and subtotal villous atrophy on jejunal biopsy. A man aged 63 developed a rapidly progressive tetraplegia with weakness of the trunk and neck muscles, the latter being described as stiff. The weakness was predominantly proximal but also severe in the distal extensor muscles. There was no dysphagia or ophthalmoplegia. The tendon reflexes were depressed in the upper limbs and absent in the legs. There were no sensory signs. He was found to be grossly hypokalaemic (serum potassium 1·9 mEq/l) with a metabolic alkalosis, hypophosphataemia (1·5 mg/100 ml) and hypocalcaemia (8·6 mg/100 ml). Rapid correction of the hypokalaemia induced a temporary but severe state of tetany. The patient improved slowly over a period of several weeks. Muscle biopsies were taken on the third and 38th day of his illness. The initial specimen showed a low mean fibre diameter with vacuolar changes in about 25 per cent of the muscle fibres, disorganisation of myofibrils and rod-shaped bodies. 'Complete disappearance' of these histological changes had occurred by the time of the second biopsy, chemical analysis of the specimen revealing, however, a persistently low potassium and abnormally high sodium and chloride content, at a time when the patient had made 'a nearly complete recovery from motor weakness'.

An EMG examination carried out on the day of admission showed increased insertion activity, movements of the needle often producing high frequency discharges. There was also spontaneous activity with rhythmic, low frequency, short-duration potentials resembling fibrillation. During weak voluntary activity, highly polyphasic, long-duration potentials were obtained. Motor nerve conduction velocity and distal latencies were normal. The amplitude of directly evoked muscle potentials was initially low (suggesting unexcitability of many muscle fibres) and there was also evidence of impaired neuromuscular transmission.

Proximal muscle weakness in coeliac disease had earlier been reported by Hall (1968). It is doubtful, however, whether the disturbance in the two patients described could adequately be designated as a myopathy. The first patient was a woman aged 41 with melanosis, panhyperlipidaemia, cholestatic jaundice and hepatomegaly of unknown aetiology. She had steatorrhoea, and peroral jejunal biopsy revealed subtotal villous atrophy. Neurological examination showed severe proximal weakness and wasting with normal sensation, retained reflexes and a 'myopathic' type of gait. Nerve conduction studies were normal. Power improved remarkably, she gained weight, and the jejunal biopsy appearances improved after several months on a gluten-free diet. Muscle biopsy showed no inflammatory changes but there was grouped fibre atrophy, interpreted as being of neurogenic origin.

Hall's second patient was a man aged 49 with muscle weakness of four years' duration, originally thought to be due to muscular dystrophy. There was wasting of the deltoids, thighs and paraspinal muscles and a waddling gait, although power was said to be normal in the upper limbs. The ankle jerks were reduced and there was impairment of vibration sense and postural sense in the feet with a positive Romberg sign. Electromyography revealed a reduction of mean potential duration, and muscle biopsy was interpreted as showing features both of myopathy and of neurogenic atrophy. Although the patient had had no gastrointestinal symptoms, three small-bowel biopsies revealed a 'totally' flat mucosa. There was steatorrhoea and a flat glucose tolerance curve. A gluten-free diet improved the steatorrhoea but had no effect on the neurological signs. The author stressed that in proximal muscular atrophy of unknown cause, the possibility of malabsorption should routinely be ruled out.

When osteomalacia complicates coeliac disease there is not infrequently an associated myopathy. The subject is discussed in detail in Chapter 9.

Peripheral neuropathy

Paraesthesiae are commonly experienced in patients with coeliac disease, particularly in the early stages of the disease. Benson, Kowlessar and Sleisenger (1964) found that 33 per cent of their patients with adult coeliac disease had experienced paraesthesiae. Thirty-one (25 per cent) of the 124 patients with 'non-tropical sprue' reviewed by Green and Wollaeger (1960) had complained of paraesthesiae, considered by the authors to be due to hypocalcaemia.

Morris, Ajdukiewicz and Read (1970) studied neurological disorders, both clinical and latent, in 30 patients with adult coeliac disease. Paraesthesiae were complained of by nine. Only one patient had signs of involvement of the peripheral nervous system—muscle wasting, areflexia and mild sensory deficit. Motor nerve conduction velocity was measured in 26 of the 30 patients and was within the normal range in all but one, while lateral popliteal nerve action potentials were normal in every case examined.

Binder, Solitare and Spiro (1967) described four patients with massive, persistent steatorrhoea and unusual neuromuscular complications, which were severe, progressive and irreversible in three cases, overshadowing the clinical picture and at times even preceding the clinical suspicion or detection of the gastroenterological disorder. Malabsorption was probably due to coeliac disease in two cases, and to jejunal diverticulosis and pancreatic insufficiency in the others. The neurological disturbances were unusual, combining clinical features of a predominantly sensory peripheral neuropathy in all four patients with histological features suggestive of myopathy in two. The authors suggested that steatorrhoea should be looked for and excluded in any patient with an unexplained peripheral neuropathy, particularly a sensory neuropathy.

Telerman-Toppet, Coërs and Desneux (1969) reported a patient who at the age of four had developed a slowly progressive external ophthalmoplegia.

At the age of 25 he had developed a chronic diarrhoea, alleged (on the basis of impaired absorption of glucose and xylose) to be due to coeliac disease. A little later, signs of a predominantly sensory but relentlessly progressive polyneuropathy had appeared, with considerable trophic disturbances in the limbs. He had also developed mild bilateral nerve deafness. The serum lipoproteins were normal and there were no acanthocytes in the peripheral blood. The CSF protein was raised, at 98 mg/100 ml. Nerve conduction studies revealed slowing of motor conduction in the lower limbs and muscle biopsy changes attributed to denervation. The authors felt that the neurological signs and symptoms were probably related to the absorptive defect, which they did not seek, however, to particularise in greater detail.

A similar case associating chronic diarrhoea, progressive external ophthalmoplegia, raised CSF protein and peripheral neuropathy was documented by Direkze (1973), and we await the appearance of further case reports to ascertain whether this is a new neurological syndrome associated with malabsorption.

The pathological basis of the neuropathy complicating coeliac disease has not been studied in any depth. Cooke, Johnson and Woolf (1966), using vital staining techniques and electron-microscopy of intramuscular nerve endings, reported findings suggestive of a 'dying-back' motor neuropathy in patients with adult coeliac disease. A patchy focal demyelination of peripheral nerves without cellular response or leucocyte infiltrate was seen in two of the four cases reported by Binder et al (1967).

Myelopathy and encephalo-myelo-radiculopathy

Woltman and Heck (1937) in a review of posterolateral degeneration of the spinal cord in conditions other than pernicious anaemia had reported in detail a personally observed case in which a severe macrocytic anaemia and a neurological disorder (suggestive of SCD, except for very brisk ankle jerks) had complicated a chronic, relapsing diarrhoea (attributed to non-tropical sprue). A good clinical response followed intensive treatment with liver extract. Both the gastroenterological and the neurological aspects of the numerous other cases of myelopathy in 'non-tropical sprue' reported by these authors are insufficiently documented for adequate analysis.

Richmond and Davidson (1958) reported a case, much quoted in the literature, alleged to illustrate the occurrence of B_{12} deficiency myelopathy in a patient with a chronic steatorrhoea, finally attributed to coeliac disease. In our opinion the case cannot be accepted as such, either on clinical or on pathological grounds.

After eight years of intermittent abdominal symptoms, a man aged 45 (who had served overseas) had developed weakness of the legs and paraesthesiae in the hands and forearms. A macrocytic anaemia had been detected at an early stage of his illness. The knee and ankle jerks could not be elicited but there were apparently 'no other abnormalities in the nervous system' (i.e. presumably no sensory signs). He had had an earlier attack of overt tetany, and low blood calcium levels had frequently been detected. Oral calcium did not relieve the paraesthesiae. He subsequently received continuous treatment with folic acid, cyanocobalamin and dietary supplements, including a B-complex preparation.

On admission to hospital four years later he was found to be emaciated with clubbing and a distended abdomen. There was generalised weakness, and the tendon reflexes were absent in all four limbs. There was slight impairment of tactile sense in the upper limbs, of 'glove' distribution. In the lower limbs there was 'slight impairment of vibration, touch and pain sensation, in a "stocking" distribution, and of positional sensation'. The plantar responses were flexor. There was steatorrhoea, a histamine-fast achlorhydria, gross malabsorption of folic acid and moderately impaired absorption of vitamin B_{12}. There were no haematological abnormalities. He was treated with cortisone which resulted in a transient improvement of his diarrhoea. He died a few weeks later.

Necropsy revealed tuberculous bronchopneumonia although a chest x-ray, one month earlier, had been normal. The stomach showed atrophic gastritis and multiple acute ulcers. There was no evidence of intestinal tuberculosis or of any other specific intestinal disease. The spinal cord showed marked atrophy and gliosis of the posterior columns at all levels but no changes in anterior or lateral columns.

It is worth stressing that although this patient may have exhibited some impairment of vitamin B_{12} absorption, he had been receiving regular injections of vitamin B_{12} during the last six years of his life, during which time the neurological deficit had developed and progressed. We prefer to consider this a case of myelopathy of uncertain aetiology, related to those later reported by Cooke and Smith (1966). The use of a gluten-free diet in coeliac disease was popularised in Britain in the early 1950s (Anderson et al, 1952; Sheldon and Lawson, 1952) but this was not tried in this case. It is therefore impossible to be dogmatic as to whether the myelopathy (whatever its exact nature) was complicating chronic sprue or coeliac disease.

In 1966 Cooke and Smith reported the clinical and pathological findings in 16 patients with adult coeliac disease in whom severe neurological complications had developed. Each patient fulfilled strict criteria for the diagnosis of adult coeliac disease with a characteristic history and laboratory findings and a flat mucosa on jejunal biopsy (Cooke et al, 1963). Necropsy findings were described in nine cases and data obtained on peripheral nerve or muscle biopsy in the other seven. Two patients were found to have 'neuropathy' at the time of original referral for their gastrointestinal symptoms. Four patients were referred on account of the neuropathy complicating their primary disorder and nine developed neurological complications while under treatment for adult coeliac disease.

The patients usually presented with symptoms affecting the lower limbs and sensory ataxia soon dominated the clinical picture in nearly all cases. Posterior column deficit and distal impairment of pain and tactile sense with absent ankle jerks were frequently encountered. Weakness was often marked but wasting relatively slight. One patient developed an extensor plantar response shortly before death, three had cerebellar signs and five had suffered from unexplained episodes of loss of consciousness. One patient presented with neurological signs and symptoms suggestive of motor neurone disease (in our view, the likely diagnosis).

In 10 patients the 'neuropathy' proved steadily progressive, the rate of progression varying considerably from case to case. Of the nine fatal cases, 'neuropathy' was considered the main cause of death in four. Among the neuropathological findings reported were demyelination (often of spongiform type) of the posterior and lateral columns of the spinal cord, producing a SCD-like picture, dorsal column degeneration alone, and cerebellar cortical degeneration. Not surprisingly in view of the rarity of the condition, there has been no comparable case-series to substantiate these dramatic findings, though occasional reports have described predominantly posterior column degeneration (Hansen and von Staa, 1936, Case 2; Hotz and Lüthy, 1939) in coeliac disease.

The possible role of vitamin B_{12} deficiency in the production of these clinical and pathological findings was discussed in some detail by Cooke and Smith. One patient developed neurological signs while receiving parenteral liver extract and another while receiving injections of vitamin B_{12}. Vitamin B_{12} absorption was normal in a further six patients. Two patients with impaired absorption had persistently normal serum levels. Only one patient is reported as having a low level of serum B_{12}. His neurological disease progressed relentlessly while he was receiving injections of cyanocobalamin. No patient improved while receiving injections of vitamin B_{12} but the neurological signs virtually disappeared in two patients who had not received such therapy. On the basis of these findings the authors argued convincingly that the 'neuropathy' of coeliac disease was unlikely to be related to hypovitaminosis B_{12}. The administration of folic acid did not appear to have played any part in producing the 'neuropathy'. The five patients who made almost complete recoveries had received a variety of treatments, the most consistent being the administration of large quantities of water-soluble vitamins by injection.

Thus the cause of myelopathy in coeliac disease is obscure. Multiple nutritional deficiency, on the basis of malabsorption, is possibly a factor. Despite the resemblance to SCD of the changes in the spinal cord in some of the reported cases, vitamin B_{12} deficiency can probably be ruled out.

References

Definitions

Baker, S. J. (1957). Idiopathic tropical steatorrhoea: a report of 60 cases. *Indian Journal of Medical Sciences*, **11**, 687–703.

Baker, S. J. & Mathan, V. I. (1968). Syndrome of tropical sprue in south India. *American Journal of Clinical Nutrition*, **21**, 984–993.

Carroll, L. (1865). *Alice's Adventures in Wonderland*. London: Macmillan.

England, N. W. J. (1968). Intestinal pathology of tropical sprue. *American Journal of Clinical Nutrition*, **21**, 962–975.

Gent, A. E. & Creamer, B. (1968). Faecal fats, appetite, and weight-loss in the coeliac syndrome. *Lancet*, **1**, 1063–1064.

Jeejeebhoy, K. N., Desai, H. G., Noronha, J. M., Antia, F. P. & Parekh, D. V. (1966). Idiopathic tropical diarrhea with or without steatorrhea (tropical malabsorption syndrome). *Gastroenterology*, **51**, 333–344.

Jeejeebhoy, K. N., Desai, H. G., Borkar, A. V., Deshpande, V. & Pathare, S. M. (1968). Tropical malabsorption syndrome in west India. *American Journal of Clinical Nutrition*, **21**, 994–1006.

Klipstein, F. A. (1968). Tropical sprue. *Gastroenterology*, **54**, 275–293.

Klipstein, F. A. & Baker, S. J. (1970). Regarding the definition of tropical sprue. *Gastroenterology*, **58**, 717–721.

Klipstein, F. A., Samloff, I. M., Smarth, G. & Shenk, E. A. (1968). Malabsorption and malnutrition in rural Haiti. *American Journal of Clinical Nutrition*, **21**, 1042–1052.

Manson, P. (1880). Notes on sprue. *Chinese Imperial Maritime Customs Medical Reports for 1879–80*, 19th issue. pp. 33–37.

Napier, L. E. (1943). *The Principles and Practice of Tropical Medicine*. New York: Macmillan.

Stewart, J. S., Pollock, D. J., Hoffbrand, A. V., Mollin, D. L. & Booth, C. C. (1967). A study of proximal and distal intestinal structure and absorptive function in idiopathic steatorrhoea. *Quarterly Journal of Medicine*, **N.S. 36**, 425–444.

Tandon, B. N., Iyenger, K. P., Deo, M. G. & Saraya, A. K. (1966). A study of 'sprue syndrome in adults' in northern India. *Journal of the Association of Physicians of India*, **14**, 197–202.

Truelove, S. C. & Reynell, P. C. (1972). *Diseases of the Digestive System.* 2nd edition, p. 299. Oxford: Blackwell.

Wellcome Trust (1972). *Tropical Sprue and Megaloblastic Anaemia: Wellcome Trust Collaborative Study*, 1961–1969. London: Churchill.

Coeliac disease: general aspects

Asquith, P., Housley, J. & Cooke, W. T. (1970). Cell-mediated immune response to dietary antigens in adult coeliac disease. In *Coeliac Disease: Proceedings of an International Conference held at the Royal Postgraduate Medical School, London, 1969*, ed. Booth, C. C. & Dowling, R. H., pp. 144–149. London: Churchill Livingstone.

Asquith, P., Thompson, R. A. & Cooke, W. T. (1970). Serum and intestinal immunoglobulins in adult coeliac disease. In *Coeliac Disease: Proceedings of an International Conference held at the Royal Postgraduate Medical School, London, 1969*, ed. Booth, C. C. & Dowling, R. H., pp. 157–161. London: Churchill Livingstone.

Cooke, W. T., Peeney, A. L. P. & Hawkins, C. F. (1953). Symptoms, signs and diagnostic features of idiopathic steatorrhoea. *Quarterly Journal of Medicine*, **22,** 59–77.

Crabbé, P. A., Douglas A. P. & Hobbs, R. J. (1970). Immunopathology and coeliac disease. In *Coeliac Disease: Proceedings of an International Conference held at the Royal Postgraduate Medical School, London, 1969*, ed. Booth, C. C. & Dowling, R. H., pp. 134–142. London: Churchill Livingstone.

Douglas, A. P., Peters, T. J., Hoffbrand, A. V. & Booth, C. C. (1970). Studies of intestinal peptidases with special reference to coeliac disease. In *Coeliac Disease: Proceedings of an International Conference held at the Royal Postgraduate Medical School, London, 1969*, ed. Booth, C. C. & Dowling, R. H., pp. 115–122. London: Churchill Livingstone.

Gent, A. E. & Creamer, B. (1968). Faecal fats, appetite and weight-loss in the coeliac syndrome. *Lancet*, **1,** 1063–1064.

Paulley, J. W. (1954). Observations on aetiology of idiopathic steatorrhoea, jejunal and lymph-node biopsies. *British Medical Journal*, **2,** 1318–1321.

Rubin, C. E., Brandborg, L. L., Flick, A. L., Phelps, P., Parmentier, C. & Van Niel, S. (1962). Studies of celiac sprue. III. The effect of repeated wheat instillation into the proximal ileum of patients on a gluten free diet. *Gastroenterology*, **43,** 621–641.

Spiro, H. M. (1970). *Clinical Gastroenterology*, p. 441. Toronto: Macmillan.

Tropical sprue: general aspects

Baker, S. J., Mathan, V. I. & Joseph, I. (1962). Epidemic tropical sprue. *American Journal of Digestive Diseases*, **7,** 959–960.

Green, P. A. & Wollaeger, E. E. (1960). The clinical behavior of sprue in the United States. *Gastroenterology*, **28,** 399–418.

Klipstein, F. A. (1968). Tropical sprue. *Gastroenterology*, **54,** 275–293.

Klipstein, F. A., Samloff, I. M. & Schenk, E. A. (1966). Tropical sprue in Haiti. *Annals of Internal Medicine*, **64,** 575–594.

Mathan, V. I. & Baker, S. J. (1968). Epidemic tropical sprue and other epidemics of diarrhea in south Indian villages. *American Journal of Clinical Nutrition*, **21,** 1077–1087.

Rodriguez-Molina, R. (1954). Fundamental concepts in the diagnosis of sprue. *Annals of Internal Medicine*, **40,** 33–41.

Sencer, W. (1957). Neurological manifestations in malabsorption syndrome. *Journal of the Mount Sinai Hospital*, **24,** 331–345.

Sprinz, H., Sribhibhadh, R., Gangarosa, E. J., Benyajati, C., Kundel, D. & Halsted, S. (1962). Biopsy of small bowel of Thai people. *American Journal of Clinical Pathology*, **38,** 43–51.

Swanson, V. L. & Thomassen, R. W. (1965). Pathology of the jejunal mucosa in tropical sprue. *American Journal of Pathology*, **46,** 511–551.

Neurological features of coeliac disease and tropical sprue

Benson, G. D., Kowlessar, O. D. & Sleisenger, M. H. (1964). Adult celiac disease with emphasis upon response to the gluten-free diet. *Medicine (Baltimore)*, **43,** 1–40.

Butterworth, C. E. Jr, Nadel, H., Perez-Santiago, E., Santini, R. Jr & Gardner, F. H. (1957). Folic acid absorption, excretion and leukocyte concentration in tropical sprue. *Journal of Laboratory and Clinical Medicine*, **50**, 673–681.

Chanarin, I. (1963). Urocanic acid and formiminoglutamic acid excretion in megaloblastic anaemia and other conditions: the effect of specific therapy. *British Journal of Haematology*, **9**, 141–157.

Chanarin, I. (1969). *The Megaloblastic Anaemias*. Oxford & Edinburgh: Blackwell.

Chanarin, I., Bennett, M. C. & Berry, V. (1962). Urinary excretion of histidine derivatives in megaloblastic anaemia and other conditions and a comparison with the folic acid clearance test. *Journal of Clinical Pathology*, **15**, 269–273.

Cooke, W. T., Cox, E. V., Fone, D. J., Meynell, M. J. & Gaddie, R. (1963). The clinical and metabolic significance of jejunal diverticula. *Gut*, **4**, 115–137.

Hoffbrand, A. V., Newcombe, B. F. A. & Mollin, D. L. (1966). Method of assay of red cell folate activity and the value of the assay as a test for folate deficiency. *Journal of Clinical Pathology*, **19**, 17–28.

Jeejeebhoy, K. N., Desai, H. G., Noronha, J. M., Antia, F. P. & Parekh, D. V. (1966). Idiopathic tropical diarrhea with or without steatorrhea (tropical malabsorption syndrome). *Gastroenterology*, **51**, 333–344.

Klipstein, F. A. (1966). Folate deficiency secondary to disease of the intestinal tract. *Bulletin of the New York Academy of Medicine*, **42**, 638–653.

McCarthy, C. F., Borland, J. L. Jr, Kurtz, S. M. & Ruffin, J. M. (1964). The value of the dissecting microscope in the diagnosis of non-tropical sprue. *American Journal of Pathology*, **44**, 585–595.

Mollin, D. L., Booth, C. C. & Baker, S. J. (1957). The absorption of vitamin B_{12} in control subjects, in Addisonian pernicious anaemia and in the malabsorption syndrome. *British Journal of Haematology*, **3**, 412–428.

O'Brien, W. & England, N. W. J. (1964). Folate deficiency in acute tropical sprue. *British Medical Journal*, **2**, 1573–1575.

O'Brien, W. & England, N. W. J. (1966). Military tropical sprue from South-east Asia. *British Medical Journal*, **2**, 1157–1162.

Rubin, C. E., Brandborg, L. L., Flick, A. L., Phelps, P., Parmentier, C. & Van Niel, S. (1962). Studies of celiac sprue. III. The effect of repeated wheat instillation into the proximal ileum of patients on a gluten-free diet. *Gastroenterology*, **43**, 621–641.

Stewart, J. S., Pollock, D. J., Hoffbrand, A. V., Mollin, D. L. & Booth, C. C. (1967). A study of proximal and distal intestinal structure and absorptive function in idiopathic steatorrhoea. *Quarterly Journal of Medicine*, **36**, 425–444.

Waters, A. H. (1963). Folic acid metabolism in the megaloblastic anaemias. Ph.D. thesis, University of London.

Williams, J. A., Hall, G. S., Thompson, A. G. & Cooke, W. T. (1969). Neurological disease after partial gastrectomy. *British Medical Journal*, **2**, 210–212.

Neurological complications of tropical sprue

Adams, R. D., Denny-Brown, D. & Pearson, C. M. (1962). *Diseases of Muscle. A Study in Pathology*. 2nd edition, p. 581. New York: Hoeber.

Ekbom, K. Hed, R., Kirstein, L. & Åström, K. E. (1964). Weakness of proximal limb muscles, probably due to myopathy after partial gastrectomy. Preliminary report. *Acta medica scandinavica*, **176**, 493–496.

Fairley, N. H. (1934). Tropical sprue and its modern treatment. *British Medical Journal*, **2**, 1192–1194.

Floch, M. H., Thomassen, R. W., Cox, R. S. Jr & Sheehy, T. W. (1963). The gastric mucosa in tropical sprue. *Gastroenterology*, **44**, 567–577.

Green, P. A. & Wollaeger, E. E. (1960). The clinical behavior of sprue in the United States. *Gastroenterology*, **28**, 399–418.

Hall, W. H. (1968). Proximal muscle atrophy in adult celiac disease. *American Journal of Digestive Diseases*, **13**, 697–704.

Harriman, D. G. F. (1966). Muscle cachexia. Some aspects of its pathology and clinical features. Proceedings of the Fifth International Congress of Neuropathology, Zurich, 1965. *Excerpta Medica International Congress Series*, **100**, 677–683.

Hotz, H. W. & Lüthy, F. (1939). Funikuläre Spinalerkrankung bei einheimischer Sprue; Mitteilung eines Falles mit pathologisch-anatomischem Befund. *Helvetica medica acta*, **6,** 415–426.

Iyer, G. V., Taori, G. M. Kapadia, C. R., Mathan, V. I., & Baker, S. J. (1973). Neurological manifestations in tropical sprue: A clinical and electrodiagnostic study. *Neurology* (Minneapolis), 23, 959–966.

Jeejeebhoy, K. N., Desai, H. G., Noronha, J. M., Antia, F. P. & Parekh, D. V. (1966). Idiopathic tropical diarrhea with or without steatorrhea (tropical malabsorption syndrome). *Gastroenterology*, **51,** 333–344.

Jeejeebhoy, K. N., Wadia, N. H. & Desai, H. G. (1967). Role of vitamin B_{12} deficiency in tropical 'nutritional' neuromyelopathy. *Journal of Neurology, Neurosurgery and Psychiatry*, **30,** 7–12.

Jeejeebhoy, K. N., Desai, H. G., Barkar, A. V., Deshpande, V. & Pathare, S. M. (1968). Tropical malabsorption syndrome in west India. *American Journal of Clinical Nutrition*, **21,** 994–1006.

Jensen, A. P. J. (1965). Myopati og andre neurologiske folgetilstande efter ventrikelresektion. *Ugeskrift for Laeger*, **127,** 823–829.

Mackie, F. P. & Fairley, N. H. (1929). The morbid anatomy of sprue. *Indian Journal of Medical Research*, **16,** 797–826.

Mollin, D. L. & Booth, C. C. (1972). Chronic tropical sprue in London. In *Tropical Sprue and Megaloblastic Anaemia: Wellcome Trust Collaborative Study, 1961–1969*. London: Churchill.

Prineas, J. W., Mason, A. S. & Henson, R. A. (1965). Myopathy in metabolic bone disease. *British Medical Journal*, **1,** 1034–1036.

Rodriguez-Molina, R. (1954). Fundamental concepts in the diagnosis of sprue. *Annals of Internal Medicine*, **40,** 33–41.

Sachdev, K. K., Taori, G. M. & Pereira, S. M. (1971). Neuromuscular status in protein-calorie malnutrition. *Neurology*, **21,** 801–805.

Sheehy, T. W., Perez-Santiago, E. & Rubini, M. E. (1961). Tropical sprue and vitamin B_{12}. *New England Journal of Medicine*, **265,** 1232–1236.

Smith, R. & Stern, G. (1967). Myopathy, osteomalacia and hyperparathyroidism. *Brain*, **90,** 593–602.

Stefanini, M. (1948). Clinical features and pathogenesis of tropical sprue. Observations on series of cases among Italian prisoners of war in India. *Medicine (Baltimore)*, **27,** 379–427.

Tomlinson, B. E., Walton, J. N. & Rebeiz, J. J. (1969). The effect of ageing and of cachexia upon skeletal muscle. A histopathological study. *Journal of Neurological Sciences*, **9,** 321–346.

Wye, P. F. & Khoo, O. T. (1969). Malabsorption syndrome in Singapore. *Singapore Medical Journal*, **10,** 198–210.

Neurological complications of coeliac disease

Anderson, C. M., Frazer, A. C., French, J. M., Gerrard, J. W., Sammons, H. G. & Smellie, J. M. (1952). Coeliac disease: gastro-intestinal studies and effect of dietary wheat flour. *Lancet*, **1,** 836–842.

Benson, G. D., Kowlessar, O. D. & Sleisenger, M. H. (1964). Adult celiac disease with emphasis upon response to the gluten-free diet. *Medicine (Baltimore)*, **43,** 1–40.

Binder, H. J., Solitare, G. B. & Spiro, H. M. (1967). Neuromuscular disease in patients with steatorrhoea. *Gut*, **8,** 605–611.

Coërs, C., Telerman-Toppet, N. & Cremer, M. (1971). Regressive vacuolar myopathy in steatorrhea. *Archives of Neurology*, **24,** 217–227.

Coërs, C., Telerman-Toppet, N. & Cremer, M. (1972). Acute quadriparesis with muscle spasms related to electrolyte disturbance in steatorrhea. *American Journal of Medicine*, **52,** 849–856.

Cooke, W. T., Fone, D. J., Cox, E. V., Meynell, M. J. & Gaddie, R. (1963). Adult coeliac disease. *Gut*, **4,** 279–291.

Cooke, W. T., Johnson, A. G. & Woolf, A. L. (1966). Vital staining and electron microscopy of the intramuscular nerve endings in the neuropathy of adult coeliac disease. *Brain*, **89,** 663–682.

Cooke, W. T., Peeney, A. L. P. & Hawkins, C. F. (1953). Symptoms, signs and diagnostic features of idiopathic steatorrhoea. *Quarterly Journal of Medicine*, **22**, 59–77.

Cooke, W. T. & Smith, W. T. (1966). Neurological disorders associated with adult coeliac disease. *Brain*, **89**, 683–722.

Direkze, M. (1973). Progressive external ophthalmoplegia: some clinical associations. *Acta neurologica scandinavica*, **49**, 195–204.

Green, P. A. & Wollaeger, E. E. (1960). The clinical behavior of sprue in the United States. *Gastroenterology*, **28**, 399–418.

Hall, W. H. (1968). Proximal muscle atrophy in adult celiac disease. *American Journal of Digestive Diseases*, **13**, 697–704.

Hansen, K. & von Staa, H. (1936). *Die einheimische Sprue*. Leipzig: Thieme.

Hotz, H. W. & Lüthy, F. (1939). Funikuläre Spinalerkrankung bei einheimischer Sprue; Mitteilung eines Falles mit pathologisch-anatomischem Befund. *Helvetica medica acta*, **6**, 415–426.

Morris, J. S., Ajdukiewicz, A. B. & Read, A. E. (1970). Neurological disorders and adult coeliac disease. *Gut*, **11**, 549–554.

Richmond, J. & Davidson, S. (1958). Subacute combined degeneration of the spinal cord in non-Addisonian megaloblastic anaemia. *Quarterly Journal of Medicine*, **27**, 517–531.

Sencer, W. (1957). Neurological manifestations in malabsorption syndrome. *Journal of the Mount Sinai Hospital*, **24**, 331–345.

Sheldon, W. & Lawson, D. (1952). Management of coeliac disease. *Lancet*, **2**, 902–905.

Telerman-Toppet, N., Coërs, C. & Desneux, J. J. (1969). Ophtalmoplégie externe progressive associée à une polyneuropathie sensitivo-motrice chez un patient atteint de maladie coeliaque. *Revue neurologique*, **121**, 57–70.

Thaysen, T. E. H. (1932). *Non-Tropical Sprue*. London: Oxford University Press.

Woltman, H. W. & Heck, F. J. (1937). Funicular degeneration of the spinal cord without pernicious anemia. *Archives of Internal Medicine*, **60**, 272–300.

CHAPTER NINE

Osteomalacia, Myopathy and other Complications

Osteomalacia may complicate several gastrointestinal disorders. Two of its main clinical associations—bone pain and muscle weakness—may bring the gastrectomised patient (or the patient with coeliac disease) to the attention of a neurologist. In this chapter we wish (a) briefly to review the main facts concerning the effect of gastrectomy upon the skeleton, (b) to discuss the general subject of muscle weakness in metabolic bone disease, (c) to record the occurrence of a proximal myopathy following certain gastric operations, and (d) to assess the significance of disorders resembling motor neurone disease alleged to complicate certain types of gastric resection. Our main theme will be that osteomalacia may underlie many of the vague 'aches and pains' complained of by these patients, and that an abnormality of vitamin D metabolism probably accounts for the syndrome of predominantly proximal muscle weakness not infrequently observed in patients with malabsorption.

OSTEOMALACIA FOLLOWING PARTIAL GASTRECTOMY

Osteomalacia following partial gastrectomy, with complete recovery following treatment with vitamin D, was described by Ask-Upmark as far back as 1939. Since then postgastrectomy bone disease has been well documented on many occasions (Ask-Upmark, 1953; Pyrah and Smith, 1956; Baird and Oleesky, 1957; Melick and Benson, 1959; Harvald, Krogsgaard and Lous, 1962; Hall and Neale, 1963). So common was postgastrectomy osteomalacia at one time that an authority on vitamin D deficiency could say (Thompson, 1970) that there had been two major 'outbreaks' of vitamin D deficiency in Europe this century. The first and major one had occurred in Vienna, just after World War I, and was clearly of nutritional origin (Chick et al, 1923). The second 'outbreak' appeared in Europe during World War II, among persons who had previously undergone gastric surgery for peptic ulcer.

By 1956 over 22 000 gastrectomies were being performed each year in

Britain, this figure corresponding roughly to one third of all patients admitted to hospital with peptic ulcer (Stammers, 1963). The reported prevalence of osteomalacia among these patients varies widely according to the criteria adopted for diagnosis. Clinicians (thinking in terms of bone pain), radiologists (searching for Looser's zones or densitometric changes), clinical pathologists (estimating alkaline phosphatase and deciding whether or not it is of osseous origin), clinical physiologists (devising ever more sophisticated tests of the body's avidity for calcium), and bone microscopists (investigating the intricacies of the calcification front in iliac crest biopsies), each see only part of the problem. A combined approach might be expected to help ascertain the real facts, but such approaches have themselves at times shown discrepancies and raised more problems than they have solved. Jones, Williams and Nicholson (1963) described some of the difficulties and reviewed some of the earlier reports. Analysing their own figures they found a raised serum alkaline phosphatase in 22 per cent of patients who had undergone partial gastrectomy. On the other hand, Morgan et al (1965a), surveying over 1000 gastrectomised patients, found an incidence of clinical osteomalacia, subsequently proven on histological grounds, of less than 0·6 per cent. The experience of our colleagues at the Royal Postgraduate Medical School, originally summarised by Thompson et al (1966), is that in the absence of Paget's disease or hepatic dysfunction a raised serum alkaline phosphatase, after partial gastrectomy, is usually indicative of overt or subclinical osteomalacia.

How does postgastrectomy osteomalacia arise? There is no evidence that it is due to an acquired resistance to the action of vitamin D and it is now generally agreed to be the result of simple deficiency of the vitamin. Thompson et al (1966), showed that there was no detectable vitamin D-like activity in the plasma of patients with this condition. Such patients certainly respond to treatment with very small intramuscular doses of vitamin D (Morgan et al, 1965b).

Why are gastrectomised patients vitamin D deficient? During the summer months, in Northern latitudes, ultraviolet irradiation by sunlight may produce vitamin D_3 from 7-dehydrocholesterol in the skin. The effect is reduced throughout the winter when the diet probably becomes the main source of vitamin D (Smith, Rizek and Frame, 1964). Dietary deficiency certainly seems to play a role in the genesis of postgastrectomy osteomalacia. Gastrectomised patients often have a poor appetite. A reduced intake of eggs or dairy produce, particularly among those not venturing out much in the open, would predispose to reduced availability of vitamin D and hence to osteomalacia. In addition, there is evidence that malabsorption of vitamin D may also play a role (Thompson, Lewis and Booth, 1966a). This role is a minor one, however, unless the patient also has marked steatorrhoea; and even then there does not seem to be any direct relationship between the prevalence of osteomalacia and the severity of steatorrhoea. This is in striking contrast to the significant part played by malabsorption of vitamin D in the pathogenesis of osteomalacia in coeliac disease (Thompson, Lewis and Booth, 1966b). Another factor contributing to postgastrectomy osteomalacia may be an increased requirement of vitamin D, itself related to a low net phosphate intake (Dalgarno, Hill and McDonald, 1962) such as might occur in patients taking aluminium hydroxide as an antacid, because of abdominal distress persisting after gastrectomy (Lotz, Ney and Bartter, 1964). Yet further factors, about which we know little, may play a role.

The intake of calcium is also often reduced after partial gastrectomy. Moreover, there may be malabsorption of what inadequate amounts of calcium are ingested, either as a result of hypoacidity (hydrochloric acid normally renders less soluble calcium salts more soluble and diffusible) or because of removal of the reservoir and triturating functions of the body and antrum of the stomach. The duodenal by-pass may also contribute to malabsorption of calcium. Clark et al (1964) found disorders of calcium metabolism in up to 28 per cent of patients examined several years after partial gastrectomy. Some patients were in negative calcium balance, as previously reported by Nicolaysen and Ragard (1955). Protein maldigestion may also occur in these patients (Neale et al, 1967).

The metabolic bone disease following partial gastrectomy may present classical features of osteomalacia but in a number of cases there are radiological and histological changes more suggestive of osteoporosis. On many occasions there are features of both conditions and there seem to be good reasons for treating each case as if it were a combination of osteoporosis and osteomalacia, using anabolic steroids in addition to calcium and vitamin D (Jones et al, 1963).

Two main aspects of postgastrectomy osteomalacia are of importance to the neurologist:

(a) Gastrectomised patients may present with *multiple aches and pains*, sometimes of radicular distribution but more often indefinable in their multiplicity and fluctuation. Many such patients are probably attending rheumatology and orthopaedic clinics but some will doubtless find their way to a neurologist. There can be few neurologists so committed to their art that their heart does not sink when some thin and depressed patient attends for follow-up complaining of yet another pain, at yet another site—particularly if there are no associated neurological signs. A misdiagnosis of psychoneurosis is more than possible under these circumstances. Yet this is exactly the way osteomalacia may present. Examination of the anterior abdominal wall for a laparotomy scar, enquiry for a history of long-standing bowel irregularity, estimation of the serum alkaline phosphatase, calcium and phosphate, and radiology of hands, chest and pelvis should be mandatory in this context. Osteomalacia is a treatable condition and failure to diagnose it is tantamount to negligence.

(b) Patients with osteomalacia may present as a *myopathy*. It is not that the osteomalacia itself causes myopathy but that vitamin D deficiency (the most significant aetiological factor in nearly all types of osteomalacia) probably interferes with muscle function. This type of muscle weakness may cause considerable problems in diagnosis, particularly if the metabolic bone disease is not associated with prominent bone pain. It may be missed altogether unless specifically sought for—or if found attributed to other neurological disease. The reflexes will often be brisk and more serious disorders such as motor neurone disease may be misdiagnosed. Before reporting the known instances in which myopathy followed gastrectomy we would like to discuss what is known, in more general terms, of the association between osteomalacia and myopathy. A full discussion of the multiple functions of vitamin D is beyond the scope of this monograph and readers are referred to full reviews by DeLuca (1967, 1970) and to an interesting short article by Thompson (1970).

OSTEOMALACIA AND MYOPATHY

In Western societies it has been known for over four decades that osteomalacia might be associated with considerable muscle weakness (Milkman, 1930). Albright and Reifenstein (1948) found muscle power reduced in many of their patients with metabolic bone disease to a degree that could not be accounted for by pain. Dent (1956) stressed that muscular weakness might at times antedate all other manifestations of osteomalacia. Other important early accounts of this particular association are those of Vicale (1949) and of Murphy, ReMine and Burbank (1960). The subject has recently received considerable attention, following recognition of how often patients with coeliac disease show evidence of proximal muscle weakness.

The story really goes back much earlier, however, and its origins are in the East, not in the West. Agnes Scott (1916) appears to have been the first to give a good account of proximal muscle weakness in osteomalacic women in India. Osteomalacia of nutritional origin has for years been a well-established entity, the bulk of the patients being women of child-bearing age, drawn from undernourished communities, and subjected to the stress of repeated childbirth and lactation. It is often assumed that tropical sunshine—acting on the skin—would more than compensate for both an inadequate dietary intake and an excessive demand for vitamin D. This is not in fact the case as anyone familiar with the social customs—and in particular the clothing habits—of certain sections of the population at risk will readily attest. Reporting from Bombay, Singhal (1966) and Wadia and Swami (1970) found 'myopathy' to be present in the majority of their patients with osteomalacia of nutritional origin.

In a careful and very detailed survey of 11 women with nutritional osteomalacia, Dastur, Wadia and Bharucha (1972) encountered a fairly constant neurological syndrome. Their study is particularly informative as all the techniques used were carefully listed and control observations given for most of the data. There was no evidence of gastrointestinal disease, the absorption of D-xylose being normal in seven of the eight patients in which it was tested. Nine of the 11 patients were Muslim women who reported staying indoors most of the time and wearing a 'burkha' on the rare occasions they ventured out. All had experienced pain, usually in the pelvis, lumbar spine, ribs and long bones, and all exhibited bone tenderness. Squeezing the pelvis produced exquisite pain in seven cases. All the patients suffered from weakness, initially affecting the pelvic and truncal muscles, with resultant difficulties in climbing stairs and in rising from a supine or squatting posture. They all had a classical waddling gait. Proximal upper limb weakness was present in seven cases. There was no appreciable wasting and no weakness of the distal musculature. The authors do not comment on whether the patients most disabled by pain were also the 'weakest'. No patients had experienced tetany. Electromyographic evaluation of eight of these patients showed a normal trace in six. A 'myopathic' record, with an excess of short-duration small-amplitude potentials was encountered in two instances. Nerve conduction studies were normal. Biopsies of the gluteus maximus in six patients showed no typical myopathic changes although in all cases there appeared to be a mild, diffuse, non-specific fibre atrophy. Fibre diameters varied from 17 to 69 μm, with a mean diameter of 36·5 μm. The authors infer the probable occurrence in osteomalacic 'myopathy' of an element of disuse atrophy. They consider this secondary to the limitation of movement, consequent upon the severe bone pains so characteristic of the disorder. In other series, as we shall show, osteomalacic myopathy occurred in patients virtually free of pain.

The biochemical observations are discussed further on. Under treatment with vitamin D there was early improvement in bone pain and later in muscle power in all cases.

A few years before this large-scale study had been undertaken in India, Prineas, Mason and Henson (1965) had described two patients with osteomalacia and long-standing muscle weakness, which they attributed to myopathy. In one instance (a patient with parathyroid adenoma) the osteomalacia was associated with renal tubular acidosis and with both osteosclerosis and the more classical bone changes of hyperparathyroidism.* The other patient had developed osteomalacia as a complication of gluten-sensitive enteropathy. In both patients the muscle weakness improved following treatment of the underlying condition.

The common denominator of these two cases was the presence of osteomalacia, confirmed by iliac crest biopsy and by the finding of raised levels of serum alkaline phosphatase. The main neurological features were proximal weakness and wasting, discomfort on movement, hypotonia and brisk reflexes. Electromyography showed abnormalities of myopathic type without evidence of denervation. Muscle biopsy was performed only in the first case, revealing scattered atrophic fibres with crowding of sarcolemmal nuclei. In both patients muscle weakness was pronounced over a period of several weeks during which time total serum calcium levels were either normal or very nearly normal. The authors suggested that the muscular weakness in their cases was probably due to a disturbance of vitamin D metabolism. They shrewdly queried whether the waddling gait, lordosis and delay in walking encountered in classical vitamin D deficiency rickets—usually attributed to 'hypotonia'—might in fact be due to metabolic myopathy.

In 1967 Smith and Stern reported a detailed survey of the prevalence of myopathy in patients with osteomalacia and with hyperparathyroidism attending University College Hospital, London. All instances where weakness might conceivably be attributed to causes other than metabolic bone disease (such as old age, intercurrent infections or neoplasm) were excluded. The authors found unequivocal muscular weakness in 20 out of 45 patients with

* Renal tubular acidosis (Cohen et al, 1957; Wrong and Davies, 1959), osteomalacia (Ball, 1963) and osteosclerosis (Davies, Dent and Willcox, 1956; Beveridge, Vaughan and Walters, 1959) are all recognised, if rare, complications of primary hyperparathyroidism.

proven osteomalacia, of varying aetiology. For instance, of 14 patients with osteomalacia due to gluten-sensitive enteropathy six had proximal myopathy. Of five patients with postgastrectomy osteomalacia, four were affected. Both their patients with nutritional osteomalacia had weak proximal muscles. On the other hand, of 91 patients with hyperparathyroidism only six showed evidence of muscle weakness, and of these half were found to have osteomalacia.

In some respects the clinical picture presented by these London patients differed strikingly from that seen in India. Muscular weakness was the first symptom (or among the presenting symptoms) in 15 cases. The other patients had been driven to seek assistance for symptoms attributable to the underlying disease: diarrhoea, bone pain or abnormal thirst. The neurological features were fairly similar, however. The weakness was proximal in all cases, with early complaints of heaviness in the legs and difficulty in negotiating kerb-stones, arising from a chair or climbing out of a bath. The gait was usually abnormal. Examination often revealed more extensive weakness in the muscles of the trunk and limb girdles than the history suggested. For instance, upper limb weakness was often demonstrable where none had been complained of. Although some of the patients were thin as a result of their underlying disease, focal atrophy of paresed muscles was never conspicuous. Anaemia and finger clubbing at times proved useful pointers to underlying malabsorption, while recent loss of height and bone tenderness suggested osteomalacia.

All five patients examined electromyographically showed myopathic features (short-duration polyphasic potentials). In this they differed from the Indian cases. No significant abnormalities were found in two muscle biopsies. All patients with proximal muscular weakness and osteomalacia were given vitamin D and showed definite improvement, 16 making a complete recovery. Patients with osteomalacic myopathy secondary to gluten-sensitive enteropathy required much larger doses of vitamin D to induce improvement than did patients with nutritional or postgastrectomy osteomalacia.

The authors stressed that proximal muscle weakness might occur, in osteomalacic patients, in the absence of symptoms or signs of bone disease and that it might deceptively simulate primary myopathy such as muscular dystrophy, or polymyositis. They discussed the possible role of secondary hyperparathyroidism but concluded that 'a vitamin D disorder would seem the most acceptable explanation for the proximal myopathy'.

In a later report, based on a prospective study of 44 hyperparathyroid and 11 osteomalacic patients, Smith and Stern (1969) again found proximal muscle weakness to be much more frequent in various types of osteomalacia than in hyperparathyroidism. The myopathy was not related to the concentration of any plasma electrolyte measured and the response to oral vitamin D was 'the most impressive of all the known clinical features of the condition'. The circulating vitamin D, as determined by biological assay, was normal in a few of these cases. The authors reiterated their former view that the myopathy was probably 'a direct or indirect result of disordered vitamin D metabolism'.

Mechanism of weakness in osteomalacia

It was long believed that muscular weakness in metabolic bone disease was related to alterations in the level of ionised calcium on excitability and transmission at the neuromuscular junction (Payne, 1959; Murphy et al, 1960; Shy, 1960). More recent reports have tended to incriminate a disturbance of vitamin D metabolism. It is worth reviewing the scanty available facts.

In the patients reported by Dastur et al (1972) there appeared to be no correlation between the level of ionised calcium and the severity of bone pain or muscle weakness. The mean serum calcium and ionised calcium were not significantly altered,* but the serum inorganic phosphate levels were usually low. The serum alkaline phosphatase was elevated in every case. Mean urinary calcium and phosphate excretion was normal. The serum vitamin D level was assessed in only one case and found to be normal.

Both of the patients reported by Prineas et al (1965) had prominent weakness over a period of several weeks during which time total serum calcium levels were normal. (In the first patient the plasma ionised calcium was 6·9 mg/100 ml† at the only estimation made, but the authors endorsed the view that much higher levels are known to occur without comparable weakness.) In the large series reported by Smith and Stern (1967) no relationship could be established between the presence of proximal myopathy and the plasma calcium concentration. In five cases plasma ionised calcium concentrations were found to vary between 5·6 and 8·8 mg/100 ml (method of measurement not specified). The plasma alkaline phosphatase was markedly raised in 18 of the 20 cases. In four patients plasma vitamin D activity was measured before treatment and low values found in three.

These facts would lead one to suspect that vitamin D deficiency is in some way related to the myopathy. Indirectly supporting this suggestion is the observation that muscle weakness is not a feature in sex-linked type I hypophosphataemic rickets (Williams, Winters and Burnett, 1966), a condition in which there is proven osteomalacia in the presence of normal blood levels of vitamin D. There are indications, however, that the problem is not quite as simple as this. Patients with coeliac disease and proximal muscle weakness do not respond to vitamin D therapy in the usual dosage, even when administered parenterally, until they are also put on a gluten-free diet (Smith and Stern, 1967). Moreover, patients with osteomalacia may develop secondary (or even tertiary) hyperparathyroidism and an effect of parathormone on muscle function cannot be excluded.

There are hints that both vitamin D and parathormone may have an action on muscle but very little is as yet known about this. Kodicek (1963) observed the autoradiographic localisation of tritiated vitamin D on the muscle membrane of rachitic rats. DeLuca et al (1960) had shown that vitamin D deficiency produced morphological changes in kidney mitochondria and DeLuca and Sallis (1965) later described how vitamin D influenced the release of calcium from mitochondria. This action of vitamin D on mitochondria seems to be influenced by parathormone (Rasmussen and Ogata, 1966). The clinical

* The ionised calcium was not directly estimated by these authors but read off from nomograms relating total calcium to total plasma protein (McLean and Hastings, 1935).

† Fowler, Fone and Cooke (1961) in a study of the plasma calcium fractions in normal individuals, in hypercalcaemic conditions and in coeliac disease found the mean ionised calcium in normal adults to be 5·85 mg/100 ml with a range (±2SD) of 5·45 to 6·23 mg/100 ml.

significance—or indeed relevance to muscle disease—of these observations remain, for the time being, obscure.

MYOPATHIC COMPLICATIONS OF PARTIAL GASTRECTOMY

If partial gastrectomy is often associated with osteomalacia and if osteomalacia may be associated with a myopathy, it would not be surprising if myopathy were occasionally encountered in gastrectomised patients. Recent reports suggest that this is a real and not just a theoretical hazard. What is really surprising is that the association is not encountered more often.

Ekbom et al (1964) described three middle-aged patients in whom severe proximal muscle weakness developed between two and eight years after Billroth II gastrectomies for peptic ulcer. The symptoms progressed slowly to complete incapacity. The degree of wasting was variable, being severe in the first case. No fasciculations were observed. Sensory examination was normal in each instance and the tendon reflexes were retained. Electromyographic examination was said to show a typical myopathic pattern with a marked excess of short-duration polyphasic potentials. No significant abnormalities were detected, in any of the three cases, on biopsy of the quadriceps muscle, the authors commenting that in their experience this was not unusual in myopathies of metabolic or endocrine origin. There was steatorrhoea in each instance, with hypocalcaemia, hypocalciuria, a raised serum alkaline phosphatase and radiological evidence of 'decalcification of the skeleton'. Two of the patients showed remarkable improvement in muscle weakness following treatment with vitamin D.

The following year the same authors reported a further case, occurring 15 years after Billroth II gastrectomy and also responding well to vitamin D. They commented that gastrectomised patients seemed particularly prone to develop the myopathy of metabolic bone disease 'in view of the high frequency of calcium disorders after gastric operations', although they admitted that recovery might follow treatment with vitamin D alone.

D'Eramo (1965) reported the development of a proximal myopathy in a 45-year-old man who had undergone gastric resection for a duodenal ulcer five years earlier. The patient, who had anaemia, oedema and hypoproteinaemia, differs from those previously recorded in that biopsy was said to have confirmed the diagnosis of 'progressive myopathic muscular atrophy', as indicated by thinning of muscle fibres with degeneration, fragmentation, and the presence of nuclear chains. No comments were made about the possibility of an associated osteomalacia, which does not seem to have been looked for. It is impossible to say whether, in this case, the development of a myopathy was fortuitous or not.

We are under the impression that late myopathic complications of partial gastrectomy may be more frequent than is believed, having ourselves seen two cases since we became aware of the association. Both responded well to vitamin D. 'Weakness' following partial gastrectomy is too frequently attributed to 'anaemia' or to 'protein malnutrition' and insufficient attention is paid to its occasionally strikingly proximal distribution. Any patient in a gastrectomy clinic noticed to have difficulty in arising from a chair should certainly have an estimation of his serum alkaline phosphatase, and this whether or not there are complaints of bone pain.

OTHER NEUROLOGICAL COMPLICATIONS OF PARTIAL GASTRECTOMY

There have been occasional reports that a neurological disorder resembling *motor neurone disease* may occasionally be encountered in patients who have undergone partial gastrectomy. Whether there is a direct relationship between these two conditions, or whether their association in a given individual is purely fortuitous remains, for the moment, uncertain. It seems, however, simplistic to believe that a deficiency state, induced by gastrectomy, can be the cause of a system degeneration the progression of which is unaffected by any sort of replacement therapy.

The occurrence of motor neurone disease in gastrectomised patients seems to be rare. It was not reported in reviews of the sequelae of gastrectomy by Wells and MacPhee (1954), Harvey (1957) or Stammers and Williams (1963). Nor was the association recognised in a review by Stiehl (1967) of 125 patients with motor neurone disease, specially screened for evidence of previous gastric surgery. Anyone familiar with the usual practice of medical or surgical gastroenterological clinics, however, will admit that a careful search for fasciculation (or detailed testing for hyperreflexia) is seldom, if ever, part of established follow-up routine. Insidiously developing neurological disorders, especially if not associated with sensory symptoms, could conceivably go unrecognised, at least for a time. Failure to gain weight following gastrectomy is far more likely to be attributed by surgeons or gastroenterologists to malnutrition than to developing anterior horn cell disease, and in this they are undoubtedly correct.

There is a handful of reports that suggest a possibly significant association between the two conditions. Ask-Upmark (1950) described four male patients, aged between 41 and 68 years, who after partial gastrectomy and a Billroth II type of anastomosis developed a clinical syndrome resembling motor neurone disease. The interval between surgery and the onset of symptoms varied from 1 to 12 years. Because of the association of distal wasting of the upper limbs and pyramidal signs in the legs the cases were described as instances of amyotrophic lateral sclerosis. Electrophysiological data and the results (if any) of muscle biopsy (if performed) were not reported. Later, Ask-Upmark and Meurling (1955) reported three further cases and raised the question of whether a deficiency state, secondary to malabsorption, might be relevant to the aetiology of certain cases of motor neurone disease.

Kniffen and Quick (1969) published a detailed study of six patients, five of them women, who had developed various neuromuscular disorders following partial gastrectomy (this had consisted of partial gastrectomy with a Billroth II type of anastomosis in five instances, and a Billroth I type in a single case). The ages of these patients ranged from 45 to 75 years.

Neurological symptoms had appeared at intervals varying from six months to 18 years after surgery. All patients except one had visible fasciculations, described as prominent in three instances. The distribution of muscle atrophy was proximal in three patients, distal in one, and combined distal and bulbar in the remaining two. Pyramidal signs were present in three patients. In two patients the reflexes were described as hypoactive and in one patient they were normal. Electromyography, performed in five of the six patients showed evidence of denervation. Muscle biopsy was also performed in five of the patients. In four it showed grouped atrophy of muscle fibres, indicating a neurogenic aetiology. In one patient there were features suggesting both myopathy and neurogenic atrophy.

Evaluation of these cases is difficult. Review of the individual protocols shows that one 51-year-old patient had absent ankle jerks, without distal motor or sensory symptoms or signs in the lower limbs. One 75-year-old woman with bilateral carotid bruits showed Parkinsonian features and evidence of mild organic dementia. Another female patient, aged 59, had well-established diabetes. One patient, not evaluated in any detail, had a serum B_{12} of only 64 pg/ml. Apart from the overtly diabetic patient, two others were considered diabetic on the basis of an intravenous glucose tolerance test and another two considered 'borderline' diabetic. Two patients showed malabsorption of vitamin B_{12} correctable by the simultaneous administration of intrinsic factor. Mild steatorrhoea, hypocarotinaemia, hypoalbuminaemia and impaired xylose excretion were encountered in various patients.

The authors considered both of the patients with bulbar signs and symptoms to have motor neurone disease and we cannot quarrel with this diagnosis. It is of interest that these are the cases with the longest latent periods (13·5 and 18 years respectively) between surgery and the onset of neurological complaints.

The patient with well-established diabetes was considered to have diabetic amyotrophy. (We find this diagnosis untenable: symmetrical wasting predominated in the hands, there was no history of pain in the thighs and no comment about proximal atrophy in the lower limbs.) In two patients no precise neurological diagnosis could be made. (In our opinion these might conceivably have been instances of the proximal type of spinal muscular atrophy.)

The authors speculated as to whether postgastrectomy absorptive defects, present in varying degree in all their patients, might be the basis of the observed neurological disorders. In this context they pointed to the occurrence of pancreatic dysfunction, with consequent malabsorption in some cases of motor neurone disease (Quick and Greer, 1967; Quick, 1968). It is doubtful in our opinion whether this analogy is meaningful, as malnutrition (so often encountered in cases of chronic bulbar palsy) may itself be a cause of impaired pancreatic function (Neale et al, 1967).

References

Albright, F. & Reifenstein, E. C. (1948). *The Parathyroid Glands and Metabolic Bone Disease*. London: Baillière, Tindall & Cox.

Ask-Upmark, E. (1939). Osteomalacia hepatica. *Acta medica scandinavica*, **99**, 204–227.

Ask-Upmark, E. (1950). Amyotrophic lateral sclerosis observed in five persons after gastric resection. *Gastroenterology*, **15**, 257–259.

Ask-Upmark, E. (1953). Disturbances of fluid and electrolyte balance—Discussion. *Acta medica scandinavica*, **146**, 55.

Ask-Upmark, E. & Meurling, S. (1955). On the presence of a deficiency factor in the pathogenesis of amyotrophic lateral sclerosis. *Acta medica scandinavica*, **152,** 217–222.

Baird, I. M. & Oleesky, S. (1957). Osteomalacia following gastric surgery. *Gastroenterology*, **33,** 284–292.

Ball, J. (1963). Histological diagnosis in metabolic bone disease. In *Bone Metabolism in Relation to Clinical Medicine*, ed. Sissons, H. A., pp. 31–35. London: Pitman.

Beveridge, B., Vaughan, B. F. & Walters, M. N. I. (1959). Primary hyperparathyroidism and secondary renal failure with osteosclerosis. *Journal of the Faculty of Radiologists (London)*, **10,** 197–200.

Chick, H., Dalyell, E. J., Hume, M., MacKay, H., Henderson Smith, H. & Wimberger, H. (1923). Studies of rickets in Vienna 1919–22. *Medical Research Council Special Report Series* No. 77. London: H.M.S.O.

Clark, C. G., Crooks, J., Dawson, A. A. & Mitchell, P. E. G. (1964). Disordered calcium metabolism after Polya type partial gastrectomy. *Lancet*, **1,** 734–738.

Cohen, S. I., Fitzgerald, M. G., Fourman, P., Griffiths, W. J. & de Wardener, H. E. (1957). Polyuria in hyperparathyroidism. *Quarterly Journal of Medicine*, **26,** 423–431.

Dalgarno, A. C., Hill, R. & McDonald, I. (1962). Vitamin D in the blood of sheep. *British Journal of Nutrition*, **16,** 91–97.

Dastur, D. K., Wadia, N. H. & Bharucha, E. P. (1972). *Studies of Nutritional Disorders of the Nervous System* (NIH project 01-011-1: Interim Report) Neuropathology Unit, Grant Medical College and JJ Group of Hospitals, Bombay 8.

Davies, D. R., Dent, C. E. & Willcox, A. (1956). Hyperparathyroidism and steatorrhoea. *British Medical Journal*, **2,** 1133–1137.

DeLuca, H. F. (1967). Mechanism of action and metabolic fate of vitamin D. *Vitamins and Hormones*, **25,** 315–367.

DeLuca, H. F. (1970). Vitamin D: mode of action. In *Symposium Proceedings: The Biochemistry, Metabolism and Chemical Analysis of Vitamin D and Related Compounds.* Chicago: Association of Vitamin Chemists.

DeLuca, H. F., Reiser, S., Steenbock, H. & Kaesberg, P. (1960). Vitamin D and the structure of kidney mitochondria. *Biochimica et biophysica acta*, **40,** 526–530.

DeLuca, H. F. & Sallis, J. D. (1965). Parathyroid hormone: its subcellular actions and its relationship to vitamin D. In *The Parathyroid Glands: Ultrastructure, Secretion and Function*, ed. Gaillard, P. J., Talmage, R. V. & Budy, A. M., pp. 181–196. Chicago: University of Chicago Press.

Dent, C. E. (1956). Discussion on surgical aspects of disordered calcium metabolism. *Proceedings of the Royal Society of Medicine*, **49,** 715–722.

D'Eramo, N. (1965). Progressive myopathic muscular atrophy after gastric resection. *Lancet*, **1,** 1277–1278.

Ekbom, K., Hed, R., Kirstein, L. & Åström, K. E. (1964). Weakness of proximal limb muscles, probably due to myopathy after partial gastrectomy. *Acta medica scandinavica*, **176,** 493–496.

Ekbom, K., Hed, R., Kirstein, L. & Åström, K. E. (1965). Myopathy in metabolic bone disease. *British Medical Journal*, **1,** 1670–1671.

Fowler, D. I., Fone, D. J. & Cooke, W. T. (1961). The calcium fractions in plasma in hypercalcaemic conditions and in adult coeliac disease. *Lancet*, **2,** 284–287.

Hall, G. H. & Neale, G. (1963). Bone rarefaction after partial gastrectomy. *Annals of Internal Medicine*, **59,** 455–463.

Harvald, B., Krogsgaard, A. R. & Lous, P. (1962). Calcium deficiency following partial gastrectomy. *Acta medica scandinavica*, **172,** 497–503.

Harvey, H. D. (1957). The nutritional status of patients after partial gastrectomy with gastro-jejunostomy for duodenal ulcer. *Surgery, Gynecology and Obstetrics*, **105,** 559–564.

Jones, C. T., Williams, J. A. & Nicholson, G. (1963). Disturbances of bone metabolism after partial gastrectomy. In *Partial Gastrectomy: Complications and Metabolic Consequences*, ed. Stammers, F. A. R. & Williams, J. A., pp. 190–226. London: Butterworth.

Kniffen, J. C. & Quick, D. T. (1969). Neuromuscular disorder following gastric resection. *Archives of Internal Medicine*, **124,** 336–340.

Kodicek, E. (1963). Turnover and distribution of vitamin D and its mode of action. In *The Transfer of Calcium and Strontium across Biological Membranes*, ed. Wasserman, R. H., pp. 185–196. New York: Academic Press.

Lotz, M., Ney, R. L. & Bartter, F. C. (1964). Osteomalacia and debility resulting from phosphorus depletion. *Transactions of the Association of American Physicians*, **77**, 281–295.

McLean, F. C. & Hastings, A. B. (1935). Clinical estimation and significance of calcium-ion concentration in the blood. *American Journal of Medical Sciences*, **189**, 601–613.

Melick, R. A. & Benson, J. A. (1959). Osteomalacia following partial gastrectomy. *New England Journal of Medicine*, **260**, 976–978.

Milkman, L. A. (1930). Pseudofractures (hunger osteopathy, late rickets, osteomalacia); report of case. *American Journal of Roentgenology*, **24**, 29-37.

Morgan, D. B., Paterson, C. R., Woods, C. G., Pulvertaft, C. N. & Fourman, P. (1965a). Search for osteomalacia in 1228 patients after gastrectomy and other operations on the stomach. *Lancet*, **2**, 1085–1088.

Morgan, D. B., Paterson, C. R., Woods, C. G., Pulvertaft, C. N. & Fourman, P. (1965b). Osteomalacia after gastrectomy. A response to very small doses of vitamin D. *Lancet*, **2**, 1089–1091.

Murphy, T. R., ReMine, W. H. & Burbank, M. K. (1960). Hyperparathyroidism: report of a case in which parathyroid adenoma presented primarily with profound muscular weakness. *Proceedings of the Staff Meetings of the Mayo Clinic*, **35**, 629–634.

Neale, G., Antcliffe, A. C., Welbourn, R. B., Mollin, D. L. & Booth, C. C. (1967). Protein malnutrition after partial gatrectomy. *Quarterly Journal of Medicine*, **36**, 469–494.

Nicolaysen, R. & Ragard, R. (1955). The calcium and phosphorus metabolism in gastrectomised patients. *Scandinavian Journal of Clinical and Laboratory Investigation*, **7**, 298–299.

Payne, W. W. (1959). Calcium and phosphorus metabolism in nervous disorders. In *Biochemical Aspects of Neurological Disorders*, ed. Cummings, J. N. & Kremer, M., pp. 73–85. Oxford: Blackwell.

Prineas, J. W., Mason, A. S. & Henson, R. A. (1965). Myopathy in metabolic bone disease. *British Medical Journal*, **1**, 1034–1036.

Pyrah, L. N. & Smith, I. B. (1956). Osteomalacia following gastrectomy. *Lancet*, **1**, 935–937.

Quick, D. (1968). Pancreatic dysfunction in amyotrophic lateral sclerosis. In *Contemporary Neurology Symposia. Vol. II—Motor Neuron Diseases—Research on Amyotrophic Lateral Sclerosis and Related Disorders*, ed. Norris, F. H. & Kurland, L. T. New York: Grune & Stratton.

Quick, D. & Greer, M. (1967). Pancreatic dysfunction in patients with amyotrophic lateral sclerosis. *Neurology*, **17**, 112–116.

Rasmussen, H. & Ogata, E. (1966). Parathyroid hormone and the reactions of mitochondria to cations. *Biochemistry (Washington)*, **5**, 733–745.

Scott, A. C. (1916). A contribution to the study of osteomalacia in India. *Indian Journal of Medical Research*, **4**, 140–168.

Shy, G. M. (1960). Some metabolic and endocrinological aspects of disorders of striated muscle. *Proceedings. Association for Research in Nervous and Mental Diseases*, **38**, 274–317.

Singhal, B. S. (1966). Muscle weakening simulating myopathy in metabolic bone disease. *Neurology (India)*, **14**, 194–196.

Smith, R. W., Rizek, J. & Frame, B. (1964). Determinants of serum antirachitic activity. Special reference to involutional osteoporosis. *American Journal of Clinical Nutrition*, **14**, 98–108.

Smith, R. & Stern, G. (1967). Myopathy, osteomalacia and hyperparathyroidism. *Brain*, **90**, 593–602.

Smith, R. & Stern, G. (1969). Muscular weakness in osteomalacia and hyperparathyroidism. *Journal of the Neurological Sciences*, **8**, 511–520.

Stammers, F. A. R. (1963). Introduction. In *Partial Gastrectomy: Complications and Metabolic Consequences*, ed. Stammers, F. A. R. & Williams, J. A., p. 2. London: Butterworth.

Stammers, F. A. R. & Williams, J. A. (1963). *Partial Gastrectomy: Complications and Metabolic Consequences*. London: Butterworth.

Stiehl, J. (1967). The incidence of gastrectomy and gastric secretion in motor neurone disease. *Australian Annals of Medicine*, **16**, 176–177.

Thompson, G. R. (1970). Vitamin D deficiency after gastrectomy. *Scientific Basis of Medicine Annual Reviews*, 260–275. London: Athlone Press.

Thompson, G. R., Lewis, B. & Booth, C. C. (1966a). Vitamin D absorption after partial gastrectomy. *Lancet*, **1**, 457–458.

Thompson, G. R., Lewis, B. & Booth, C. C. (1966b). Absorption of vitamin D_3-^3H in control subjects and patients with intestinal malabsorption. *Journal of Clinical Investigation*, **45**, 94–102.

Thompson, G. R., Neale, G., Watts, J. M. & Booth, C. C. (1966). Detection of vitamin D deficiency after partial gastrectomy. *Lancet*, **1**, 623–626.

Vicale, C. T. (1949). Diagnostic features of muscular syndrome resulting from hyperparathyroidism, osteomalacia owing to renal tubular acidosis, and perhaps to related disorders of calcium metabolism. *Transactions of the American Neurological Association*, **74**, 143–147.

Wadia, N. H. & Swami, R. K. (1970). Pattern of nutritional deficiency disorders of the nervous system in Bombay. *Neurology* (*India*), **18**, 203–219.

Wells, C. & MacPhee, I. W. (1954). Partial gastrectomy: ten years later. *British Medical Journal*, **2**, 1128–1132.

Williams, T. F., Winters, R. W. & Burnett, C. H. (1966). Familial (hereditary) vitamin D-resistant rickets with hypophosphataemia. In *Metabolic Basis of Inherited Disease*, ed. Stanbury, J. B., Wyngaarden, J. B. & Fredrickson, D. S., 2nd edition, pp. 1179–1204. New York: McGraw-Hill.

Wrong, O. & Davies, H. E. F. (1959). The excretion of acid in renal disease. *Quarterly Journal of Medicine*, **28**, 259–313.

CHAPTER TEN

Central Pontine Myelinolysis

A book dealing with the borderland between neurology and gastroenterology may or may not be a good place to discuss the mysterious condition of central pontine myelinolysis, first described in 1959. We feel that little can be added to the original account of Adams, Victor and Mancall or to the excellent recent reviews of Monseu and Flament-Durand (1971) and of Goebel and Zur (1972). Yet the condition remains pathologically so striking, and its clinical manifestations often so widely at variance with what might have been expected, that a further brief discussion may be justified. Over 100 cases have now been documented. Inasmuch as a nutritional disturbance of one kind or another has been implicated in the majority of affected patients, we feel that some comment is here appropriate.

Central pontine myelinolysis (CPM) appears to be a new pathological entity. One or two doubtful descriptions, but no really convincing accounts, have been found prior to 1959, when Adams and his colleagues published their report. Case 1 of Lüthy (1931) is one of these possible early instances. That CPM is a new condition seems inherently unlikely, and the unearthing of earlier descriptions is a task awaiting some future neurological historian. However, until such cases are discovered there is nothing to refute the view of Aleu and Terry (1963) that CPM might be linked to some new environmental hazard, such as a cytotoxic or antimicrobial drug. The lesson of subacute myelo-opticoneuropathy (SMON) (see p. 180) should be kept in mind.

In this brief survey we shall review the pathological and clinical features and try to evaluate the significance of various associated factors, in particular the relationship of CPM to gastrointestinal disorder and impaired nutrition.

Pathological features

CPM is strikingly homogeneous from the pathological angle. All reported cases show a more or less symmetrical demyelination in the central part of the basis pontis, maximal in width at the level of the trigeminal nerves, and sparing both mesencephalon and medulla. The area involved may appear discoloured, granular or necrotic macroscopically. It may resemble an infarct.

Yet with appropriate stains and under the microscope, the lesion is seen to be selective. The zone of myelin loss is always sharply defined, although its edges are often irregular. It may involve an area a few millimetres across, or almost the whole of the basis pontis. Microscopically there is loss of myelin sheaths and of oligodendrocyte nuclei. In cases that survive long enough myelin *débris* become incorporated in lipid macrophages and fibrous gliosis appears. In contrast, axons are relatively preserved (though often damaged in the centre of the affected region). Neurones are usually only slightly affected. There is no evidence of inflammation or vascular disease.

Some cases have shown extrapontine lesions, but for these an alternative explanation can nearly always be found. When the condition is encountered in alcoholics the brain may show features of Wernicke's encephalopathy. Histological evidence of anoxia may be found in patients who were deeply comatose and had suffered severe hypotension or cardiac arrest. Coincidental brain lesions may be found, but the specific feature remains the single, central, predominantly demyelinating pontine lesion.

Clinical features

It is remarkable that this gross abnormality, occurring in a well-defined locus tightly packed with important neuronal structures and pathways, should have no regular clinical correlate other than a lethal outcome. While many neurologists during the last 10 years or so must at some time or other have considered CPM in the differential diagnosis of a patient with an obscure, rapidly evolving brainstem disorder, the fact remains that only two of the 100 or more documented cases were diagnosed during life (Boudin et al, 1963; Paguirigan and Lefken, 1969). The clinical picture associated with CPM may range from no neurological abnormality to 'what it should be' (a florid syndrome resembling basilar artery occlusion). Among the signs noted are confusion, coma, mutism, incontinence, external ocular palsies, abnormal pupils, dysarthria, dysphagia, para- or tetraparesis, hyper- or hyporeflexia, tremors and convulsions. When clinical histories of patients with CPM are reviewed retrospectively, a number could be said to have shown initial confusion, subsequent weakness and pyramidal signs in the legs, and late bulbar signs and coma. Recognising this progression of events might perhaps enable further cases to be diagnosed ante mortem.

Of 69 cases collected by McCormick and Danneel (1967) one-third were dead within two weeks of admission to hospital. Nearly all the survivors died within three months. One case survived for two years (Green, Sung and Wolf, 1962) though of course the relationship of the initial neurological events to the finding of CPM at autopsy in this case must remain speculative. Most of the patients were aged between 35 and 60 years, the extremes being 7 and 72. Several reports of CPM in children have appeared in recent years. The lower age limit has now dropped to 20 months (Cadman and Rorke, 1969; Valsamis, Peress and Wright, 1971).

Aetiology

Of reported adult cases, well over half were either alcoholic, malnourished or suffering from liver disease. These three factors have obviously been the favourites in the list of possible causes. Many of the reported cases, however, had suffered from neither alcoholism or liver disease, and were perfectly well nourished. Severe electrolyte disturbance is reported to have been present in many patients with CPM, usually a consequence of severe vomiting or diarrhoea.

Vomiting seems to precede the onset of other symptoms in a proportion of cases. Although often related to alcoholic excess, it may be due to a variety of other causes such as appendicitis (Mathieson and Olszewski, 1960), pyloric carcinoma (Adams, 1962: Case 1), volvulus (Adams, 1962: Case 2) and scleroderma of the oesophagus (Adams et al, 1959: Case 4). Prolonged intravenous feeding and extensive burns have also been reported as immediate antecedents (Tihen, 1972; McCormick and Danneel, 1967). In one patient (Conger, McIntyre and Jacoby, 1969) diuretic-induced hyponatraemia appeared to be the precipitating factor. In others, CPM has appeared after head injury (Minauf and Jellinger, 1970; Seitelberger and Jonasch, 1970) or neurosurgery (Kepes, Reece and Oxley, 1965), again with profound electrolyte imbalance. Many patients had had adequate vitamin therapy, although others could well have been vitamin deficient. Neoplasia, especially leukaemia in children, is another significant association (Cadman and Rorke, 1969). Several cases of CPM have occurred in patients submitted to renal transplantation (Schneck, 1966; Monseu and Flament-Durand, 1971). Clearly no single aetiological agent can be singled out, yet it is hard to escape the conclusion that some (undefined) nutritional deficiency in association with some (also undefined) alteration in blood chemistry is responsible for the development of CPM. But try as we may, we currently find ourselves unable to define these factors further.

From time to time authors have questioned the role of disturbed brainstem circulation in the aetiology of CPM. One severely dehydrated, hypernatraemic patient with CPM (Landers, Chason and Samuel, 1965) was found at autopsy to have thrombosis of the tributaries of the great vein of Galen. It was suggested that obstructed pontine venous drainage might be a causal factor. There is no evidence for this hypothesis though it should be remembered that the central pontine area is unusually susceptible to vascular damage, as shown by the occurrence of haemorrhage at this site in patients with raised intracranial pressure (Klintworth, 1965) or following a severe acute rise of serum osmolality (Cameron and Dayan, 1966). The cases of Cameron and Dayan died after therapeutic abortion, induced by replacement of amniotic fluid with hypertonic saline, and showed striking haemorrhagic softening in the central brainstem. While this is topographically analogous to CPM, it cannot be inferred that CPM may be produced by haemorrhage following acute dehydration. As already stated, no vascular changes are ever seen in CPM. Nevertheless, these cases point to the possible vulnerability of the central pontine area to marked alterations in ionic concentration, and may offer a clue to the causation of CPM.

Adams et al (1959) regarded alcoholism as the possible cause of CPM, assuming either a direct toxic effect or an induced deficiency of vitamin B. A proportion of CPM patients are, it is true, alcoholics. Such patients may show such neuropathological stigmata of alcoholism and hypovitaminosis B as Wernicke's encephalopathy, atrophy of the cerebellar vermis, Morel's laminar cortical sclerosis (Monteiro, 1971), and pellagrous neuronal change (Cole, Richardson and Segarra, 1964). However, the fact remains that the majority of CPM patients are not alcoholic, and that many received vitamins in large doses. Alcohol, if ever directly responsible, cannot be the sole cause.

Severe hepatic disease, caused either by alcoholism or by hepatolenticular degeneration, has been reported in about 30 per cent of cases of CPM (Monseu and Flament-Durand, 1971). The degree of liver failure has been variable, some cases showing only minor laboratory evidence of impaired liver function. Quite apart from this, hepatic failure cannot seriously be considered as the cause of CPM. Extensive demyelination of the brainstem is not one of the neuropathological features of liver failure, whether acute or chronic, human or experimentally induced.

The aetiology of CPM remains unknown. The disorder may well represent the effect, on a susceptible region of the brain, of a combination of insults, including altered serum osmolality and nutritional deprivation. This, however, is speculation. An exogenous toxic cause may eventually be incriminated. For the present we need only remind both gastroenterologists and internists —in whose wards further cases are most likely to occur—of the existence of this mysterious and lethal neurological condition.

References

Adams, J. H. (1962). Central pontine myelinolysis. In *Proceedings of 4th International Congress of Neuropathology, München*, 1961, ed. Jacob, H., vol. 3, pp. 303–308. Stuttgart: Thieme.

Adams, R. D., Victor, M. & Mancall, E. L. (1959). Central pontine myelinolysis. A hitherto undescribed disease occurring in alcoholic and malnourished patients. *Archives of Neurology and Psychiatry*, **81**, 154–172.

Aleu, F. P. & Terry, R. D. (1963). Central pontine myelinolysis. A report of two cases. *Archives of Pathology*, **76**, 140–146.

Boudin, G., Labet, R., Lyon, G. & Brunet, P. (1963). La myélinolyse centrale de la protubérance. *Presse médicale*, **71**, 2080–2082.

Cadman, J. E. & Rorke, L. B. (1969). Central pontine myelinolysis in childhood and adolescence. *Archives of Disease in Childhood*, **44**, 342–350.

Cameron, J. M. & Dayan, A. D. (1966). Association of brain damage with therapeutic abortion induced by amniotic fluid replacement: report of two cases. *British Medical Journal*, **1**, 1010–1013.

Cole, M., Richardson, E. P. & Segarra, J. M. (1964). Central pontine myelinolysis. Further evidence relating lesion to malnutrition. *Neurology (Minneapolis)*, **14**, 165–170.

Conger, J. D., McIntyre, J. A. & Jacoby, W. J. (1969). Central pontine myelinolysis associated with inappropriate antidiuretic hormone secretion. *American Journal of Medicine*, **47**, 813–817.

Goebel, H. H. & Zur, P. H. B. (1972). Central pontine myelinolysis. A clinical and pathological study of 10 cases. *Brain*, **95**, 495–504.

Green, D., Sung, J. H. & Wolf, A. (1962). Central pontine myelinolysis (abstracted). *Neurology (Minneapolis)*, **12**, 302.

Kepes, J. J., Reece, C. A. and Oxley, D. K. (1965). Central pontine myelinolysis in a 7 year old boy. *Journal of Neurology, Neurosurgery and Psychiatry*, **28**, 39–47.

Klintworth, G. K. (1965). The pathogenesis of secondary brainstem haemorrhages as studied in an experimental model. *American Journal of Pathology*, **47**, 523–536.

Landers, J. W., Chason, J. L. & Samuel, V. N. (1965). Central pontine myelinolysis. A pathogenetic hypothesis. *Neurology (Minneapolis)*, **15**, 968–971.

Lüthy, F. (1931). Über die hepato-lentikuläre Degeneration (Wilson–Westphal–Strümpell). *Deutsche Zeitschrift für Nervenheilkunde*, **123**, 101–181.

Mathieson, G. & Olszewski, J. (1960). Central pontine myelinolysis with other cerebral changes. *Neurology*, **10**, 345–354.

McCormick, W. F. & Danneel, C. M. (1967). Central pontine myelinolysis. *Archives of Internal Medicine*, **119**, 444–478.

Minauf, M. & Jellinger, K. (1970). Zentrale pontine Myelinolyse bei einem Kind mit protrahiertem posttraumatischen Koma. *Neuropädiatrie*, **2**, 107–111.

Monseu, G. & Flament-Durand, J. (1971). Pathogenesis of central pontine myelinolysis. A clinical and pathological description of three cases. *Pathologia europaea*, **6**, 75–94.

Monteiro, L. (1971). La myélinolyse du centre du pont dans le cadre d'un nouveau syndrome histopathologique de topographie systématisée. A propos d'un cas anatomo-clinique. *Journal of the Neurological Sciences*, **13**, 293–314.

Paguirigan, A. & Lefken, E. B. (1969). Cental pontine myelinolysis. *Neurology (Minneapolis)*, **19**, 1007–1011.

Schneck, S. A. (1966). Neuropathological features of human organ transplantation. Central pontine myelinolysis and neuroaxonal dystrophy. *Journal of Neuropathology and Experimental Neurology*, **25**, 18–39.

Seitelberger, F. & Jonasch, G. (1970). Zentrale pontine Myelinolyse nach Schädeltrauma. Klinisch-anatomische und pathogenetische Studie. *Deutsche Zeitschrift für Nervenheilkunde*, **197**, 28–41.

Tihen, W. S. (1972). Central pontine myelinolysis and Rosenthal fibers of the brainstem. Association with emaciation and prolonged intravenous hyperalimentation. *Neurology (Minneapolis)*, **22**, 710–716.

Valsamis, M. P., Peress, N. P. & Wright, L. D. (1971). Central pontine myelinolysis in childhood. *Archives of Neurology*, **25**, 307–312.

CHAPTER ELEVEN

Neurological Complications of Infective Diarrhoeas

A number of severe bacterial and protozoal infections of the alimentary tract, uncommon to-day in Northern Europe and North America but widespread in many other parts of the globe, will be discussed here. Their nervous complications have been largely ignored, even in those standard textbooks of neurology printed and read in the 'Third World'. Arbitrarily perhaps, the neurological problems arising from treatment with the antidiarrhoeal remedy, clioquinol, will also be briefly considered.

BACILLARY DYSENTERY

An earlier generation of neurologists, anxious to find causes for obscure diseases, often inculpated the infectious diarrhoeas. Turning the pages of Kinnier Wilson's textbook (1954), we find dysentery or cholera named as a frequent cause of encephalitis and as an occasional cause of transverse myelitis, spinal arachnoiditis, ulnar neuritis, tetany and myoclonus. Yet if we consult the writings of contemporary physicians who dealt with large numbers of dysenteric or choleraic patients, we find no mention of these alleged sequelae. Neurologists seem to be as capable as most other people in papering over the cracks in their knowledge.

Polyneuropathy

The only neurological complication of bacillary dysentery that can be said to be well-documented is polyneuropathy. Manson-Bahr (1939) wrote that 'peripheral neuropathy may follow bacillary dysentery, as it does many other specific infections. This has been doubted, but the author has seen so many cases following on dysentery epidemics that he is inclined to believe there is some connection between the two. The legs are usually affected, with loss of knee-jerks, glossy, atrophic skin, oedema of the ankles, and hyperaesthesia of the calves. This condition may persist for several months.'

Other authors describe similar cases. Predominantly sensory symptoms, including cramp-like pains in the calf muscles, affected 1 per cent of patients in one epidemic (Bittorf, 1918). The patient reported by Biggam (1929) as having 'peripheral neuritis' as a complication of bacillary dysentery is interesting; he appears to be an early case of neuralgic amyotrophy following the administration of serum, coeval with Foster Kennedy's (1929) report but antedating Parsonage and Turner's (1948) classic description of the syndrome by some 19 years.

Until an adequate number of new cases comes under expert scrutiny, we can only speculate on the pathogenesis of dysenteric neuropathy. Multiple nutritional deficiencies, exacerbated by the acute illness in a poorly nourished population, probably play a part. Some of the older writers on the subject implicate a 'secondary toxic process', i.e. one unrelated to the local effects on the bowel of the heat-stable Shigella endotoxins. This takes us into an area of bacteriological controversy, for one antigenic variety of Shigella, *S. dysenteriae* Type 1, does produce a toxin with severe systemic effects, particularly marked on the nervous system. The existence of this toxin in vivo, and its role in the production of dysentery in man, has been hotly disputed. The Shigella neurotoxin was discovered by Conradi (1903), who found that autolysates of 18-hour cultures of *S. dysenteriae* produced paralysis, diarrhoea, collapse and death within 48 hours when injected intravenously into rabbits. Dopter (Vaillard and Dopter, 1903; Dopter, 1905) showed a clear neuropathological basis for the paralysis. The anterior horn cells of his rabbits were chromatolytic, with foci of grey matter necrosis and many small interstitial haemorrhages. Subsequent workers demonstrated that the potent bacterial autolysate contained a mixture of toxins. The neurotoxin was ultimately categorised as a highly antigenic, relatively heat-labile protein, with a molecular weight of about 75 000 (Engley, 1952). It produces lesions in the central nervous system of mice as well as rabbits (Cavanagh, Howard and Whitby, 1956), and is a natural tool, neglected by neuropathologists in recent years, in the experimental study of postexanthematous encephalitis. There is no evidence, however, that this toxin, or *S. dysenteriae* Type 1, bears any relation to the occurrence of encephalitis in man.

Encephalopathy

A proportion of patients with shigellosis do in fact develop an encephalopathy. This is especially liable to occur in children, and it has been reported that as many as 30 per cent of dysenteric children under the age of seven may have febrile convulsions (Kowlessar and Forbes, 1958). These may appear at the same time as abdominal symptoms, or even antedate them by a few hours, creating a diagnostic problem. The onset of encephalopathic symptoms and signs—irritability, vertigo, headache, neck stiffness and fits—may be dramatic, and in the pre-chemotherapeutic era this form of the disease had a grave prognosis. Tanaka (1924) reported that dysentery was a frequent cause of encephalopathy in Japanese infants in the summer months, death generally occurring within three days of the fulminating onset. In his series, 106 out of 400 children with dysentery were so affected.

In adults similar but less severe manifestations occur, including confusion, delirium, drowsiness, and even coma (Alexander and Wu, 1934; Zellweger,

1943). Recovery is the rule and there is no convincing evidence that recognisable central nervous lesions occur.

Evanescent Parkinsonism, reported from time to time in typhoid fever (see p. 179) has been seen in association with bacillary dysentery. Pott Hofstede (1928) described a case occurring in a young Chinese male, with onset of neurological symptoms five days after the start of abdominal symptoms.

CHOLERA

Like bacillary dysentery, cholera is a disease which primarily affects the alimentary tract. Death results from intestinal fluid loss, hypovolaemia and anuria. The major clinical features are so self-evident, and treatment of such overriding importance, that relatively minor neurological signs and symptoms might well escape recognition. Physicians experienced in dealing with the disease have however reported occasional nervous manifestations. Seizures may occur in the acute stage of the illness and after rehydration, while in young children a picture of pyrexial convulsions, meningeal irritation and encephalopathy has been reported (Gavino, 1927). Muscle weakness, occasionally described, may well be related to hypokalaemia. 'Psychiatric' disturbances are said to occur in the recovery phase but are presumably linked to the severe biochemical changes which follow fluid loss; they are rather more frequently seen than neurological abnormalities, and include sleep disorders, apathy and severe delirium. Prolonged depression in the convalescent period has been seen in some cases. No clear neuropathological picture emerges from the study of the brains of patients dead from cholera, and the minor changes which have been noted are of dubious significance (Choudhury, 1969).

As with typhoid vaccination, occasional neurological complications may follow *anticholera vaccination*, an important point to remember at times of epidemics and mass prophylaxis. Georgiev, Yordanov and Chukova Bojinova (1971) described the neurological symptoms and signs in six cases following such vaccination, both first and second injections and revaccination being responsible in one or other of their patients. In three cases central nervous symptoms and signs indicating brainstem encephalitis were noted. An associated psychosis was present. One patient developed a facial palsy, another had signs of involvement of the nervus intermedius and eighth cranial nerve, while another had a Guillain–Barré polyneuritis. Full recovery occurred within a few weeks.

AMOEBIASIS

Entamoeba histolytica, the protozoon causing amoebic dysentery, is an uncommon cause of neurological disease. Meningoencephalitis due to other genera of amoeba (especially Naegleriae which are free-living and do not primarily affect the alimentary tract) is, however, being increasingly recognised (Dos Santos Neto, 1970).

Amoebic abscess of the brain is almost always secondary to amoebic abscesses of lung or liver, themselves complications of the primary intestinal infection. Amoebic brain abscess is, nevertheless, a rare development, for while liver abscesses may be present in as many as 50 per cent of cases of amoebic dysentery coming to autopsy, no more than 3 per cent of these cases show cerebral involvement (Clark, 1925). The highest reported incidence in amoebiasis is only 8 per cent (Lombardo et al, 1964).

Surgical operation on an amoebic liver abscess is sometimes directly responsible for spread to the brain, as in the patient of Stout and Fenwick (1918) who died three months after abdominal exploration and excision of a liver abscess. Amoebic brain abscess should usually be suspected when patients with amoebiasis and evidence of liver and lung lesions develop a picture of meningitis, with raised intracranial pressure and focal cerebral symptoms or signs. Fever, in this condition, is said to be moderate rather than severe. The early literature on the subject was reviewed by Armitage (1919) who noted that in the majority of patients death occurred six to eight days after the onset of pyrexia.

Pathologically, amoebic brain abscesses show a gliotic capsule in the more chronic cases and a necrotic core containing many lipid-laden macrophages and easily recognisable organisms. Stein and Kozan (1942) recommend Best's carmine as an aid to the identification of amoebae, though the latter are readily seen in ordinary preparations stained with haematoxylin and eosin.

Occasionally *Entamoeba histolytica* produces a purulent meningoencephalitis without abscess formation. Villegas-González (1970) reported the case of a two-month-old boy with massive amoebic invasion of the brain. Four days after birth he developed bloody diarrhoea, fever and meningitis. By the time of death motile forms of *Entamoeba histolytica* had been recovered from faeces and from pus draining from a liver abscess. At autopsy the meninges showed a dense, mixed acute and chronic inflammatory infiltrate and many organisms, and the choroid plexus showed vascular necrosis in association with amoebic colonisation. Such cases, although rare, illustrate the lethal effects of brain invasion by an organism normally restricted to the gut, liver or lung.

TYPHOID FEVER

In contrast to bacillary dysentery and cholera, typhoid fever is a septicaemic illness. It is hardly surprising that neurological complications are often seen.

The most common of these complications are 'psychiatric'. Although often appearing in the first few days of fever they sometimes develop later in the course of the disease or may even appear during convalescence. They include acute toxic confusional states and transient psychoses of various types which usually clear up during recovery. Meningeal involvement is seen in many patients. It often presents as a relatively mild disturbance with headache, photophobia and slight neck stiffness (in which case the cerebrospinal fluid is likely to be normal). Occasionally there is a severe meningitis. Such meningeal infection may be due to a combination of bacteria. The patient may become comatose and show focal and long-tract neurological signs, the cerebrospinal fluid then usually containing many pus cells and organisms.

Parenchymatous central nervous involvement by *Salmonella typhi* produces a multiplicity of neurological abnormalities, including (Albos, 1957) aphasia, epilepsy, hemiplegia, disorders of movement (both extrapyramidal and cerebellar) and disturbances of autonomic function suggesting pathological changes at both brainstem and hypothalamic levels. Visual failure has also been described. Spinal cord infection may result in paraplegia: this may be an immediate consequence of the disease or a long-delayed sequel. Some cases of chronic spinal arachnoiditis have been attributed to previous typhoid infection (Elkington, 1936).

Peripheral neuropathy has also been reported from time to time. Facial palsy occurring with typhoid fever has been described, while other patients have had a mononeuritis or polyneuritis. The latter is predominantly sensory, involves the legs and is accompanied by much calf tenderness. Occasionally, it is of the Guillain–Barré type (Chanmugam and Waniganetti, 1969).

The reported prevalence of neurological and psychiatric complications of typhoid fever has varied widely. This is hardly surprising when one takes into account the differences, from country to country, in affected populations and in standards of medical care. However, it seems that a confusional state is seen in about half of all typhoid patients (Stuart and Pullen, 1946; Ikeme and Anan, 1966), while marked impairment of consciousness occurs in up to 15 per cent of patients (Stuart and Pullen, 1946; Rowland, 1961).

In recent years many useful observations have come from West Africa (e.g. Ikeme and Anan, 1966; Lafaix et al, 1968). Of these, the largest and best-documented series is that of Osuntokun and his colleagues (1972). These authors found that in 959 Nigerian patients confusional states occurred in 57 per cent, meningism in 5 per cent, coma in 3·6 per cent, meningitis in 0·2 per cent, convulsions in 1·7 per cent, and generalised myoclonus in 0·5 per cent. Evanescent Parkinsonism was observed in 1 per cent of their patients and short-lived symmetrical spasticity of all limbs in 3·1 per cent. Seven patients had a sensorimotor polyneuropathy without abnormality of the cerebrospinal fluid. One patient developed an unusual picture resembling motor neurone disease two months after recovery from typhoid: follow-up examination showed no deterioration in the ensuing nine months. Cases with neurological abnormalities who came to autopsy failed to show significant lesions in the central nervous system. The pathogenesis of these manifestations is still obscure.

NEUROLOGICAL COMPLICATIONS OF CLIOQUINOL THERAPY

Clioquinol, a halogenated hydroxyquinoline compound (5-chloro-7-iodo-8-quinolinol) is taken in many parts of the world in the hope of preventing gastrointestinal infections. The drug is also used in the treatment of diarrhoea. The major part of any ingested dose passes through the alimentary tract unabsorbed, where it is supposed to have a local antiseptic effect. A proportion is absorbed, some being rapidly excreted in a conjugated form, but the remainder persisting in the body for months. It is this absorbed fraction which may be responsible for the clinical syndromes here described.

There is doubt as to whether clioquinol has any significant prophylactic or therapeutic action (Martindale, 1972; Schultz, 1972). Less doubtful seem to be its neurotoxic effects. Circumstantial evidence has accumulated to link it with a disease seen in Japan and known as subacute myelo-optico-neuropathy or SMON.

At the time of writing it is difficult to survey this field without a sense of being caught up in wider issues. These include the deep need, felt in Japan, to define the cause of a new and disabling disease of sizeable proportion—but also some significant objections, put forward by the pharmaceutical interests concerned. We have tried to be as objective as possible in this developing controversy, but recognise that such objectivity may only be possible with hindsight.

SMON was first noted in Japan in the mid-1950s. More than 10 000 cases were estimated to have occurred there up to the end of 1970. Very few similar cases have been reported outside Japan, although Scandinavian, other European, and Australian occurrences have been convincingly described.

One of the largest and best-documented series is that of Sobue et al (1971a, b). Significantly, 84 per cent of the 1090 cases seen by these authors at Nagoya between 1956 and 1970 had suffered from a pre-existing chronic gastrointestinal disorder. In about two-thirds of these diarrhoea had been the main feature, while the remainder had suffered from abdominal pain. In most cases these symptoms were of long standing, having been present for over six years in 60 per cent and for over 11 years in 40 per cent. Sobue and his colleagues submitted their paper (1971a) for publication in May 1970. At that time the relationship of SMON to antidiarrhoeal therapy had not been fully explored, and the report makes no mention of any treatment the patients might have been receiving for their abdominal complaints.

The initial symptoms of SMON were claimed also to be abdominal, consisting either of severe, deep, burning *pain*—without features of colic or peritonitis—or *diarrhoea*, bloody in a proportion of patients. In two-thirds of all cases diarrhoea and pain persisted after the development of neurological disease. It is not clear to what extent these alleged prodromata were premonitory of SMON, or simply exacerbations of a pre-existing and unrelated gastroenterological disorder. It is likely that burning abdominal pain was a true prodromal symptom in many cases, since it often disappeared before neurological signs developed, while diarrhoea usually persisted.

The neurology of SMON is the result of damage to the spinal cord, and to the optic and peripheral nerves. The disease developed acutely in 60 per cent of the patients described by Sobue et al (1971a), subacutely in the remainder. The first symptoms were numbness or unpleasant paraesthesiae in the feet, numbness and weakness of the legs, pain in the legs and feet, paraesthesiae of the hands, and blurring of vision. Sensory disturbances often ascended from the lower extremities, reaching an indefinite upper level at about groin level. Objective sensory impairment, most marked distally, was almost always found. Touch, pain and vibratory sensation were equally affected. Two out of three SMON patients had an ataxic gait, but only one in two had objective weakness of the lower limbs, usually mild to moderate in degree. In some of the most severe cases there was a complete flaccid paraplegia. Reflexes in the lower limbs were usually abnormal, a combination of exaggerated knee jerks and reduced or absent ankle jerks being found in 23 per cent of cases. Extensor plantar responses were elicitable in 8 per cent.

Impaired bladder function was present in 16 per cent of patients. A few had weakness of the hands, or symptoms and signs of involvement of the lower cranial nerves. In contrast, the optic nerves were frequently involved, and 28 per cent of cases had decreased visual acuity from optic neuritis. Several patients had encephalopathic manifestations, such as convulsions and disturbances of consciousness.

After the acute stage, the illness followed a chronic course, with relapses in a proportion of cases. Sobue et al (1971a) observed 684 patients for periods of six months to 10 years; 6·6 per cent died, 7·4 per cent deteriorated and 24·8 per cent remained in an unchanged condition; 54·3 per cent showed some improvement, although sensory symptoms, especially unpleasant paraesthesiae, almost always persisted. Only 6·6 per cent of the patients recovered completely.

Standard laboratory investigations other than electrophysiological studies (which showed denervation in muscle and impaired conduction in peripheral nerves) were unhelpful.

Sural nerve biopsies (Sobue et al, 1971a; Miyakawa et al, 1970, 1971) revealed evidence of both axonal and Schwann cell damage. The neuropathological findings at autopsy have been well described by Shiraki (1971). In more acute cases axonal damage predominates. Chronic cases show myelin loss and gliosis of dorsal columns, and to a lesser extent, anterior and lateral columns. Distal parts of long tracts are selectively involved, suggesting an initial Wallerian degeneration. Optic nerves are demyelinated and neurones of Sommer's sector and olivary nuclei unequivocally damaged.

Little attention has been devoted to the study of the abdominal, as distinct from the neurological, symptomatology of SMON. Noda et al (1970) in a detailed review of this subject point out that, in the 36 patients they had studied, the duration of abdominal symptoms had 'ranged from less than a day to several years'. Symptoms had usually been present for less than a month. Many patients had shown features of paralytic ileus in addition to pain and diarrhoea. Abdominal pain was usually epigastric, occasionally spreading through to the back. These patients have repeatedly been described as having a low pain threshold and of being of an introspective nature—although no one has suggested in so many words that these characteristics might be associated with a tendency to self-medication. Ten of the 36 patients reported by Noda and his colleagues had previously undergone abdominal surgery for conditions as diverse as cholelithiasis, peptic ulcer, appendicitis and endometritis.

Changes in the intestinal mucosa, detected at necropsy or biopsy (Noda et al, 1970) have consisted of marked cellular infiltration, mainly with plasma cells and lymphocytes, shortening and degeneration of the villi, and degeneration and necrosis of the mucosal epithelium. On electron microscopy the cytoplasm of the enterocytes contained small vesicles, droplets and virus-like particles, 130–180 μm [sic] in diameter, 'covered with a membranous structure'. Similar findings, predominating in the colon, were reported by Takeuchi et al (1971).

The extraordinary clinical variability of this gastroenterological syndrome raises serious doubts, in our minds, as to whether we are dealing with a single entity. The implication of these doubts is that one must look for some factor, or factors, other than the gastroenterological disorder itself, as being responsible for the development of the neuropathy. Drugs used in the treatment of the diarrhoea should clearly be considered.

Doubt also arises as to the neurological homogeneity of SMON. Japanese authors repeatedly discuss multiple sclerosis and SCD in the differential diagnosis of the condition. Myelopathy and neuropathy due to vitamin B_{12} deficiency can readily be excluded by appropriate tests although multiple sclerosis may, in some cases, be more difficult to disprove. It seems probable that some patients with alleged 'SMON' may in fact have been suffering from multiple sclerosis. As late as 1970 Japanese neurologists were faced by the problem of an obscure disease, characterised by the combination of lesions of the posterior and lateral columns, and of peripheral and optic nerves. Parallel (although far from identical) situations had been encountered in the West Indies (Montgomery et al, 1964) and in West Africa (Osuntokun, 1968). In Japan the position was suddenly and radically to be changed by the inculpation of an exogenous toxic agent.

Through 1971, the correspondence columns of the *Lancet* contained a series of letters increasingly implicating clioquinol therapy in the genesis of SMON. Tsubaki, Honma and Hoshi (1971) studied 263 patients with various gastroenterological complaints given 0·6 to 1·5 g clioquinol daily, and compared their neurological symptoms and signs with those in 706 similar patients not receiving this drug. No neurological symptoms were observed in the larger group, but in 44 (16·7 per cent) of the patients taking clioquinol neurological symptoms were present. Of 110 patients given clioquinol for more than 14 days, 40 (35·4 per cent) developed such symptoms, while of 153 patients receiving this treatment for a shorter period only four (2·6 per cent) had evidence of a neurological disturbance. A diagnosis of SMON was suspected in two-thirds of the neurologically affected cases and clinically confirmed in one-third.

The authors went on to conduct an epidemiological survey of clioquinol ingestion in cases of SMON. They found that 166 of 171 patients with SMON had taken clioquinol, mainly for digestive disorders, before the onset of their neurological symptoms. The cases had occurred in patients under treatment in many hospitals and clinics throughout Japan, where it appears that clioquinol is certainly administered more freely and in possibly larger dosage than elsewhere in the world. Nakae et al (1973) later pointed out that during the period of peak prevalence of the disease 184 drugs containing clioquinol could be purchased over the counter in Japan. The average daily dose ingested by SMON cases had risen from 1·1 g (in 1964) to 1·3 g (in 1969). In relation to body weight this is considerably more than in other countries. In Japan 90 per cent of prescribed hydroxyquinolines had been dispensed in powder form, whereas in other countries these drugs were usually taken as tablets. Tsubaki et al (1971) also noted that the increasing incidence of SMON in the late 1950s and 1960s paralleled the increasing production and sale of clioquinol in Japan. After the Japanese Ministry of Health prohibited the drug in September 1970 there was an abrupt and striking fall in the incidence of new cases.

Further evidence implicating clioquinol was reported by Igata (1971). In 1970, SMON patients were noted often to have a greenish, hairy tongue and at times to pass green faeces. Some patients also passed green urine. The abnormal colour was found to be due to an iron chelate of clioquinol. In addition, the urine contained large amounts of free (unconjugated) clioquinol. Igata presented other evidence incriminating clioquinol in the genesis of SMON, including observations on the production of SMON in previously healthy patients by the 'prophylactic' administration of the drug, and the induction of peripheral nerve lesions experimentally in rabbits. Construction of a time–dose curve indicated that a daily dose below 0·5 g could be continued indefinitely without risk of nervous damage, while a dose over 1 g was likely to be neurotoxic if maintained for a fortnight. Daily doses approaching 2 g were toxic within a shorter period (Igata, 1971; Igata and Toyokura, 1971a, b; Nakae et al, 1971).

Cases with features similar to SMON have now been reported from Switzerland (Kaeser and Wüthrich, 1970), Sweden (Osterman, 1971), Great Britain (McEwen, 1971; Spillane, 1972) and the Netherlands (Bron et al, 1972). Eight cases have been reported from Australia (Selby, 1972, 1973) in patients receiving daily doses of clioquinol of the order of 1·5 g. A case has also been described in North America (Kean, 1972).

Other syndromes of clioquinol neurotoxicity have been documented. Ataxia was reported in a few American patients taking 750 mg daily for one and a half to four years, as prophylaxis against amoebiasis and shigellosis (Gholz and Arons, 1964). Polyneuropathy occurred in another patient described by Kaeser and Wüthrich (1970). Optic atrophy developed in an infant with severe acrodermatitis enteropathica who received the drug in a dose of more than 1·2 g daily for 11 months (Berggren and Hansson, 1966). and possibly in a 47-year-old woman subsequently reported by the same authors (Berggren and Hansson, 1968). Acute encephalopathy with retrograde amnesia, perhaps due to selective temporal lobe damage, has also been described in patients taking large doses over short periods (Kaeser and Scollo-Lavizzari, 1970; Kjaersgaard, 1971).

Tateishi and his co-workers (Tateishi et al, 1971; Tateishi et al, 1972a, b, c) claim to have produced acute and chronic neurological disturbances in mongrel dogs, beagles, cats and one monkey following the administration of a wide variety of doses of clioquinol, for very variable periods. The authors claim that their findings were 'well in accord with the changes observed in SMON in man' (Tateishi et al, 1971) and that they had produced a 'myeloneuropathy identical clinically as well as pathologically with SMON' (Tateishi et al, 1972a). In their more acute cases, however, 'optic and peripheral neuropathies were not obvious' at necropsy, the changes predominating in the *central* nervous system. Igata (1971) briefly reported the production of peripheral neuropathy in rabbits following the administration of clioquinol.

On the other hand, Hess et al (1972) described experiments in rats, cats, rabbits and beagles which failed to furnish evidence that clioquinol was neurotoxic. Pharmacokinetic studies in beagles showed that the repeated oral administration of 30 mg/kg/day of clioquinol—for seven days—did not lead to any increase in the blood or tissue concentrations of the substance compared with the concentration determined after a single dose. While the methodology of many of the Japanese experiments is suspect, we feel that much of this animal work is of limited relevance to the occurrence of SMON *in man*. Of greater significance might be information concerning the absorption of clioquinol from the inflamed human intestinal mucosa. As far as we know such information is lacking.

Not all patients developing SMON can be shown to have ingested clioquinol. Shimada and Tsuji (1971) examined 113 patients with the disease, whose drug intake was definitely known, and found that 21·2 per cent had not taken this particular drug. Inoue (1971) claimed that 14·8 per cent of patients with SMON had not taken clioquinol. Sobue and Ando (1971), in a special report prepared for the SMON Research Unit, studied the time relationship between the onset of neurological and gastroenterological symptoms, with special reference to the administration of clioquinol. Adequate data were available on 256 cases. In 25 patients abdominal symptoms developed simultaneously with or subsequent to the development of neurological symptoms. Although clioquinol was eventually given in such cases it is difficult to see how it could be implicated in the pathogenesis of the neurological disorder (unless, of course, it had previously been taken 'prophylactically'). If one believes that clioquinol intoxication is the cause of SMON, one is confronted with an embarrassing dilemma. The occurrence of those cases of SMON who have apparently not taken clioquinol must represent either the proportion of cases misdiagnosed as SMON or the proportion of cases of SMON who, for some reason or another, were reluctant to admit to their 'prophylactic' use of clioquinol. Familiar though we are with problems of purgative addiction in the West, we are totally ignorant of the customs and attitudes determining the continuous ingestion, in Japan, of substances known as 'sei-cho-zai', roughly translatable as drugs 'active in normalising enteric function' (Nelson, 1972).

Agents other than clioquinol have been incriminated in the aetiology of SMON. Inoue, Nishibe and Nakamura (1971) reported the isolation of a virus from the stools and spinal fluid of most SMON patients in whom it had been sought. The virus was grown in BAT 6 (hamster tumour cell) cultures, had a weak cytopathic effect and was pathogenic to mice, the pathological changes including spongy degeneration of the brain. A few weeks later Shimada and Tsuji (1971) reported the examination of the spinal cords of five patients who had died of SMON. Using rabbit antiserum to the virus previously isolated by Inoue et al (1971) they demonstrated fluorescence in the cytoplasm of anterior horn cells, in spinal ganglia and in the pia mater of four of the five spinal cords examined, suggesting the presence of virus antigen at these sites. The significance of this virus in the aetiology of SMON remains conjectural.

It has been suggested (*Lancet*, 1971) that some environmental pollutant might have caused diarrhoea and then SMON, the taking of clioquinol being an unrelated intermediate event. No such chemical poison, however, has as yet been identified. The possibility of genetic predisposition to SMON has been voiced, it being suggested that the Japanese may be more susceptible to the toxic effects of the drug by being less efficient at inactivating the absorbed fraction. No enzyme deficiency has as yet been demonstrated. However carefully one considers these various 'alternative' interpretations, one cannot escape the crucial fact that the vast majority of patients developing SMON have ingested large doses of clioquinol, an agent which may be neurotoxic to man.

In summary, it is our opinion that the large number of cases in Japan did not result from some genetic predisposition, abnormal enzyme, or locally endemic virus, but from the vast quantities of clioquinol ingested there. The cultural determinant of this dietary habit will doubtless be fruitful subject matter for future sociological study. The only significant objection to this view stems from the fact that clioquinol has been widely consumed, sometimes apparently on as large a scale and in as high a dosage as in Japan, in other countries—where, however, its presumed neurotoxic effects have largely eluded detection. Be this as it may, we think there may be a parallel between SMON and phenacetin-induced nephropathy, where a well-established drug, without obvious toxic effects in animals, produced disease of epidemic proportions, in some parts of the world.

In our opinion clioquinol is a compound probably capable of producing extensive and irreversible nerve damage. Until the matter is settled its continued sale for self-administration—in the dubious hope of preventing infectious diarrhoea—can have no medical justification.

References

Bacillary dysentery

Alexander, L. & Wu, T. T. (1934). Symptomatic involvement of the nervous system in different forms of dysentery. *Chinese Medical Journal*, **48**, 1–19.

Biggam, A. G. (1929). Peripheral neuritis as a complication of bacillary dysentery associated with treatment by antidysenteric serum. *Journal of the Royal Army Medical Corps*, **53**, 367–371.

Bittorf, A. (1918). Die Ruhrneuritis. *Deutsche medizinische Wochenschrift*, **44**, 567–568.

Cavanagh, J. B., Howard, J. G. & Whitby, J. L. (1956). The neurotoxin of *Shigella shigae*. A comparative study of the effects produced in various laboratory animals. *British Journal of Experimental Pathology*, **37**, 272–278.

Conradi, H. (1903). Ueber lösliche, durch aseptische Autolyse erhaltene Giftstoffe von Ruhr—und Typhus-bazillen. *Deutsche Medizinische Wochenschrift*, **29**, 26–28.

Dopter, C. (1905). Effets experimentaux de la toxine dysenterique sur le système nerveux central. *Comptes rendus de la Société de Biologie*, **58**, 400–402.

Engley, F. B. Jr (1952). The neurotoxin of *Shigella dysenteriae* (Shiga). *Bacteriological Reviews*, **16**, 153–178.

Kennedy, F. (1929). Certain nervous complications following the use of therapeutic and prophylactic sera. *The American Journal of the Medical Sciences*, **177**, 555–559.

Kowlessar, M. & Forbes, G. B. (1958). The febrile convulsion in shigellosis. *New England Journal of Medicine*, **258**, 520–526.

Manson-Bahr, P. (1939). *The Dysenteric Disorders*, p. 75. London: Cassell.

Parsonage, M. J. & Turner, J. W. A. (1948). Neuralgic amyotrophy. The shoulder-girdle syndrome. *Lancet*, **1**, 973–978.

Pott Hofstede, G. W. (1928). Een geval von Parkinsonisme bij bacillaire dysenterie. *Psychiatrische en neurologische bladen*, **32**, 394–397.

Tanaka, T. (1924). Über die Hirnsymptome bei der foudroyant verlaufenden Kinder-dysenterie und Ekiri. *Mitteilungen aus der medizinischen Fakultät der Kaiserl. Universität, Kyushu*, **9**, 139–171.

Vaillard, L. & Dopter, C. (1903). La dysenterie épidémique. *Annales de l'Institut Pasteur*, **17**, 463–491.

Wilson, S. A. K. (1954). *Neurology*, 2nd edition. London: Butterworth.

Zellweger, H. (1943). Ueber die neurologische Komplikationen der Dysenterie. *Praxis*, **32**, 707–712.

Cholera

Gavino, C. (1927). Cholera cases admitted in San Lazaro Hospital from September 1 to November 30 1925. *Journal of the Philippine Islands Medical Association*, **7**, 3–7.

Choudhury, R. P. (1969). Effects of cholera on the human hypothalamus and hypophysis. II. *Journal of Tropical Medicine and Hygiene*, **72**, 185–192.

Georgiev, I., Yordanov, B. & Chukova Bojinova, T. (1971). [Nervous system complications following anticholera vaccination.] (in Bulgarian) *Neurologia, psihiatria, neurochirurgia*, **10**, 380–383.

Amoebiasis

Armitage, F. L. (1919). Amoebic abscess of the brain: with notes on a case following amoebic abscess of the lung. *Journal of Tropical Medicine*, **22**, 69–76.

Clark, H. C. (1925). The distribution and complications of amebic lesions found in 186 post mortem examinations. *American Journal of Tropical Medicine and Hygiene*, **5**, 157–171.

Dos Santos Neto, J. G. (1970). Fatal primary amebic meningoencephalitis: a retrospective study in Richmond, Virginia. *American Journal of Clinical Pathology*, **54**, 737–742.

Lombardo, L., Alonso, P., Saénz-Arroyo, L., Brandt, H. & Mateos, J. H. (1964). Cerebral amebiasis. Report of 17 cases. *Journal of Neurosurgery*, **21**, 704–709.

Stein, A. & Kozan, A. (1942). Brain abscess due to *Entameba histolytica*. *Journal of Neuropathology and Experimental Neurology*, **1**, 32–41.

Stout, T. D. M. & Fenwick, D. E. (1918). A case of amoebic abscess of the liver and brain with no previous history of dysentery. *Lancet*, **1**, 769.

Villegas-González, J. (1970). Invasion cerebral por Entamoeba histolytica en el lactante. *Archivos de Investigación medica*, **1**, 109–120.

Typhoid fever

Albos, J. (1957). Encéphalopathies typhiques infantiles. *Archives françaises de Pédiatrie*, **14**, 526–531.

Chanmugam, D. & Waniganetti, A. (1969). Guillain-Barré syndrome associated with typhoid fever. *British Medical Journal*, **1**, 95–96.

Elkington, J. St. C. (1936). Meningitis serosa circumscripta spinalis (spinal arachnoiditis). *Brain*, **59**, 181–203.

Ikeme, A. C. & Anan, C. O. (1966). A clinical review of typhoid fever in Ibadan, Nigeria. *Journal of Tropical Medicine and Hygiene*, **69**, 15–21.

Lafaix, C., Rey, M., Diop Mar, I. & Alihonou, E. (1968). Manifestations encéphalitiques de la fièvre typhoïde (dix-sept observations). *Bulletin de la Société médicale de l'Afrique noire de langue française*, **13**, 517–524.

Osuntokun, B. O., Bademosi, O., Ogunremi, K. & Wright, S. G. (1972). Neuropsychiatric manifestations of typhoid fever in 959 patients. *Archives of Neurology*, **27**, 7–13.

Rowland, H. A. K. (1961). The complications of typhoid fever. *Journal of Tropical Medicine and Hygiene*, **64**, 143–152.

Stuart, B. M. & Pullen, R. L. (1946). Typhoid: clinical analysis of three hundred and sixty cases. *Archives of Internal Medicine*, **78**, 629–661.

Neurological complications of clioquinol therapy

Berggren, L. & Hansson, O. (1966). Treating acrodermatitis enteropathica. *Lancet*, **1**, 52.

Berggren, L. & Hansson, O. (1968). Absorption of intestinal antiseptics derived from 8-hydroxyquinolines. *Clinical Pharmacology and Therapeutics*, **9**, 67–70.

Bron, H., Korten, J. J., Pinckers, A. & Majoor, G. (1972). Subacute myelo-optico neuropathie na het gebruik van grote hoelveelheden joodchloorhydroxychinoline (enterovioform). *Nederlands Tijdschrift voor geneeskunde*, **116**, 1615–1618.

Gholz, L. M. & Arons, W. L. (1964). Prophylaxis and therapy of amebiasis and shigellosis with iodochlorhydroxyquin. *American Journal of Tropical Medicine and Hygiene*, **13**, 396–401.

Hess, R., Keberle, H., Koella, W. P., Schmid, K. & Belzer, J. (1972). Clioquinol: absence of neurotoxicity in laboratory animals. *Lancet*, **2**, 424–425.

Igata, A. (1971). Halogenated oxyquinoline derivatives and neurological syndromes. *Lancet*, **2**, 42–43.

Igata, A. & Toyokura, Y. (1971a). Subakute Myelo-Optiko-Neuropathie (SMON) in Japan. Zur Frage der Chinoform-Vergiftung. *Münchener medizinische Wochenschrift*, **113**, 1062–1066.

Igata, A. & Toyokura, Y. (1971b). Clioquinol as causative agent of subacute myelo-optico-neuropathy (SMON) in Japan. *Third Asian and Oceanian Congress of Neurology Bombay, 29th November to 3rd December*, 1971. Abstracts of papers, p. 108.

Inoue, Y. K. (1971). The aetiology of SMON. *Lancet*, **2**, 869.

Inoue, Y. K., Nishibe, Y. & Nakamura, Y. (1971). Virus associated with S.M.O.N. in Japan. *Lancet*, **1**, 853–854.

Kaeser, H. E. & Scollo-Lavizzari, G. (1970). Akute zerebrale Störungen nach hohen Dosen eines Oxychinolinderivatives. *Deutsche medizinische Wochenschrift*, **95**, 394–397.

Kaeser, H. E. & Wüthrich, R. (1970). Zur Frage der Neurotoxizität der Oxychinoline. *Deutsche medizinische Wochenschrift*, **95**, 1685–1688.

Kean, B. H. (1972). Subacute myelo-optic-neuropathy. A probable case in the United States. *Journal of the American Medical Association*, **220**, 243–244.

Lancet (1971). Only in Japan? **1**, 690–691 (Editorial).

Kjærsgaard, K. (1971). Amnesia after clioquinol. *Lancet*, **2**, 1086.

McEwen, L. M. (1971). Neuropathy after clioquinol. *British Medical Journal*, **4**, 169–170.

Martindale, W. (1972). *The Extra Pharmacopoeia*, ed. Blacow, N. W., 26th edition, pp. 94–95. London: The Pharmaceutical Press.

Miyakawa, T., Sumiyoshi, S., Murayama, E., Deshimaru, M., Goto, K. & Tatetsu, S. (1971). Electron microscopical study of a nerve biopsy from a case in the chronic state of 'subacute myelo-optico-neuropathy'. *Acta neuropathologica*, **19**, 323–330.

Miyakawa, T., Sumiyoshi, S., Murayama, E., Ishikawa, H., Miyakawa, K. & Tatetsu, S. (1970). Ultrastructural study of a nerve and muscle biopsy from a case of 'subacute myelo-optico-neuropathy'. *Acta neuropathologica*, **16**, 17–24.

Montgomery, R. D., Cruickshank, E. K., Robertson, W. B. & McMenemey, W. H. (1964). Clinical and pathological observations on Jamaican neuropathy. *Brain*, **87**, 425–462.

Nakae, K., Yamamoto, S. & Igata, A. (1971). Subacute myelo-optic-neuropathy (SMON) in Japan. A community survey. *Lancet*, **2**, 510–512.

Nakae, K., Yamamoto, S., Shigematsu, I. & Kono, R. (1973). Relation between subacute myelo-optico-neuropathy (SMON) and clioquinol: nationwide survey. *Lancet*, **1**, 171–173.

Nelson, E. (1972). Subacute myelo-optico-neuropathy (SMON). *Annals of Internal Medicine*, **77**, 468–470.

Noda, A., Toda, Y., Hayakawa, T., Hitokawa, S., Hattori, T., Nagura, H., Nakano, S. & Nakamura, M. (1970). Gastroenterological approach to the abdominal symptoms of so-called subacute myelo-optic-neuropathy (SMON). *Saishin-Igaku*, **25**, 2542–2554. (In Japanese.)

Osterman, P. O. (1971). Myelopathy after clioquinol treatment. *Lancet*, **2**, 544.

Osuntokun, B. O. (1968). An ataxic neuropathy in Nigeria. A clinical, biochemical and electrophysiological study. *Brain*, **91**, 215–248.

Schultz, M. G. (1972). Enterovioform for preventing traveller's diarrhea (editorial). *Journal of the American Medical Association*, **220**, 273–274.

Selby, G. (1972). Subacute myelo-optic neuropathy in Australia. *Lancet*, **1**, 123–125.

Selby, G. (1973). Subacute myelo-optic neuropathy (SMON). Neurotoxicity of clioquinols. *Proceedings of the Australian Association of Neurologists*, **9**, 23–30.

Shimada, Y. & Tsuji, T. (1971). Halogenated oxyquinoline derivatives and neurological syndromes. *Lancet*, **2**, 41–42.

Shiraki, H. (1971). Neuropathology of subacute myelo-optico-neuropathy, 'SMON'. *Japanese Journal of Medical Science and Biology*, **24**, 217–243.

Sobue, I. & Ando, K. (1971). Time relationship between onsets of neurological symptoms and abdominal symptoms which are specific to SMON. *Proceedings of the SMON Research Unit of the Specific Diseases Research Unit*. Tokyo. (In Japanese.)

Sobue, I., Ando, K., Iida, M., Takayanagi, T., Yamamura, Y. & Matsuoka, Y. (1971a). Myelopathy with abdominal disorders in Japan. *Neurology (Minneapolis)*, **21**, 168–173.

Sobue, I., Ando, K., Iida, M., Takayanagi, T., Mukoyama, M. & Matsuoka, Y. (1971b). Subacute myelo-optico-neuropathy in Japan. *Third Asian and Oceanian Congress of Neurology, Bombay, 29th November to 3rd December* 1971. Abstracts of papers, p. 107.

Spillane, J. D. (1972). SMON. *Lancet*, **1**, 154.

Takeuchi, T., Sakurama, N., Etoh, N. & Miyayama, T. (1971). Pathological changes in the intestines of patients with SMON. *Annual Report of the SMON Research Committee, 1970*. Book no. 4: Reports of the Pathology Group.

Tateishi, J., Ikeda, H., Saito, A., Kuroda, S. & Otsuki, S. (1972a). Myeloneuropathy in dogs induced by iodoxyquinoline. *Neurology*, **22**, 702–709.

Tateishi, J., Kuroda, S., Saito, A. & Otsuki, S. (1971). Myelo-optic-neuropathy induced by clioquinol in animals. *Lancet*, **2**, 1263–1264.

Tateishi, J., Kuroda, S., Saito, A. & Otsuki, S. (1972b). Strain-differences in dogs for neurotoxicity of clioquinol. *Lancet*, **1**, 1289–1290.

Tateishi, J., Kuroda, S., Saito, A. & Otsuki, S. (1972c). Neurotoxicity of clioquinol in laboratory animals. *Lancet*, **2**, 1095.

Tsubaki, T., Honma, Y. & Hoshi, M. (1971). Neurological syndrome associated with clioquinol. *Lancet*, **1**, 696–697.

CHAPTER TWELVE

The Pancreas and the Nervous System

THE PANCREAS, HYPOGLYCAEMIA AND THE NERVOUS SYSTEM

Hypoglycaemia and its neurological effects are far too big a theme to be covered here. 'Non-pancreatic' causes, such as essential and postgastrectomy reactive hypoglycaemia, endocrine hypoglycaemia, and hypoglycaemia in inborn errors of metabolism, are in any event beyond the scope of this chapter. We propose here to look at some pancreatic causes of a low blood sugar, and to consider briefly certain extrapancreatic intestinal neoplasms which may produce the same effect.

A variety of neurological and neuropathological changes are seen in association with severe hypoglycaemia, whatever its cause. The clinical alterations are undoubtedly the result of an inadequate supply of glucose to the nervous system. Since glucose itself does not directly participate in any mechanism involved in neural activity, some alteration of a glucose-dependent metabolic process must be implicated as the ultimate cause of depressed nerve cell function. Because of the important role of glucose in making energy available (through the production of ATP) the neurological manifestations of hypoglycaemia are commonly ascribed to a failure of energy-supplying mechanisms (Lawrence, Meyer and Nevin, 1942). There is some experimental evidence, however, that this explanation is inadequate (Tarr, Brada and Samson, 1962; Ferrendelli and Chang, 1973). A disturbance of some other metabolic pathway utilising glucose has to be postulated. This biochemical lesion has yet to be worked out.

When hypoglycaemia affects the nervous system it produces a number of more or less recognisable clinical effects. In adults three distinct, but not mutually exclusive, syndromes can be defined (Marks and Rose, 1965). *Acute* hypoglycaemia results in tachycardia, sweating, flushing, confusion and coma, and is familiar to every clinician. *Subacute* hypoglycaemia may be harder to recognise, with its more subtle changes of diminished spontaneous activity, increasing somnolence and lethargy, and deterioration of social behaviour patterns and speech. Both of these syndromes are immediately and fully reversed by glucose. The third pattern, easily overlooked, is *chronic* hypoglycaemia. Patients suffering from this condition show a slow deterioration of higher mental function, resembling presenile dementia. On this may be superimposed a wide variety of neurological abnormalities including episodic, sometimes transient coma (due to acute hypoglycaemia) and such motor abnormalities as extrapyramidal rigidity and tremor, cerebellar ataxia and (rarely) lower motor neurone signs. Treatment will never restore such patients to normal because irreversible pathological changes have taken place.

The cellular alterations in the brain in the more acute forms of hypoglycaemia are said to be indistinguishable from those of anoxia (Lawrence et al, 1942; Jetter and Sheflen, 1952). Provided the patient survives for a few days damage to cortical neurones becomes apparent, while if survival is prolonged widespread necrosis of inner and outer cortical laminae, or even of the full thickness of the cortex, will be seen. Ischaemic and homogenising neuronal change will be found in some of the regions most vulnerable to anoxic insult, notably Ammon's horn. Neurones of the caudate nucleus and putamen are also often severely affected. In those cases which survive for long enough, reactive glial and vascular changes will be present in the damaged areas. Widespread glial fibrosis of cerebral white matter is a peculiar change sometimes observed.

Chronic hypoglycaemic encephalopathy presents a varied histological picture, though basically little different from that seen in death after acute insulin overdosage. Striatal and cerebellar signs and symptoms can clearly be related to neuronal alterations in the caudate nucleus, putamen and in the Purkinje cell and molecular layers of the cerebellum. Chronic hypoglycaemia may affect spinal as well as cerebral neurones and widespread degeneration of anterior horn cells was found in one patient with an islet cell tumour and a clinical picture of dementia, cortical visual loss, hemichorea, dysphagia and amyotrophy (Tom and Richardson, 1951).

For more information on the biochemical, neuropathological and endocrine aspects of hypoglycaemia the reader is referred to the monograph by Marks and Rose (1965) and to a companion volume in the present series.

Chronic pancreatitis and hypoglycaemia

Pancreatitis is a familiar cause of diabetes but a less well recognised cause of hypoglycaemia. Nevertheless, this association was first described 40 years ago (Holman and Railsback, 1933; Judd, Allan and Rynearson, 1933) and a number of cases have subsequently been reported. Most of these (e.g. Friedlander, 1961; Joyeux et al, 1963) are very poorly documented, but in one at least (Marks and Rose, 1965) the connexion seems clearly established. Those cases with chronic pancreatitis and hypoglycaemia have shown atrophy of the exocrine tissue in the pancreas and sometimes apparent enlargement of the islets of Langerhans. However, increased numbers or volumes of β-cells have not been demonstrated (an impossible task, probably) and the suggestion that hypoglycaemia is due to hyperinsulinism secondary to islet hypertrophy is only speculative. Other proposed explanations implicate increased insulin secretion, yet in one case in which insulin levels were measured hyperinsulinism could at no time be demonstrated (Marks and Rose, 1965).

Islet-cell tumours of the pancreas

Small islet-cell adenomas are alleged to be present in 1 to 2 per cent of all autopsies (Lopez-Kruger and Dockerty, 1947; Spencer, 1955). The number of functional islet-cell tumours producing hyperinsulinism is very much smaller, and insulinomas are a clinical and pathological rarity. They can develop at any age but are most frequent in the fifth decade. There is no sex preponderance. They may occur in any part of the pancreas, or in ectopic pancreatic tissue, and may be multiple. They are rarely large enough to cause local pressure effects. A few are well encapsulated but most have ill-defined margins: this is not in itself evidence of malignancy, though a proportion of them are infiltrative and may metastasise. The histological appearance is usually remarkably uniform, with trabeculae of islet cells separated by a vascular connective tissue stroma which may become hyalinised. Cytoplasmic granulation can sometimes be demonstrated ultrastructurally or by special stains, and assays of tumour tissue extracts may reveal a high insulin content. Nevertheless the staining reactions of the tumour cells are often less well marked than those of the normal β-cells in adjacent islets.

Gastrointestinal carcinomas producing hypoglycaemia

Carcinomas of the alimentary system are a well-recognised, if rare, cause of hypoglycaemia. Connective tissue tumours ('fibrous mesotheliomas') are a commoner cause than epithelial tumours, but the most frequent epithelial neoplasm associated with hypoglycaemia is *hepatocellular carcinoma.* This association seems first to have been described by Nadler and Wolfer (1929), who reported the case of a 30-year-old man with a hepatoma who had repeated episodes of coma with a low blood sugar. McFadzean and Yeung (1956) showed that persistent hypoglycaemia was present in 7 of 23 Chinese patients with primary hepatocellular carcinoma. A possible mechanism for this phenomenon was demonstrated by Schonfeld, Babbott and Gundersen (1961) in a patient with a hepatoma, profound intractable hypoglycaemia and severe neuroglycopenic symptoms: a high insulin-like activity was present in an extract of the tumour, though not in the patient's serum.

Carcinoma of the stomach associated with hypoglycaemia was first noted by Bielschowsky (1932), and cases have since been reported by Gonzales, Gold and Shnider (1963) and Marks, Auld and Barr (1965). The last of these was a woman aged 52 with recurrent hypoglycaemic coma in whom normal plasma insulin and low growth hormone levels were found when the blood glucose was very low. One of the cases of Gonzales et al had very little insulin-like activity in a tumour extract. Whether these gastric carcinomas release a substance with actions of insulin remains to be proven.

One case of carcinoma of the caecum with hypoglycaemia has been described (Tranquada, Bender and Bergelman, 1962). Here neurological manifestations were severe and the patient died in coma with bilateral extensor plantar responses. Assays of an acid-alcohol extract of the caecal adenocarcinoma showed a highly significant insulin-like activity, in contrast to the cases of gastric carcinoma already noted. The tumour protein had about 10 per cent of the potency of pancreatic protein; nevertheless, it was distinct from insulin, for no insulin could be identified immunologically.

PANCREATIC ENCEPHALOPATHY

Acute pancreatitis is occasionally followed, within a period of days, by a delirious or confusional state which may be associated with diffuse or focal neurological signs and widespread disturbances in the EEG. Patients exhibiting these symptoms and signs have been labelled as suffering from 'pancreatic encephalopathy'. The condition is not widely known, probably because of its rarity, possibly because of its dubious nosological status. The label should not be appended to cases of pancreatitis complicated by encephalopathy when the latter is due to such concomitants of pancreatitis as alcohol withdrawal, cerebral circulatory disturbance, diabetic acidosis, hypokalaemia, hypo- or hyper-calcaemia, the hyperosmolarity syndrome or the effects of renal failure.

The term 'pancreatic encephalopathy' was coined in 1941 by Rothermich and von Haam. The authors described eight elderly patients who had developed a remarkably uniform neurological syndrome against a surprisingly variable background of abdominal symptoms. The 'encephalopathy' consisted of an agitated hallucinatory state, clouding of consciousness, dysarthria and cog-wheel rigidity of the limbs. The tendon reflexes were brisk. There was variable ankle clonus, but no patient had unequivocally extensor plantar responses. Stretching of various muscle groups was painful. The authors appeared to regard a strong grasp reflex, reported in one case, as an integral part of the disorder. The illness showed a tendency to spontaneous remissions and relapses. The patients often obstinately refused to take anything by mouth, even water. Most gave a history of previous abdominal complaints, present either for some years, or immediately antedating the neurological disorder.

Only one of the eight patients was an alcoholic. One (Case 6) died following acute pancreatitis. In four (Cases 1, 2, 3 and 8) the neurological symptoms were prominent but there was no clinical evidence of acute pancreatitis. The remaining three (Cases 4, 5 and 7) had suffered from chronic psychiatric disorders, and again clinical evidence of acute pancreatic disease was strikingly absent.

Necropsy was performed on seven of the eight patients. Examination of the brain, carried out in five cases, revealed gross vascular lesions in two (Cases 7 and 8), microscopic haemorrhages in four (Cases 2, 5, 6 and 7), and perivascular demyelination in one (Case 5). The pancreatic lesions were severe in one patient (Case 6), who had typical acute haemorrhagic pancreatitis. In each of the remaining seven cases small foci of fat necrosis were found: none had evidence of old haemorrhage, massive necrosis or fibrosis. In at least three, the pancreatic weight was normal. Minor inflammatory change was seen in two instances.

Because of the clinical similarity of this syndrome to the syndrome of acute nicotinic acid deficiency encephalopathy, described shortly before by Jolliffe et al (1940), Rothermich and von Haam (1941) suggested that their cases migh have arisen on a similar basis. This may or may not have been the case. A more serious defect in their argument, however, is their failure to show significant pancreatic lesions in the majority of their patients. It is known that 15 per cent of routine autopsies may show minor fibrosis or inflammatory changes in the pancreas, while foci of fat necrosis are often found with a completely normal pancreas (Czernobilsky and Mikat, 1964). Even if the changes reported do represent subclinical pancreatitis, it is difficult to envisage such attacks as responsible for some of the florid neurological syndromes described. Critical assessment of Rothermich and von Haam's findings leaves us in considerable doubt that they were dealing with a clinicopathological entity.

Little progress was made in eliciting the possible relationship of pancreatic disorder to brain disease until Vogel (1950) showed that purified lipase, extracted from hog pancreas, appeared to produce focal areas of demyelination (without noteworthy inflammation) when injected intracerebrally into rabbits. Damage to myelin sheaths also seemed to be produced when segments of normal spinal cord, from various species, were incubated with solutions containing purified lipase. Trypsin and chymotrypsin were without effect. Vogel (1951a) later showed that, in rabbits, the intravascular injection of lipase also produced small focal areas of demyelination in the cerebrum, brainstem and cerebellum. Demyelination did not result when heat-inactivated pancreatic lipase was injected intracerebrally. The intracerebral injection of trypsin or chymotrypsin produced necrosis of all cerebral tissues (i.e. of nerve cells and their axons as well as of their myelin sheaths). These findings appeared to provide a rational biochemical basis for 'pancreatic encephalopathy', for the explanation of which several hypotheses had earlier been put forward. For instance, Lovell (1923, 1937), in his early accounts of psychiatric symptoms related to pancreatitis, mentioned cerebral oedema and alterations of the surface tension of the blood as possible mechanisms. Edelmann (1936) had discussed the problem of how pancreatic lesions caused death. Just as components of the bile might enter the blood in cases of biliary obstruction, so might pancreatic juice, under the appropriate conditions of mechanical obstruction. Edelmann and Leidler (1938) later described psychiatric symptoms resembling Korsakoff psychosis in cases of 'hepato-pancreatitis'. The cerebral lesions recorded in their single autopsied case resembled those of Wernicke's encephalopathy (numerous petechiae and marked capillary proliferation in the region of the quadrigeminal plate and around the aqueduct of Sylvius). The basis of these changes is clear from their report: their patient did not have pancreatic disease but gallstones, ascending cholangitis, peritonitis, intractable vomiting and presumably acute thiamine deficiency.

Vogel (1951b) later published a clinicopathological report which appeared to substantiate his views. A severely hypertensive woman aged 44 failed to recover from anaesthesia following thoracolumbar sympathectomy and died three days later. At autopsy she was found to have acute haemorrhagic pancreatitis, and massive cerebral oedema. Histological examination of the brain showed patchy pallor of myelin staining, often at the junction of cerebral cortex and white matter, together with variable neuronal alterations. Although

Vogel's case is often referred to as one of demyelination, there was no evidence of myelin breakdown. Small areas of necrosis (probably ischaemic but attributed by the author to circulating trypsin) were found in the myocardium; foci of necrosis were also found in the adrenals and ovaries. The author interpreted the changes in the brain as due to the release of pancreatic lipase, although it seems to us rather more likely that cerebral anoxia was responsible.

Current status of pancreatic encephalopathy

In recent years several cases (Bertrand, Cerbonnet and Godet-Guillain, 1958; Delarue et al, 1965; Sherins and Verity, 1968) have been published, adequately documented from both clinical and pathological angles, which suggest a relationship between pancreatic disease and brain pathology. The main clinical features will be summarised first and the pathological features then reviewed together:

Bertrand et al (1958). A man aged 48 developed acute abdominal symptoms, later shown to be due to acute haemorrhagic pancreatitis. The serum amylase was 1030 Somogyi units/100 ml. Neurological symptoms developed four days after an exploratory laparotomy, in the context of increasing leucocytosis and persisting pyrexia. He became confused and lapsed into a muttering delirium. The eyeballs exhibited jerky movements and the hands irregular twitching. Tone was increased in all four limbs and there were periodic attacks of rigidity in which the neck would be retracted and the arms and legs extended. There were no lateralising signs and no pathological reflexes could be elicited. The patient developed slight hyperosmolarity (328 mEq/l), hypocalcaemia (7·1 mg/100 ml) and a blood urea which at one stage reached 180 mg/100 ml. He died 24 hours after a second laparotomy.

Delarue et al (1965). A woman aged 60 died of an 'acute necrotizing and haemorrhagic pancreatitis', which followed a relapsing course over a period of four weeks. About a fortnight after the appearance of the first abdominal symptoms, she became confused and delirious and developed dysarthria and a left facial weakness, without obvious pyramidal signs.

Sherins and Verity (1968). An alcoholic Negro aged 48 died 35 days after admission to hospital for severe acute haemorrhagic pancreatitis. The serum amylase was 2300 Somogyi units/100 ml, the blood glucose 420 mg/100 ml and there was marked hypercholesterolaemia and hyperlipaemia with lipaemia retinalis but no cutaneous xanthomata. Twelve hours after admission the patient became febrile and very restless and a positive Chvostek sign led to the recognition of slightly reduced levels of serum calcium (4·3 mEq/l) and magnesium (0·9 mEq/l). These were readily corrected. On the third day the patient became confused and on the eighth day, in a context of persisting pyrexia, icterus and migratory thrombophlebitis, he lapsed into a state of akinetic mutism. The hyperglycaemia proved difficult to control, even with insulin, and hypernatraemia developed. The CSF was normal. The patient died of a Pseudomonas septicaemia.

In all three of these cases necropsy revealed acute haemorrhagic pancreatitis and severe brain lesions, summarised in Table 12.1. In the first and third cases a resemblance to the condition of central pontine myelinolysis (Adams, Victor and Mancall, 1959) is apparent, though the brainstem lesions in the cases here reported showed substantial neuronal alterations, and extensive lesions were found in other parts of the neuraxis, in contradistinction to the stereotyped picture described by Adams et al. The case of Delarue et al (1965) seems to us to be essentially of the same nature, although most of the lesions affected the cerebrum.

Table 12.1

Pathological Findings in Three Cases of Pancreatic Encephalopathy

	Cerebral hemispheres	Cerebellum	Brainstem
Bertrand et al (1958)	+ Focal neuronal loss and myelin pallor	++ Extensive loss of myelin and axons; neuronal loss in cortex and dentate nuclei	++ Massive pontine demyelination with relative preservation or neuronal elements Medulla showed marked neuronal changes in olives
Delarue et al (1964)	++ Small areas of softening and oedema in thalami, frontal white matter and parietal cortex	+ Small area of necrosis in right dentate nucleus	+ Multiple small areas of axonal and myelin destruction, with some neuronal loss, concentrated in central pons
Sherins and Verity (1968)	+ Demyelination of central part of corpus callosum	+ Demyelination of middle cerebellar peduncles and cerebellar white matter	++ Central pontine softening with myelin and axonal loss and neuronal changes

+ = affected
++ = severely affected

Other, purely clinical, accounts of alleged 'pancreatic encephalopathy' stress either psychiatric features (Poilleux and Couzinet, 1963) or more complex episodes where agitated or delirious states were associated with dysarthria (Brion et al, 1968), extrapyramidal rigidity (Goulon et al, 1967), or even seizures (Kuntz, 1961; Sharafeev, 1961; Gaultier et al, 1964). Of the rarer manifestations, encountered in single cases, we must mention unilateral cerebellar disturbance (Edelmann, 1936), and bilateral pyramidal signs, with extensor plantar responses, described by Brion et al (1968). A recent report by Sharf and Bental (1971) mentions a patient who, after presenting with a focal neurological deficit (aphasia and right hemiparesis) developed a state of akinetic mutism.

The nature of the cerebral lesions has been the subject of much controversy. Ever since Vogel's (1950, 1951a) original experiments it has been assumed, at times rather uncritically, that they are due to lipases and proteolytic enzymes liberated from the acutely inflamed pancreas. Indirect evidence for such an hypothesis is provided by (a) the occurrence of fat necrosis of bone marrow in cases of acute pancreatitis (Scarpelli, 1956; Immelman et al, 1964), (b) the occurrence of subcutaneous fat necrosis (Szymanski and Bluefarb, 1961; Schrier, Melman and Fenster, 1965; Mullin et al, 1968) which may be mistaken for erythema nodosum, in the same clinical context, and (c) the high concentrations of lipase found in the pleural fluid in some cases of acute pancreatitis complicated by pleural effusion (Roseman, Kowlessar and Sleisinger, 1960). On the other hand, normal plasma has powerful antitryptic activity and any abnormal enzyme in the blood would have to be present in considerable amount in order to remain active in the presence of this enzyme-inhibiting effect.

Prevalence

Pancreatic encephalopathy may be more common than is generally recognised. Bernard (1963) reported four cases of encephalopathy occurring in the course of 40 episodes of acute pancreatitis (10 per cent), Sharafeev (1961) 42 attacks in the course of 283 episodes (14·9 per cent), Hoffman, Perez and Somera (1959) four cases out of 17 (23·5 per cent), Savage, Butcher and Noble (1952) 11 cases out of 45 (24·4 per cent) and Lagache, Combemale and Valtille (1964) seven encephalopathic disturbances (three of them fatal) during 20 episodes of acute pancreatitis (35 per cent). In an account of 172 attacks of acute pancreatitis, Poilleux and Mouktar (1963) report 39 fatal cases of whom four had neurological signs. In many of these reports, however, the clinical documentation is so scanty that we cannot be certain that the encephalopathic episodes were not due to some of the causes listed in the following section.

Diagnosis

The clinical diagnosis of *acute pancreatitis* may be straightforward or very difficult. In a typical and severe case it is based on the sudden development (usually on a background of either biliary tract disease or alcoholism) of severe upper abdominal pain, often associated with vomiting, and upper abdominal tenderness and rigidity. Shock and ileus may supervene. The diagnosis is confirmed by the detection of a rise in the serum amylase to four or five times normal levels.* This increase in serum amylase may only last for a few hours and may readily be missed if the first estimation is made 48 hours or more after the initial symptoms or if there has been previous extensive destruction of pancreatic tissue (Bockus, Bogoch and Roth, 1953). Slighter increases in serum amylase may be encountered in cholecystitis, perforated or penetrating peptic ulcer or intestinal obstruction (Bockus, 1965).

It is important to remember that prolonged elevations of serum amylase may result from injection of morphine for relief of pain (Bogoch, Roth and Bockus, 1954; Burke, Plummer and Bradford, 1950; Gross et al, 1951). This is probably the result of increased intraductal pressure and spasm of the sphincter of Oddi. Codeine and meperidine may have the same effect. The serum amylase may also be increased following the administration of ACTH (Challis, Reid and Hinton, 1957), from defective renal clearance of amylase (Dankner and Heifetz, 1951) and in uraemia (Raffensperger, 1950, 1951; Sachar and Weinhaus, 1956). On the other hand, for reasons not yet clearly understood, normal levels of serum amylase may sometimes be encountered in cases of acute pancreatitis showing gross alcohol-induced hyperlipaemia (Greenberger et al, 1966). An increase in urinary amylase (upper limit of normal 6000 S.u./24 h) occurs later and may persist for several days but

* According to Tierney et al (1963) normal values for serum amylase range from 54 to 185 Somogyi units/100 ml. According to Bockus (1965) normal values, in 80 per cent of people, lie between 80 and 150 Somogyi units/100 ml.

considerable variations may occur in random specimens and the results may be difficult to interpret (Dozzi, 1940).

In the presence of obvious pancreatitis, *encephalopathic symptoms* should first lead to the exclusion of delirium tremens, cerebral circulatory disturbance (due to shock), renal failure, diabetic acidosis, hyperosmolarity syndrome, hypokalaemia and hypo- or hyper-calcaemia.

Recurrent pancreatitis is common in alcoholics and the occurrence of encephalopathic symptoms in a chronic alcoholic with acute abdominal pain should of course lead to a suspicion of *delirium tremens*, particularly if the patient has been admitted to hospital and the intake of alcohol abruptly curtailed. The incidence of encephalopathic symptoms seems, however, to be much higher in alcoholics admitted to hospital with acute pancreatitis than it is in alcoholics admitted with other conditions. Schuster and Iber (1965) reported a high incidence of 'acute toxic psychosis' in a prospective study of 28 alcoholic patients with chronic relapsing pancreatitis. Hallucinations, both visual and auditory, were observed more frequently in their patients (57 per cent of such cases) than any of the better-known complications of pancreatic disease, such as malabsorption (34 per cent), diabetes (30 per cent), or pancreatic calcification (17 per cent). In a control group of 30 alcoholics of equal severity, admitted with acute pneumonia, only 13 per cent had been hallucinated. The authors comment that this differential frequency of psychosis in the two groups makes it unlikely that the hallucinations were solely a manifestation of alcohol withdrawal, or of a febrile or non-specific stress. The undoubted occurrence of encephalopathic symptoms in non-alcoholic patients with acute pancreatitis—or in alcoholic patients in whom the alcohol intake has not been abruptly reduced—suggests that delirium tremens is but one of the possible causes of cerebral symptoms in acute pancreatitis.

Acute pancreatitis, particularly in the elderly, may present with *shock* (Gerber, 1963) or *coma* (Toffler and Spiro, 1962) closely mimicking myocardial infarction or a cerebrovascular accident. Confused or stuporose patients may not complain of pain. If there is associated glycosuria gross errors in diagnosis may be made. Moreover, *acute tubular necrosis due to hypotension* may complicate acute pancreatitis (Frey, 1965) and the subsequent renal failure will induce its own train of neurological complications.

Diabetic acidosis (Tully and Lowenthal, 1958) has been well documented as a rare complication of pancreatitis, and transient hyperglycaemia may occur in 35 per cent of cases of acute pancreatitis (Bockus, 1965). Davidson (1964) recorded a case of 'diabetic coma without ketoacidosis' complicating acute pancreatitis (almost certainly a case of *hyperosmolarity syndrome*, in view of a blood sugar of over 900 mg/100 ml). *Hypokalaemia* has also been incriminated (Doubilet and Mulholland, 1956; Bockus and Raffensperger, 1948; Zollinger, Keith and Ellison, 1954) as the cause of excitement, hallucinations and disorientation in acute pancreatitis. *Hypocalcaemia* may be encountered in severe acute pancreatitis (Edmondson et al, 1952). It has been attributed to soap formation consequent upon diffuse necrosis (and hydrolysis) of retroperitoneal fat. The hypocalcaemia may lead to tetany and convulsions (Bertrand et al, 1958). There is also a definite association between hyperparathyroidism (with *hypercalcaemia*) and pancreatitis (Turchi et al, 1962; Mixter et al, 1962).

Thirty per cent of patients with acute hyperparathyroidism or 'parathyroid crisis' seem to have an associated acute pancreatitis (Fink and Finfrock, 1961).

Yet further possibilities have to be considered. Sometimes the cause of the pancreatitis may itself be contributing to the neurological signs. For instance, *hypothermia* (Duguid, Simpson and Stowers, 1961; Read et al, 1961) or *carbon monoxide poisoning* (Gaultier et al, 1964; Goulon et al, 1967) may themselves both have triggered off the pancreatitis and be responsible for persisting stupor. Gaultier et al (1964) question whether pancreatitis and pancreatic encephalopathy may not be commoner complications of carbon monoxide poisoning than is generally recognised. They stress the fever, leucocytosis, early hyperglycaemia and sometimes rather delayed confusional states that may complicate this form of intoxication.

Pancreatitis has also been reported following the administration of such *drugs* as corticosteroids (Baar and Wolff, 1957; Challis et al, 1957; Lindner, 1964), chlorothiazide (Cornish, McClellan and Johnston, 1961) and isoniazid (Hoffman et al, 1959; Bockus, 1965). It may also be a feature of methyl alcohol poisoning (Bennett, Nation and Olley, 1952). Neurological features encountered in any such cases might be due to the precipitating agent rather than to the pancreatitis itself. Hereditary pancreatitis with lysinuria and cystinuria (Gross, Ulrich and Jones, 1964) has not so far been associated with any neurological complications.

Other conditions entering into the differential diagnosis of pancreatic encephalopathy include infection with mumps virus (causing both pancreatitis and meningitis or meningoencephalitis). The presence of cells in the CSF does not rule out 'pancreatic encephalopathy' as defined in this chapter and there are reports of CSF pleocytosis in cases of pancreatic encephalopathy in which mumps virus was not incriminated (7 cells/mm^3 in the case reported by Gaultier et al, 1964; 16 cells/mm^3 in Case 2 of Rothermich and von Haam, 1941; 28 lymphocytes/mm^3 in the case reported by Sharf and Bental, 1971). Errors in diagnosis may also be made if it is not remembered that serum amylase (of parotid origin) is often raised in mumps, even in the absence of associated pancreatitis (Bockus, 1965). Acute porphyria should also be considered in patients presenting a combination of abdominal and cerebral symptoms.

This formidable list of conditions to be considered in the differential diagnosis should reinforce the note of scepticism sounded in our discussion of the original cases. The current situation is perhaps best summarised in the statement that although the production of effects on the brain by liberated pancreatic lipases and proteolytic enzymes is in some ways an attractive hypothesis, encephalopathic symptoms in acute pancreatitis will, in the vast majority of instances, be due to other causes. This does not prejudice the issue of whether a genuine 'pancreatic encephalopathy', in Vogel's sense (1950, 1951a, b), exists or not.

Treatment

The management of acute pancreatitis is beyond the scope of this monograph: it is well reviewed by Bockus (1965) and Spiro (1970). With the introduction, a decade ago, of 'anti-enzyme' preparations there was some hope that acute pancreatitis and some of its complications (such as 'encephalopathy') might prove amenable to treatment. The use of 'anti-enzymes' is based on the assumption that some of the harmful effects of pancreatitis are due to the activation of pancreatic proteolytic enzymes and to the subsequent formation of biologically active polypeptides.

Aprotinin (Trasylol—Bayer A 128) is a low molecular weight polypeptide produced from the parotid gland or lung, and capable of inhibiting the action of trypsin, chymotrypsin, kallikrein, fibrinolysin and other proteolytic enzymes. It was initially believed to be effective in both experimental and human acute pancreatitis (Forell and Dobovicnik, 1961; Guelzow, Trettin and Diwok, 1961). Later studies (Skyring, Singer and Tornya, 1965) suggested that anti-enzymes did not modify the course of acute pancreatitis.

Gaultier et al (1964) treated their case of 'pancreatic encephalopathy' with 'Zymofren' (dose: 20 000 units/24 h, route unspecified) with satisfactory results. Goulon et al (1967) treated two well-documented cases with a preparation described as CY 66 (Iniprol). The doses administered varied from one million to 12 million units a day and were continued for about two weeks. The first patient also received 'Zymofren'. Both patients made satisfactory recoveries. Brion et al (1968) reported dramatic improvement in a case of pancreatic encephalopathy following the daily intravenous injection of three million units of CY 66 (Iniprol). Sharf and Bental (1971) finally report the successful treatment of their case with aprotinin (Trasylol—Bayer) in a dose of 200 000 units daily.

'PANCREATIC CHOLERA' AND NON-β ISLET-CELL TUMOURS

Certain islet-cell tumours—currently believed to be derived from elements of neural crest origin—give rise to a syndrome of intractable watery diarrhoea, acidosis, and reduced gastric acidity. Hypokalaemia and muscular weakness are important consequences of the diarrhoea, which may be choleraic in its severity—hence the term 'pancreatic cholera' (Matsumoto et al, 1966). The final part of this chapter on pancreatic disease and the nervous system looks into this syndrome, taking us, in the process, into the field of histochemistry and an esoteric world of acronyms.

The cells of the islets of Langerhans share with (*inter alia*) the pituitary adrenotrophs, thyroid parafollicular (C) cells, and certain cells of the foregut mucosa the ability to secrete endocrine polypeptides. Cells specialised in the production of polypeptide hormones were shown by Pearse (1966a, b) to be able to take up the amino-acid precursor of a biogenic amine and to decarboxylate it, and these cells were subsequently linked conceptually as the amine precursor uptake and decarboxylation (APUD) series (Pearse, 1968). To explain the wide dispersal in the body of the polypeptide-secreting APUD cells, a common origin (in the neural crest) was postulated. Circumstantial evidence for this hypothesis came originally from the demonstration in the embryo mouse of the extrathyroidal origin of the calcitonin-producing C cells, using the APUD–FIF method (amine precursor (L-dopa) uptake and decarboxylation; dopamine formaldehyde-induced fluorescence) of Pearse and Carvalheira (1967). Support was provided independently by Le Douarin and Le Lièvre (1970), who grafted neural tubes of Japanese quail embryos into chick embryos. The quail cells possess a large nuclear chromocentre not shared by the chick, and by following this biological marker it could be shown that a proportion of the C cells in the developing embryo chick were of quail origin. More recently, observations on formalin-induced fluorescence in the early mouse embryo have revealed that neural crest cells colonise the lateral processes of the foregut, and the foregut itself. It has been shown that the labelled cells migrate into the definitive stomach and into the duodenum, the bronchi, and the pancreas (Pearse and Polak, 1971a, b). The gastrointestinal and pancreatic endocrine polypeptide cells have been further studied by immunofluorescence, which enables cells synthesising different but chemically related hormones to be differentiated from each other (Pearse, Polak and Bussolati, 1972). It is against this background that we now consider a syndrome associated with tumours releasing such polypeptide hormones as glucagon, gastrin, secretin, gastric inhibitory polypeptide (GIP)—a hormone with a potent enterogastrone action but no cholecystokinin–pancreozymin effects (Brown, 1970)—and vasoactive intestinal polypeptide (VIP—Said and Mutt, 1972).

Clinical features

The first reports of patients with islet-cell tumours of the pancreas associated with profuse watery diarrhoea, leading to severe hypokalaemia and ultimate death from shock and dehydration, appeared in the 1950s. Moldawer, Nardi and Raker (1954), in an account of multiple endocrine adenomatosis, described the case of a woman aged 57 with an α-cell pancreatic adenoma at autopsy, whose diarrhoea had been present for four years. For one year before death her symptoms had included moderate diminution of muscle power, and she had been partially incapacitated by muscle cramps and pain and stiffness of the legs. Terminally her limbs and trunk became completely paralysed. The serum potassium level was not documented before death, but hypokalaemia seems the most likely cause of her weakness. In the next reports of the syndrome (Priest and Alexander, 1957; Verner and Morrison, 1958) 'weakness' or 'prostration' was a variable feature, though one of the cases of Verner and Morrison again had very severe loss of muscle power in the last days of life, and here marked hypokalaemia was documented.

The term 'pancreatic "cholera"' was coined by Matsumoto et al (1966), who analysed 15 case reports and characterised the syndrome. The reported cases showed no sex preponderance and ranged in age from 19 to 67 years with a peak incidence in the fifth decade. Diarrhoea, with or without symptoms of hypokalaemia and weight loss, was the presenting feature in all cases. The diarrhoea was of variable severity and duration (from several months to as long as 15 years) but generally progressive. In the more quiescent stages the stools were semi-liquid while in the fulminating phase they contained very little formed substance and had the appearance of weak tea. Abdominal cramps, nausea and vomiting appeared as the disease advanced. As progression occurred symptoms due to hypokalaemia and dehydration appeared. Patients complained of generalised muscular weakness, or even paralysis, and showed signs of developing coma. The volume of stools during exacerbations could attain 'prodigious and frightening' levels. This devastating loss of fluid and electrolytes would prove fatal unless ample replacement therapy was given.

In contrast to the Zollinger–Ellison syndrome, also occurring with non-β islet-cell tumours, gastric hypersecretion and peptic ulceration were not found in patients with pancreatic cholera. Significantly, a number of these patients were shown to have achlorhydria. The importance of reduced gastric acid secretion in this context was stressed by Marks, Bank and Louw (1967) and Zollinger et al (1968), though *increased* acid output in the syndrome has since been documented, suggesting that tumours responsible for pancreatic cholera may be releasing more than one hormone (Sircus et al, 1970).

Pathological findings

The number of reported cases has now reached 40 (Elias et al, 1972), which seems to represent about 5 per cent of all cases with hormone-producing non-β islet-cell tumours of the pancreas. About half the patients with pancreatic cholera have had (benign) adenomas and roughly the same number have had metastasising tumours. The tumours all fail to show β-granulation when appropriately stained, though cytoplasmic argyrophilia has been demonstrated in a few, and ultrastructural examination has revealed the presence of round, electron-dense secretory granules. The identification of the hormone, by implication the cause of the diarrhoea, has depended on the use of a variety of methods. Using bioassays, Kraft, Tompkins and Zollinger (1970) failed to find gastrin in extracts of seven tumours but found secretin in one. They suggested that secretin was the diarrhoeogenic hormone. Cleator et al (1970) studied the patient with hyperchlorhydria already referred to, and demonstrated secretin-like (and possibly glucagon-like) activity in a tumour extract and gastrin-like activity in plasma, indicating the probable production of multiple polypeptide hormones. Finally, Elias et al (1972) failed to show the presence of gastrin, secretin, glucagon or enteroglucagon in a tumour extract by means of radioimmunoassay, but obtained a strongly positive result for GIP using immunofluorescence. However, further investigation of this case suggests the presence of VIP-like activity in tumour and plasma (Dr Julia Polak, personal communication). Proof that any one polypeptide hormone is the cause of pancreatic cholera remains, for the time being, inconclusive.

References

The pancreas, hypoglycaemia and the nervous system

Bielschowsky, F. (1932). Zur Klinik und Pathologie der Spontanhypoglykämie. *Klinische Wochenschrift*, **11**, 1492–1494.

Ferrendelli, J. A. & Chang, M. M. (1973). Brain metabolism during hypoglycemia. *Archives of Neurology*, **28**, 173–177.

Friedlander, E. O. (1961). Hyperinsulinism in pancreatic or biliary and gastrointestinal tract disease. *Journal of the American Medical Association*, **177**, 300–303.

Gonzales, F. M., Gold, G. L. & Shnider, B. I. (1963). Gastrointestinal carcinoma and concomitant hypoglycemia. *Annals of Internal Medicine*, **58**, 149–154.

Holman, E. & Railsback, D. C. (1933). Partial pancreatectomy in chronic spontaneous hypoglycaemia with a review of cases of hypoglycaemia surgically treated. *Surgery, Gynecology and Obstetrics*, **56**, 591–600.

Jetter, W. W. & Sheflen, A. E. (1952). Delayed pathologic manifestations of hypoglycemic coma. *Journal of Neuropathology and Experimental Neurology*, **11**, 317–323.

Joyeux, R., Colin, R., Mirouze, J. & Pascal, E. (1963). Pancréatite aiguë, récidivante sur pancréatite chronique. Traitement par hemi-pancréatectomie gauche et anti-enzymes. Diabète aigu transitoire post-opératoire avec hypoglycémie et hypertension initiales. *Journal de Chirurgie (Paris)*, **85**, 149–157.

Judd, E. S., Allan, F. N. & Rynearson, E. H. (1933). Hyperinsulinism. Its surgical treatment. *Journal of the American Medical Association*, **101**, 99–103.

Lawrence, R. D., Meyer, A. & Nevin, S. (1942). The pathological changes in the brain in fatal hypoglycaemia. *Quarterly Journal of Medicine*, **11**, 181–201.

Lopez-Kruger, R. & Dockerty, M. B. (1947). Tumours of the islets of Langerhans. *Surgery, Gynecology and Obstetrics*, **85**, 495–511.

McFadzean, A. J. S. & Yeung, T. T. (1956). Hypoglycemia in primary carcinoma of liver. *Archives of Internal Medicine*, **98**, 720–731.

Marks, V., Auld, W. H. R. & Barr, J. B. (1965). Carcinoma of stomach and other non-pancreatic lesions as causes of spontaneous hypoglycaemia. *British Journal of Surgery*, **52**, 925–928.

Marks, V. & Rose, F. C. (1965). *Hypoglycaemia*. Oxford: Blackwell.

Nadler, W. H. & Wolfer, J. A. (1929). Hepatogenic hypoglycemia associated with primary liver cell carcinoma. *Archives of Internal Medicine*, **44**, 700–710.

Schonfeld, A., Babbott, D. & Gundersen, K. (1961). Hypoglycemia and polycythemia associated with primary hepatoma. *New England Journal of Medicine*, **265**, 231–233.

Spencer, H. (1955). Pancreatic islet-cell adenomata. *Journal of Pathology and Bacteriology*, **69**, 259–267.

Tarr, M., Brada, D. & Samson, F. E. (1962). Cerebral high-energy phosphates during insulin hypoglycemia. *American Journal of Physiology*, **203**, 690–692.

Tom, M. L. & Richardson, J. C. (1951). Hypoglycaemia from islet-cell tumour of pancreas with amyotrophy and cerebrospinal nerve cell changes. *Journal of Neuropathology and Experimental Neurology*, **10**, 57–66.

Tranquada, R. E., Bender, A. B. & Bergelman, P. M. (1962). Hypoglycemia associated with carcinoma of the cecum and syndrome of testicular feminization. *New England Journal of Medicine*, **266**, 1302–1306.

Pancreatic encephalopathy

Adams, R. D., Victor, M. & Mancall, E. L. (1959). Central pontine myelinolysis. A hitherto undescribed disease occurring in alcoholic and malnourished patients. *Archives of Neurology and Psychiatry*, **81**, 154–172.

Baar, H. S. & Wolff, C. H. (1957). Pancreatic necrosis in cortisone-treated children. *Lancet*, **1**, 812–815.

Bennett, I. L., Nation, T. C. & Olley, J. F. (1952). Pancreatitis in methyl alcohol poisoning. *Journal of Laboratory and Clinical Medicine*, **40**, 405–409.

Bernard, A. (1963). *Les pancréatites aiguës*. Paris: Doin Deren.

Bertrand, I., Cerbonnet, G. & Godet-Guillain, J. (1958). Contribution à l'étude des encéphalopathies d'origine pancréatique. *Revue neurologique*, **98**, 245–262.

Bockus, H. L. (1965). *Gastroenterology*, 2nd edition. Philadelphia & London: Saunders.

Bockus, H. L. & Raffensperger, E. C. (1948). Acute pancreatitis. *New York Journal of Medicine*, **48**, 2252–2259.

Bockus, H. L., Bogoch, A. & Roth, J. L. A. (1953). Acute pancreatitis; diagnosis and treatment. *Southern Medical Journal*, **46**, 388–396.

Bogoch, A., Roth, J. L. A. & Bockus, H. L. (1954). The effects of morphine on serum amylase and lipase. *Gastroenterology*, **26**, 697–708.

Brion, S., Aillet, J., Graveleau, J. & Leonardon, N. (1968). Encéphalopathie pancréatique probable guérie par les antitrypsiques. *Presse médicale*, **76**, 9–12.

Burke, J. O., Plummer, K. & Bradford, S. (1950). Serum amylase response to morphine, mecholyl and secretin as a test of pancreatic function. *Gastroenterology*, **15**, 699–707.

Challis, T. W., Reid, L. C. & Hinton, J. W. (1957). Study of some factors which influence the level of serum amylase in dogs and humans. *Gastroenterology*, **33**, 818–829.

Cornish, A. L., McClellan, J. T. & Johnston, D. H. (1961). Effects of chlorothiazide on the pancreas. *New England Journal of Medicine*, **265**, 673–675.

Czernobilsky, B. & Mikat, K. W. (1964). The diagnostic significance of interstitial pancreatitis found at autopsy. *American Journal of Clinical Pathology*, **41**, 33–43.
Dankner, A. & Heifetz, C. J. (1951). The inter-relationship of blood and urine diastase during transient acute pancreatitis. *Gastroenterology*, **18**, 207–217.
Davidson, A. I. G. (1964). Diabetic coma without ketoacidosis in a patient with acute pancreatitis. *British Medical Journal*, **1**, 356.
Delarue, J., Chomette, G., Monsaingeon, A., Pinaudeau, Y. & Brocheriou, Cl. (1965). Encéphalopathie subaiguë secondaire à une pancréatite nécrosante hémorrhagique. *Archives d'Anatomie pathologique*, **13**, 45–47.
Doubilet, H. & Mulholland, J. H. (1956). Eight year study of pancreatitis and sphincterotomy. *Journal of the American Medical Association*, **160**, 521–528.
Dozzi, D. L. (1940). Evaluation of methods for determining blood and urinary amylase, *Journal of Laboratory and Clinical Medicine*, **25**, 1303–1308.
Duguid, H., Simpson, R. G. & Stowers, J. M. (1961). Accidental hypothermia. *Lancet*, **2**, 1213–1219.
Edelmann, A. (1936). Ueber ein bisher nicht beachtetes pankreohepatisches Syndrom, bedingt durch Uebertritt des Pankreassaftes in die Blutbahn. *Wiener klinische Wochenschrift*, **2**, 1336–1339.
Edelmann, A. & Leidler, R. (1938). Ein Fall von pankreohepatischem Syndrom mit toxisch-enzephalitischen Herden in beiden hinteren Längsbündeln und im periaquäduktiellen Grau der hinteren Vierhügel. *Confinia neurologica*, **1**, 202–216.
Edmondson, H. A., Berne, C. J., Hoxmann, R. E. Jr & Wertman, M. (1952). Calcium, potassium, magnesium and amylase disturbances in acute pancreatitis. *American Journal of Medicine*, **12**, 34–42.
Fink, W. J. & Finfrock, J. D. (1961). Fatal hyperparathyroid crisis associated with pancreatitis. *American Surgeon*, **27**, 424–430.
Forell, M. M. & Dobovicnik, W. (1961). Über die Möglichkeit durch Inaktivierung des Trypsins die akute Pankreatitis kausal zu beeinflussen. *Klinische Wochenschrift*, **39** 597–598.
Frey, C. F. (1965). Pathogenesis of nitrogen retention in pancreatitis. *American Journal of Surgery*, **109**, 747–755.
Gaultier, M., Fournier, E., Gervais, P. & Bodin, F. (1964). Encéphalopathie pancréatique survenue au cours d'une intoxication oxycarbonée. *Presse médicale*, **72**, 3263–3265.
Gerber, B. C. (1963). Hereditary pancreatitis. The role of surgical intervention. *Archives of Surgery*, **87**, 70–80.
Goulon, M., Julien, C. G., Rapin, M., Nouailhat, F. & Barois, A. (1967). L'encéphalopathie pancréatique. À propos de trois observations. *Revue neurologique*, **117**, 363–373.
Greenberger, N. J., Hatch, F. T., Drummey, G. D. & Isselbacher, K. J. (1966). Pancreatitis and hyperlipemia: a study of serum lipid alterations in 25 patients with acute pancreatitis. *Medicine (Baltimore)*, **45**, 161–174.
Gross, J. B., Comfort, M. W., Mathieson, D. R. & Power, M. H. (1951). Elevated values for serum amylase and lipase following the administration of opiates. *Proceedings of the Staff Meetings of the Mayo Clinic*, **26**, 81–87.
Gross, J. B., Ulrich, J. A. & Jones, J. D. (1964). Urinary excretion of aminoacids in a kindred with hereditary pancreatitis and aminoaciduria. *Gastroenterology*, **47**, 41–48.
Guelzow, M., Trettin, H. J. & Diwok, K. (1961). Experimentelles zur Wirksamkeit des Kallikrein-Trypsin-Inaktivators (Trasylol). *Klinische Wochenschrift*, **39**, 597–598.
Hoffman, E., Perez, E. & Somera, V. (1959). Acute pancreatitis in the upper age groups. *Gastroenterology*, **36**, 675–685.
Immelman, E. J., Banks, S., Krige, H. & Marks, I. N. (1964). Roentgenologic and clinical features of intramedullary fat necrosis in acute and chronic pancreatitis. *American Journal of Medicine*, **36**, 96–105.
Jolliffe, N., Bowman, K. M., Rosenblum, L. A. & Fein, H. D. (1940). Nicotinic acid deficiency encephalopathy. *Journal of the American Medical Association*, **114**, 307–312.
Kuntz, J. Y. (1961). Contribution à l'étude des encéphalopathies d'origine pancréatique. Thèse de Médecine, Paris.
Lagache, G., Combemale, B. & Valtille, C. (1964). Les troubles psychiques des pancréatites aiguës. *Lille chirurgical*, **19**, 227–232.

Lindner, H. (1964). Akute Pankreatitis (Pankreasnekrose) infolge Glucocorticoidtherapie. *Deutsche medizinische Wochenschrift*, **89**, 833–839.

Lovell, C. (1923). The surface tension of the serum in anxiety psychoses. *Journal of Mental Science*, **69**, 497–501.

Lovell, C. (1937). Cerebral oedema in certain mental disorders. *British Medical Journal*, **2**, 656–659.

Mixter, C. G., Keynes, W. M., Chu, M. & Cope, O. (1962). Further experience with pancreatitis as a diagnostic clue to hyperparathyroidism. *New England Journal of Medicine*, **226**, 265–272.

Mullin, G. T., Erskine, M. C., Stephen, R. C. & Williams, R. C. (1968). Arthritis and skin lesions resembling erythema nodosum in pancreatic disease. *Annals of Internal Medicine*, **68**, 75–96.

Poilleux, F. & Couzinet, G. (1963). Deux observations de pancréatite aiguë avec manifestations d'encéphalopathie, traitée par les anti-enzymes. *Archives des maladies de l'appareil digestif et des maladies de la nutrition*, **52**, 1038–1045.

Poilleux, F. & Mouktar, M. (1963). Conclusions au débat sur les pancréatites aiguës traitées par les anti-ferments. *Mémoires de l'Académie de Chirurgie*, **89**, 460–468.

Raffensperger, E. C. (1950). Serum pancreatic enzyme values in abdominal lesions not originating in the pancreas. In *Postgraduate Gastroenterology*, ed. Bockus, H. L. Philadelphia: Saunders.

Raffensperger, E. C. (1951). Elevated serum pancreatic enzyme values without primary intrinsic pancreatic disease. *Annals of Internal Medicine*, **35**, 342–351.

Read, A. E., Emslie-Smith, D., Gough, K. R. & Holmes, R. (1961). Pancreatitis and accid-dental hypothermia. *Lancet*, **2**, 1219–1221.

Roseman, D. M., Kowlessar, D. & Sleisinger, M. H. (1960). Pulmonary manifestations of pancreatitis. *New England Journal of Medicine*, **263**, 294–296.

Rothermich, N. O. & von Haam, E. (1941). Pancreatic encephalopathy. *Journal of Clinical Endocrinology and Metabolism*, **1**, 872–881.

Sachar, L. A. & Weinhaus, R. (1956). Misinterpretation of elevated blood diastase due to impaired renal clearance. *Archives of Surgery*, **73**, 305–308.

Savage, C., Butcher, W. & Noble, D. (1952). Psychiatric manifestations in pancreatic disease. *Journal of Clinical and Experimental Psychopathology and Quarterly Review of Psychiatry and Neurology*, **13**, 9–16.

Scarpelli, D. G. (1956). Fat necrosis of bone marrow in acute pancreatitis. *American Journal of Pathology*, **32**, 1077–1088.

Schrier, R. W., Melman, K. L. & Fenster, L. F. (1965). Subcutaneous nodular fat necrosis in pancreatitis. *Archives of Internal Medicine*, **116**, 832–836.

Schuster, M. M. & Iber, F. L. (1965). Psychosis with pancreatitis: a frequent occurrence infrequently recognised. *Archives of Internal Medicine*, **116**, 228–233.

Sharafeev, A. G. (1961). [General cerebral disorders in acute pancreatitis.] (in Russian) *Klinicheskaia Meditsina (Moskva)*, **39**, 86–90.

Sharf, B. & Bental, E. (1971). Pancreatic encephalopathy. *Journal of Neurology, Neurosurgery and Psychiatry*, **34**, 357–361.

Sherins, R. J. & Verity, M. A. (1968). Central pontine myelinolysis associated with acute haemorrhagic pancreatitis. *Journal of Neurology, Neurosurgery and Psychiatry*, **31**, 583–588.

Skyring, A., Singer, A. & Tornya, P. (1965). Treatment of acute pancreatitis with Trasylol: report of a controlled therapeutic trial. *British Medical Journal*, **2**, 627–629.

Spiro, H. M. (1970). *Clinical Gastroenterology*. London: Macmillan.

Szymanski, F. J. & Bluefarb, S. M. (1961). Nodular fat necrosis and pancreatic disease. *Archives of Dermatology*, **83**, 224–229.

Tierney, J. M., Carter, J. F., van Goidsenhoven, G. E. & Knight, W. A. Jr (1963). Screening for pancreatic disease. *Annals of Internal Medicine*, **58**, 229–234.

Toffler, A. & Spiro, H. M. (1962). Shock or coma as the predominant manifestation of painless acute pancreatitis. *Annals of Internal Medicine*, **57**, 655–659.

Tully, G. T. & Lowenthal, J. J. (1958). The diabetic coma of acute pancreatitis. *Annals of Internal Medicine*, **48**, 310–319.

Turchi, J. J., Flandreau, R. H., Forte, A. L., French, G. N. & Ludwig, G. D. (1962). Hyperparathyroidism and pancreatitis. *Journal of the American Medical Association*, **180,** 799–804.

Vogel, F. S. (1950). Demyelinization induced experimentally by means of lipase (Abstract). *Federation Proceedings*, **9,** 347.

Vogel, F. S. (1951a). Demyelinization induced in living rabbits by means of a lipolytic enzyme preparation. *Journal of Experimental Medicine*, **93,** 297–304.

Vogel, F. S. (1951b). Cerebral demyelination and focal visceral lesions in a case of acute hemorrhagic pancreatitis with a consideration of the possible role of circulating enzymes in the causation of the lesions. *American Medical Association Archives of Pathology*, **52,** 355–362.

Zollinger, R. M., Keith, L. M. & Ellison, E. H. (1954). Pancreatitis. *New England Journal of Medicine*, **251,** 497–502.

Pancreatic cholera and non-β islet-cell tumours

Brown, J. C. (1970). A gastric inhibitory polypeptide. I. The amino acid composition and the tryptic peptides. *Canadian Journal of Biochemistry*, **49,** 255–261.

Cleator, I. G. M., Thomson, C. G., Sircus, W. & Coombes, M. (1970). Bio-assay evidence of abnormal secretin-like and gastrin-like activity in tumour and blood in cases of 'choleraic diarrhoea'. *Gut*, **11,** 206–211.

Elias, E., Bloom, S. R., Welbourn, R. B., Kuzio, M., Polak, J. M., Pearse, A. G. E., Booth, C C. & Brown, J. C. (1972). Pancreatic cholera due to production of gastric inhibitory polypeptide. *Lancet*, **2,** 791–793.

Kraft, A. R., Tompkins, R. K. & Zollinger, R. M. (1970). Recognition and management of the diarrheal syndrome caused by nonbeta islet cell tumors of the pancreas. *American Journal of Surgery*, **119,** 163–170.

Le Douarin, N. & Le Lièvre, C. (1970). Démonstration de l'origine neurale des cellules à calcitonine du corps ultimobranchial chez l'embryon du poulet. *Compte rendu de l'Académie des Sciences, Paris, Série D*, **270,** 2857–2860.

Marks, I. N., Bank, S. & Louw, J. H. (1967). Islet cell tumor of the pancreas with reversible watery diarrhea and achlorhydria. *Gastroenterology*, **52,** 695–708.

Matsumoto, K. K., Peter, J. B., Schultze, R. G., Hakim, A. A. & Franck, P. T. (1966). Water diarrhea and hypokalemia associated with pancreatic islet cell adenoma. *Gastroenterology*, **50,** 231–242.

Moldawer, P. M., Nardi, G. L. & Raker, J. W. (1954). Concomitance of multiple adenomas of the parathyroids and pancreatic islets with tumor of the pituitary: a syndrome with familial incidence. *American Journal of the Medical Sciences*, **228,** 190–206.

Pearse, A. G. E. (1966a). 5-Hydroxytryptophan uptake by dog thyroid C cells and its possible significance in polypeptide hormone production. *Nature (London)*, **211,** 598.

Pearse, A. G. E. (1966b). Common cytochemical properties of cells producing polypeptide hormones, with particular reference to calcitonin and the thyroid C cells. *Veterinary Record*, **79,** 587–590.

Pearse, A. G. E. (1968). Common cytochemical and ultrastructural characteristics of cells producing polypeptide hormones (the APUD series) and their relevance to thyroid and ultimobranchial C cells and calcitonin. *Proceedings of the Royal Society of London Series B, Biological Sciences*, **170,** 71–80.

Pearse, A. G. E. & Carvalheira, A. F. (1967). Cytochemical evidence for an ultimobranchial origin of rodent thyroid C cells. *Nature (London)*, **214,** 929–930.

Pearse, A. G. E. & Polak, J. M. (1971a). Cytochemical evidence for the neural crest origin of mammalian ultimobranchial C cells. *Histochemie*, **27,** 96–102.

Pearse, A. G. E. & Polak, J. M. (1971b). Neural crest origin of the endocrine polypeptide (APUD) cells of the gastrointestinal tract and pancreas. *Gut*, **12,** 783–788.

Pearse, A. G. E., Polak, J. M. & Bussolati, G. (1972). The neural crest origin of gastrointestinal and pancreatic endocrine polypeptide cells and their distinction by sequential immunofluorescence. *Folia histochemica et cytochemica*, **10,** 115–120.

Priest, W. M. & Alexander, M. K. (1957). Islet-cell tumour of the pancreas with peptic ulceration, diarrhoea and hypokalaemia. *Lancet*, **2,** 1145–1457.

Said, S. I. & Mutt, V. (1972). Isolation from porcine intestinal wall of a vasoactive octacosapeptide related to secretin and to glucagon. *European Journal of Biochemistry*, **28**, 199–204.

Sircus, W., Brunt, P. W., Walker, R. J., Small, W. P., Falconer, C. W. A. & Thomson, C. G. (1970). Two cases of 'pancreatic cholera' with features of peptide-secreting adenomatosis of the pancreas. *Gut*, **11**, 197–205.

Verner, J. V. & Morrison, A. B. (1958). Islet cell tumor and a syndrome of refractory watery diarrhea and hypokalemia. *American Journal of Medicine*, **25**, 374–380.

Zollinger, R. M., Tompkins, R. K., Amerson, J. R., Endahl, G. L., Kraft, A. R. & Moore, F. T. (1968). Identification of the diarrheogenic hormone associated with non-beta islet cell tumors of the pancreas. *Annals of Surgery*, **168**, 502–521.

CHAPTER THIRTEEN

Whipple's Disease and the Nervous System

Devoting a chapter to some rare manifestations of an uncommon condition is not hard to justify in the case of Whipple's disease. This is an interesting multisystem disorder and in recent years the brain and spinal cord have been added to the list of organs that may be involved. The occurrence of central nervous complications in Whipple's disease is worth emphasising since a variety of neurological presentations may occur, with or without other systems being involved. The neurological disorders thus arising are, moreover, potentially treatable.

Whipple's disease is a chronic condition characterised by weight loss, arthralgia, steatorrhoea and abdominal pain. The first reported case (Whipple, 1907) was a 36-year-old man who was found at autopsy to have deposits of fat in the intestinal mucosa and in mesenteric lymph nodes. Under the microscope, Whipple recognised foamy macrophages in the lamina propria of the small bowel mucosa, and these post-mortem findings led him to name the disorder 'intestinal lipodystrophy'.

Less than 40 possible cases had been reported up to 1949 (Russo, 1952), in which year Black-Shaffer showed that characteristic abnormal macrophages might be found in a number of tissues. These contained small particles, readily stained by the periodic acid-Schiff (PAS) technique. In 1958 Sieracki showed that the PAS-positive 'sickle-shaped particles' in these macrophages could be distinguished from other positively staining material (such as lipofuscin) which was often in droplet form. Two years later he and his colleagues (Haubrich, Watson and Sieracki, 1960) amplified this finding, pointing out that the diagnostic feature of Whipple's disease was not abnormal fat accumulation but the presence in many organs of large reticuloendothelial cells containing PAS-positive 'sickle-form particles'. These cells were especially abundant at the two sites where lesions had originally been noted: the intestinal mucosa and mesenteric lymph nodes. They were at first thought to contain an abnormally accumulated glycoprotein, synthesised within the cells. The following year two groups of workers (Chears and Ashworth, 1961;

Yardley and Hendrix, 1961) showed that the PAS-positive material resembled bacilli, and that these structures could be identified in intestinal mucosa, both inside and outside macrophages.

No subsequent progress has been made in defining the aetiology of Whipple's disease. While the condition is generally believed to be associated with bacterial infection, no single organism has been causally implicated. There is no agreement even on the most elementary points of characterisation. Some authors (Chears and Ashworth, 1961) reported Gram-positivity; others (Roberts et al, 1970) Gram-negativity. Problems of identification arise from contamination of biopsy samples and from failure to demonstrate that a cultured organism was responsible for the patient's illness (the problem is similar in fact to the one often faced by the virologist, studying a possibly infective nervous disease or a microorganism found by chance in brain tissue). Even where an organism, for instance a β-haemolytic streptococcus (Charache et al, 1966), has been successfully grown from blood and intestinal mucosal culture, has been sensitive in vitro to an antibiotic which in vivo had improved the patient's condition, and has produced an elevated agglutinin titre in the patient's blood, the proof that it caused the patient's intestinal disease is still lacking. Perhaps this could only come from the application of more sophisticated techniques than have been used in the past.

Among the organisms other than streptococci that have been implicated in Whipple's disease, on the basis of morphology or culture, are corynebacteria (Caroli et al, 1963; Dybkaer and Kok, 1965); haemophilus (Kjaerheim et al, 1966); brucella (Dybkaer and Kok, 1965); and an unusual mycobacterium (Groodt-Lasseel and Martin, 1969). Despite these reports, and despite frequent dramatic improvement of symptoms and signs with antibiotic treatment, an infective and bacterial aetiology remains unproven. The lack of evidence for the infectivity of Whipple's disease, the failure of transmission from man to experimental animals, and the virtual absence of childhood cases (unlike what is seen in almost every recognised infectious disease) are points that are hard to explain if a microorganism is indeed responsible.

General aspects of Whipple's disease

The clinical and pathological findings in Whipple's disease have been well reviewed by Maizel, Ruffin and Dobbins (1970) who studied 19 patients and analysed data on 114 others reported after Black-Shaffer's stress on PAS-positive macrophages as a diagnostic feature.

The age of the patients ranged from 20 to 67 years (mean 49), and men outnumbered women by 8·5 to 1. The symptom tetrad of weight loss, diarrhoea, abdominal pain and arthralgia was present in three-quarters of all cases, and the most frequent signs, apart from loss of weight, included fever, hypotension, lymphadenopathy, abdominal tenderness and distension, and hyperpigmentation. The majority of symptoms antedated diagnosis by less than a year, though arthralgia generally appeared long beforehand. Normocytic, hypochromic anaemia and decreased intestinal absorption of fat and D-xylose will almost always be found. Diagnosis of patients with Whipple's disease is based on the findings in jejunal biopsy. Macrophages filled with PAS-positive material will be seen in the small intestinal mucosa, and it may be possible to demonstrate bacterial invasion and degenerating bacteria in macrophages at this site by electron microscopy. Lymph nodes from the mesentery and elsewhere in the body may show prominent fatty spaces and characteristic PAS-positive macrophages, while bacterial bodies may be found here both within macrophages and free in lymph channels (Dobbins and Ruffin, 1967). Several studies agree on the size of these organisms, which average 2 μm in length and 0·25 μm in diameter.

At autopsy, macrophages containing abnormal PAS-positive material have been identified in most of the tissues of the body, although bacteria have only been convincingly shown at one site other than intestine and lymph nodes: the brain (Groodt-Lasseel and Martin, 1969; Schochet and Lampert, 1969) Sieracki and his colleagues (Sieracki, 1958; Sieracki and Fine, 1959; Sieracki et al, 1960), considering that reticuloendothelial cells with PAS-positive 'sickle-form particles' in their cytoplasm were diagnostic of the disease, found characteristic lesions not only at established sites but also in heart valves, myocardium, lungs, pleura, oesophagus, stomach, colon, spleen, pancreas, retroperitoneal tissue, adrenals and bone marrow. Focal involvement of the central nervous system was also observed, which brings us to the neurology and neuropathology of the disease.

Neurological aspects of Whipple's disease

The central nervous lesions seen by Sieracki and his colleagues (Sieracki and Fine, 1959; Sieracki et al, 1960) were in the form of microscopic cell foci containing PAS-positive histiocytes in periventricular, hypothalamic and tuberal regions. The two patients studied were neurologically asymptomatic. This finding has the implication that histological involvement of the nervous system in Whipple's disease might be fairly common, and this has been confirmed by Schochet and Lampert (1969) who found microscopic lesions in four of the 21 autopsies on file at the U.S. Armed Forces Institute of Pathology. Certainly, clinical manifestations of such involvement are far from common, and probably fewer than 10 per cent of patients with Whipple's disease develop neurological complications. Seventeen such cases, reported between 1949 and 1971, have been collected. Others could doubtless be found, where minor central nervous symptoms and signs were overshadowed by a major gastrointestinal or systemic disorder.

The data are summarised (together with those derived from neurologically asymptomatic cases with nervous involvement at autopsy) in Tables 13.1 and 13.2. No clear picture of a typical clinical syndrome emerges from an analysis of these cases. This very vagueness might be due to the fact that in some cases the neurological events and the Whipple's disease were not causally related. Nevertheless, it is worth stressing that the neurological complaints may be those first bringing the patient with Whipple's disease to medical attention.

The average age of these patients (51 years, range 33 to 68) is almost the same as that of all patients with Whipple's disease. Except in four instances, the duration of neurological symptoms was under a year. Three of these four (Lampert, Tom and Cumings, 1962; Minauf and Stochdorph, 1969; Janota, 1971) showed a similar clinical picture of *progressive dementia* over a period

Table 13.1

Central Nervous Involvement in Autopsied Cases of Whipple's Disease

	Sex	Age	Symptoms and signs	Central nervous system lesions	Histological findings in central nervous system
Jones & Paulley (1949)	M	44	Diarrhoea 1 year before death; retrobulbar neuritis and optic atrophy 6 years before death	Not recorded	
Russo (1952)	M	64	3 years weight loss; 1 year fits	None found	
Sieracki et al (1960)	M M	35 59	Gastrointestinal but no neurological features	Microscopic glial nodules: subependymal, hypothalamus, tuber cinereum	Nodules containing PAS-positive histiocytes; perivascular cuffing
Hecker & Reid (1962)	M	49	Arthritis 15 years, steatorrhoea 1 year, double hemiparesis 4 months before death	Cerebral white matter	Oedema, demyelination, abnormal astrocytes and oligodendroglia, compound granular corpuscles; no PAS-positive cells
Krücke & Stochdorph (1962)	M	49	Arthritis 1 year; myoclonus, impaired vision, apathy, coma in last 6 months	Microscopic nodules in cerebral cortex, ependyma, dentate, brainstem, retina	Nodules containing PAS-positive histiocytes; perivascular cuffing
	F	53	Arthritis 20 years, vertigo, apathy	Aqueduct stenosis, hydrocephalus	Granular ependymitis (cells PAS-positive)
Lampert et al (1962)	M	49	Dementia for 7 years, arthritis; no diarrhoea; ophthalmoplegia	Frontal atrophy, dilated ventricles with granular ependymitis	PAS-positive microglia in clumps throughout grey, diffusely in white matter; PAS-positive granular ependymitis
Koudouris et al (1963)	F	35	8 months progressive paraparesis, 2 months fits, no previous intestinal or joint symptoms	Spinal cord	PAS-positive histiocytes in demyelinated dorsal columns and pituitary stalk
Badenoch et al (1963)	M	51	Steatorrhoea for $4\frac{1}{2}$ years; 6 months dysarthria, ataxia, blurred vision, coma	Widespread microscopic lesions in grey matter, occasionally in white; granular ependymitis	Abnormal particulate PAS-positive material, mainly extracellular; glial proliferation with perivascular cuffing; histiocytes containing PAS-positive particles; similar material in ependyma and in granulations
Smith et al (1965)	M	37	2 years diarrhoea; 6 months headache, confusion, ophthalmoplegia, facial myoclonus, coma	Cerebral atrophy, dilated ventricles	Intra- and extra-cellular particulate PAS-positive material in foci throughout grey matter; similar material in ependyma and granulations

Table 13.1 (*continued*)

	Sex	Age	Symptons and signs	Central nervous system lesions	Histolgical findings in central nervous system
Smith et al (1969)	M	60	8 years steatorrhoea; 1 year facial numbness	Microscopic foci in cerebrum	As above
Tengström & Werner (1966)	F	41	Steatorrhoea; nil neurological	Microscopic	A few PAS-positive perivascular cells
Schwartzová et al (1967)	M	58	Apathy, pyramidal and extra-pyramidal signs, meningitis	Microscopic; leptomeninges, cortex, posterior pituitary	PAS-positive histiocytes
Schochet & Lampert (1969)	(No clinical details; 3 previously unreported cases)			Microscopic; random distribution of lesions in cerebrum, brainstem and cerebellum	Nodular aggregates of PAS-positive macrophages; bacteria identified in lesions
Switz et al (1969)	M	49	6 years arthralgia; 6 months blurred vision due to papilloedema; terminal lymphadenopathy, hepatomegaly, retinal haemorrhages, heart murmurs	Infarct 1·5 cm diameter in frontoparietal subcortical region	Widespread intra- and extra-cellular PAS-positive material in cerebral grey plus white matter (including optic nerves)
Minauf & Stochdorph (1969)	M	33	Fever 10 years, arthritis 18 months; mental change, myoclonus, ophthalmoplegia, coma 10 months	Ependymal granulations (both cases)	PAS-positive histiocytes in cerebral grey matter
	M	63	Arthritis 20 years; dementia and involuntary movements 18 months; coma		
Stoupel et al (1969) / Groodt-Lasseel & Martin (1969)	F	68	3 years arthritis, 2 years weight loss, 1 year trigeminal neuralgia, myoclonus, ophthalmoplegia	Microscopic in rhinencephalon, corpus luysii, tegmentum of brainstem, grey matter of cord	PAS-positive glial nodules, perivascular cuffing; degenerate bacteria identified as actinomycetes
Janota (1971)	M	56	10 years arthritis, 2 years dementia; no intestinal symptoms	Cortical atrophy; dilated ventricles; uncal gliosis	PAS-positive material in microglia, diffuse and perivascular, mainly temporal
Kodousek & Kojecky (1971)	M	43	Terminal confusion, headache	Internal hydrocephalus; leptomeningitis	PAS-positive microglial nodules mainly in deep cerebral and posterior fossa grey structures

Table 13.2

Neurological Manifestations of Whipple's Disease (17 cases)

Intellectual impairment	7
Coma	5
Visual impairment	4
Ophthalmoplegia	4
Myoclonus	5
Miscellaneous brainstem features	3
Pyramidal	2
Fits	2
Extrapyramidal	1
Cerebellar	1
Meningeal	1
Spinal cord	1

of years, suggesting a diagnosis of Alzheimer's disease. All three had arthritis but no diarrhoea. Other patients (Krücke and Stochdorph, 1962; Minauf and Stochdorph, 1969; Schwartzová, Schwartz and Marek, 1967) had features suggestive of intellectual impairment, and it is perhaps from psychiatric centres that further cases will be described. Pathologically these patients have all shown PAS-positive histiocytes in the brain, either singly and diffusely scattered, or concentrated around blood vessels. Ependymal granulations containing a few PAS-positive cells were present in two of the four. Moderate gliosis and neuronal loss in the cortex was seen by Lampert et al, while Janota's case showed accumulations of microglia, most of which contained PAS-positive granules, present as tumour-like masses in uncus and hippocampus. Bacteria could not be identified in the brain of any of these four cases. Janota showed by electron microscopy that the intracellular PAS-positive material was composed of twisted structures (partly tubular and 5 to 10 nm in diameter) and patches of finer, twisted membranes.

Among other neurological manifestations were *visual impairment, ophthalmoplegia and myoclonus*. The patient of Jones and Paulley (1949) may have had optic neuritis from an unrelated cause, since visual symptoms and optic atrophy developed five years before the onset of diarrhoea. The combination of ophthalmoplegia and myoclonus, appearing in the last year of life, was described by Smith et al (1965, Case 1), Minauf and Stochdorph (1969, Case 1) and Stoupel et al (1969). Electron-microscopic study of the brain in the latter case by Groodt-Lasseel and Martin (1969) is of particular interest because, as already noted, organisms were recognised. These were bacteria, probably intracytoplasmic, and were present in PAS-positive pericapillary inflammatory nodules, in the grey matter of the upper brainstem. They measured 2 μm or more in length by 0·25 μm in diameter, and were surrounded by an envelope 10 nm thick. Budding was observed, suggesting to the authors that the organisms were related to actinomycetes. Apart from budding, they resemble the organisms seen in intestinal biopsies in other cases and this identification must be regarded as tentative. Another electron-microscopic study (Schochet and Lampert, 1969) revealed organisms in brain lesions identical with those seen in the small bowel, and failed to show budding.

A different pathological picture, with areas of demyelination in the cerebrum and neuroglial changes resembling those of progressive multifocal leukoencephalopathy, has been reported in one patient with Whipple's disease (Hecker and Reid, 1962). Eight months before his death, this disorder was diagnosed by cervical lymph node biopsy, and in the last four months of his life the patient developed a severe left and mild right hemiparesis. At autopsy the diagnosis was confirmed by the characteristic changes in small bowel and mesenteric lymph nodes. Both cerebral hemispheres contained large areas of softening in frontal and parietal subcortical white matter. In these, bizarre astrocyte nuclei and abnormal oligodendroglia were seen under the microscope. Macrophages in the larger softened areas were filled with myelin debris but apparently contained no PAS-positive material. Whether this represents a true case of progressive multifocal leukoencephalopathy (Åström, Mancall and Richardson, 1958), with its implication of disordered immunity, or whether something else, is unclear. No similar case has as yet come to light.

References

Åström, K. E., Mancall, E. L. & Richardson, E. P. Jr (1958). Progressive multifocal leukoencephalopathy: hitherto unrecognised complication of chronic lymphatic leukaemia and Hodgkin's disease. *Brain*, **81,** 93–111.

Badenoch, J., Richards, W. C. D. & Oppenheimer, D. R. (1963). Encephalopathy in a case of Whipple's disease. *Journal of Neurology, Neurosurgery and Psychiatry*, **26,** 203–210.

Black-Shaffer, B. (1949). The tinctoral demonstration of a glycoprotein in Whipple's disease. *Proceedings of the Society for Experimental Biology and Medicine*, **72,** 225–227.

Caroli, J., Julien, C., Étévé, J., Prévot, A. R. and Sébald, M. (1963). Trois cas de maladie de Whipple. Remarques cliniques, biologiques, histologiques et thérapeutiques. Étude au microscope électronique de la muqueuse jéjunale. Démonstration de l'origine bactérienne de l'affection. Isolement et identification du germe en cause. *Semaine des hôpitaux de Paris*, **39,** 1457–1480.

Charache, P., Bayless, T. M., Shelley, W. M. & Hendrix, T. R. (1966). Atypical bacteria in Whipple's disease. *Transactions of the Association of American Physicians*, **79,** 399–408.

Chears, W. C. Jr & Ashworth, C. T. (1961). Electron microscopic study of the intestinal mucosa in Whipple's disease. Demonstration of encapsulated bacilliform bodies in the lesion. *Gastroenterology*, **41,** 129–138.

Dobbins, W. O. III & Ruffin, J. M. (1967). A light and electron microscopic study of bacterial invasion in Whipple's disease. *American Journal of Pathology*, **51,** 225–242.

Dybkaer, R. & Kok, N. (1965). Bacteria in Whipple's disease. 3. Studies in two patients of antibodies in serum and cutaneous hypersensitivity against some bacterial antigens. *Acta pathologica et microbiologica scandinavica*, **64,** 373–380.

Groodt-Lasseel, M. de & Martin, J. J. (1969). Étude ultrastructurale des lésions du système nerveux central dans la maladie de Whipple. *Pathologie et Biologie*, **17,** 121–132.

Haubrich, W. S., Watson, J. H. L. & Sieracki, J. C. (1960). Unique morphologic features of Whipple's disease. A study by light and electron microscopy. *Gastroenterology*, **39,** 454–467.

Hecker, R. & Reid, R. T. W. (1962). Cerebral demyelination in Whipple's disease. *Medical Journal of Australia*, **1,** 211–212.

Janota, I. (1971). Whipple's disease with neurological presentation. *Acta neuropathologica (Berlin)*, **18,** 361.

Jones, F. A. & Paulley, J. W. (1949). Intestinal lipodystrophy (Whipple's disease). *Lancet*, **1,** 214–216.

Kjaerheim, Å., Midtredt, T., Skrede, S. & Gjone, E. (1966). Bacteria in Whipple's disease. Isolation of a haemophilus strain from the jejunal propria. *Acta pathologica et microbiologica scandinavica*, **66,** 136–142.

Kodousek, R. & Kojecky, Z. (1971). On the basis of cerebral lesions in Whipple's disease. *Review of Czechoslovak Medicine*, **17,** 137–143.

Koudouris, S. D., Stern, T. N. & Utterback, R. A. (1963). Involvement of the central nervous system in Whipple's disease. *Neurology (Minneapolis)*, **13,** 397–404.

Krücke, W. & Stochdorph, O. (1962). Über Veränderungen im Zentralnervensystem bei Whipple'scher Krankheit. *Verhandlungen der Deutschen Pathologischen Gesellschaft*, **46,** 198–202.

Lampert, P., Tom, M. I. & Cumings, J. N. (1962). Encephalopathy in Whipple's disease. A histochemical study. *Neurology (Minneapolis)*, **12,** 65–71.

Maizel, H., Ruffin, J. M. & Dobbins, W. O. III (1970). Whipple's disease: a review of 19 patients from one hospital and a review of the literature since 1950. *Medicine (Baltimore)*, **49,** 175–205.

Minauf, M. & Stochdorph, O. (1969). Das ZNS bei Morbus Whipple. *Archiv für Psychiatrie und Nervenkrankheiten, vereinigt mit Zeitschrift fur die gesamte Neurologie und Psychiatrie*, **212,** 180–199.

Roberts, D. M., Themann, H., Knust, F. J., Preston, F. E. & Donaldson, J. R. (1970). An electron microscope study of bacteria in two cases of Whipple's disease. *Journal of Pathology*, **100,** 249–255.

Russo, F. R. (1952). Whipple's disease; review of the literature and report of two cases. *Archives of Internal Medicine*, **89,** 600–614.

Schochet, S. S. Jr & Lampert, P. W. (1969). Granulomatous encephalitis in Whipple's disease. Electron microscopic observations. *Acta neuropathologica*, **13,** 1–11.

Schwartzová, K., Schwartz, A. & Marek, J. (1967). Whipplova choroba s. neurologickou symptomatologii. *Plžensky lékarsky Sbornik*, **28,** 99–106.

Sieracki, J. C. (1958). Whipple's disease—observation on systemic involvement. I. Cytologic observations. *Archives of Pathology*, **66,** 464–467.

Sieracki, J. C. & Fine, G. (1959). Whipple's disease—observations on systemic involvement. II. Gross and histologic observations. *Archives of Pathology*, **67,** 81–93.

Sieracki, J. C., Fine, G., Horn, R. C. Jr & Bebin, J. (1960). Central nervous system involvement in Whipple's disease. *Journal of Neuropathology and Experimental Neurology*, **19,** 70–75.

Smith, W. T., French, J. M., Gottsman, M., Smith, A. J. & Wakes-Miller, J. A. (1965). Cerebral complications of Whipple's disease. *Brain*, **88,** 137–150.

Stoupel, N., Monseu, G., Pardoe, A., Heimann, R. & Martin, J. J. (1969). Encephalitis with myoclonus in Whipple's disease. *Journal of Neurology, Neurosurgery and Psychiatry*, **32,** 338–343.

Switz, D. M., Casey, T. R. & Bogaty, G. V. (1969). Whipple's disease and papilledema. *Archives of Internal Medicine*, **123,** 74–77.

Tengström, B. & Werner, I. M. (1966). Whipple's disease. A report of two cases and a review of the literature. *Acta Societatis medicorum Upsaliensis. Upsala Läkareförenings Förhandlingar*, **71,** 237–252.

Whipple, G. H. (1907). A hitherto undescribed disease characterised anatomically by deposits of fat and fatty acids in the intestinal mesenteric lymphatic tissues. *Bulletin of the Johns Hopkins Hospital*, **18,** 382–391.

Yardley, J. H. & Hendrix, T. R. (1961). Combined electron and light microscopy in Whipple's disease. Demonstration of 'bacillary bodies' in the intestine. *Bulletin of the Johns Hopkins Hospital*, **109,** 80–98.

CHAPTER FOURTEEN

Non-Metastatic Effects of Gastrointestinal Neoplasia on the Nervous System and Muscles

Although older journals contain isolated reports linking disease of the nervous system with a remote cancer (Greenfield, 1934) it is only in the last 25 years that the patterns of non-metastatic involvement of the brain, spinal cord, peripheral nerves and muscles in patients with malignant neoplasms has been well documented. This is in large part due to the enthusiasm of groups of workers in Boston and at the London Hospital, as well as to the increasing incidence of lung cancer during this period (especially of oat-cell type, most clearly implicated in this context).

The various syndromes associated with carcinomas and malignant lymphomas are discussed in a companion volume in this series. It is here proposed only to look at those neurological and muscular disorders found in patients with tumours of the gastrointestinal tract. This immediately limits the scope of this section, for a number of these syndromes have yet to be adequately described in association with such neoplasms. Gastrointestinal tumours show remarkable differences in the frequency with which they are associated with remote neurological and muscular effects.

It will be seen from Table 14.1 that the highest incidence of paraneoplastic neurological disorders occurs in carcinoma of the lung or ovary, with gastric carcinoma only a short distance behind. In contrast, carcinomas of the rectum and uterus show no increased incidence of 'neuromyopathy' in comparison with a control group. Tumours of colon, along with those of breast and prostate, fall into an intermediate group. Thus of the common malignant neoplasms of the alimentary tract, gastric carcinoma is the important tumour in relation to remote effects on the nervous system, while colonic cancer is of only secondary interest.

Table 14.1

Sites of Primary Cancer and Incidence of Non-metastatic Neurological Disease ('Neuromyopathy') in 1476 Patients (Data of Croft and Wilkinson, 1965)

Site	No. of patients	No. of patients with neuromyopathy	Percentage with neuromyopathy
Lung	319	49	15·3
Breast	250	11	4·4
Prostate	31	2	6·4
Ovary	55	9	16·4
Uterus (including cervix)	225	4	1·7
Stomach	181	18	10·0
Colon	160	7	4·4
Rectum	207	1	0·5
Double primary	48	2	4·2
Controls	200	(3)	1·5

Whether or not this association of stomach and colonic cancer with nervous disease is a significant one may be seen by analysis of the various paraneoplastic syndromes. Three main points will be stressed. First, that a number of these syndromes have not been described, or described only unconvincingly, in patients with gastrointestinal tumours. Secondly, that at least one syndrome (dermatomyositis) appears to have a close relation with gastric cancer. Finally, that in other and more common patterns of paraneoplastic disease, there seems to be no preponderance of gastrointestinal cases.

Syndromes not convincingly described in association with gastrointestinal carcinomas

The reader is referred elsewhere for details of these disorders, all of which are rare and comprise a small fraction of remote nervous effects of carcinoma and lymphoma.

'Encephalomyelitis with carcinoma' (Henson, Hoffman and Urich, 1965) or 'limbic encephalitis' (Corsellis, Goldberg and Norton, 1968) almost always occurs in patients with oat-cell carcinoma of the bronchus.

Carcinomatous cerebellar degeneration (Brain, Daniel and Greenfield, 1951). The associated neoplasm is almost always one involving the bronchus or ovary. In one case (Balla, 1968) subacute cerebellar degeneration occurred in a patient with a gastric carcinoma. Since this patient was a severe alcoholic, the association of his neoplasm with his cerebellar disease may be fortuitous. A more acceptable case report is that of Julien and Vital (1969). This described a male patient aged 42 who died of a diffusely infiltrating gastric adenocarcinoma 16 months after the onset of cerebellar and upper motor neurone signs. Further reports are needed to establish a relationship between stomach carcinoma and cerebellar degeneration.

Progressive multifocal leukoencephalopathy (Åström, Mancall and Richardson, 1958) is seen in some patients without malignant disease but is most often associated with lymphomas. It has been reported in three patients with carcinomatosis, none obviously of gastrointestinal origin (Richardson, 1961, 1965).

The carcinomatous myasthenic syndrome occurs almost always in association with oat-cell carcinoma of the bronchus (Rooke et al, 1960).

Sensory neuropathy with carcinoma requires special mention. Here there is a ganglio-radiculo-neuropathy, with gross degenerative changes in the dorsal roots, their ganglia and in the dorsal columns, sometimes accompanied by focal inflammatory lesions in cord and brainstem. There is also severe loss of myelinated fibres in peripheral nerves (Croft et al, 1965). The syndrome was first described by Denny-Brown (1948) and most cases reported subsequently have suffered from a bronchial carcinoma (21 out of 23 cases in the London Hospital series reported by Henson and Urich, 1969) and from a simultaneously evolving encephalomyelitis, of the type already mentioned.

Limited data are available about two patients with sensory neuropathy and a gastrointestinal carcinoma. Both cases are so unusual as to raise doubts about the relation of the neurological syndrome to the neoplasm. The first is that of a man aged 54, reported by Dodgson and Hoffman (1953), who developed distal sensory symptoms and signs six months before death, at the same time as a carcinoma of the pyriform fossa was diagnosed. Four weeks after local radiotherapy he was found to have left facial sensory loss and lower motor neurone signs in his hands and right forearm. At autopsy there was a squamous carcinoma of the upper end of the oesophagus. The dorsal columns showed recent, symmetrical degenerative changes and loss of neurones was observed in cervical anterior horns and in one cervical posterior root ganglion. Although these changes would fit a diagnosis of carcinomatous ganglio-radiculo-neuropathy the clinical features are atypical, and documentation of the pathological findings in this case is incomplete. Moreover, remote effects of any kind other than hypercalcaemia are virtually unknown with squamous carcinomas.

The second case is a woman mentioned by Croft and Wilkinson (1969), in whom sensory symptoms and signs anteceded a carcinoma of the caecum by nine years. No further details were recorded, and neither this nor the previous case can be said firmly to link alimentary carcinomas with sensory neuropathy.

Syndromes apparently associated with gastrointestinal carcinomas

Necrotising myelopathy associated with visceral carcinoma (Mancall and Rosales, 1964) was originally described with cancer of the bronchus. However, it is the only unusual paraneoplastic neurological (as distinct from muscular) syndrome that has been reported as having special links with gastric carcinoma. Of 14 cases of spinal cord disease associated with neoplasia described or discussed by Mancall and Rosales, stomach cancer was present in four. An authoritative review of the non-metastatic effects of malignancy (Azzopardi, 1966) takes up this point and suggests that the relationship may be a close one, but we hope to show that this is far from being the case.

The two patients described by Mancall and Rosales, a woman aged 55 and a man aged 49, both died with a bronchial carcinoma and a clinical picture of acute flaccid areflexic paraplegia, sphincter paralysis and sensory loss below a 'level' in the lower cervical or upper dorsal regions. Mild, intermittent, premonitory sensory and motor symptoms had been present for a year. One patient died five days after the onset of acute symptoms while the other survived for five weeks, during which time he developed ascending segmental signs and evidence of cervical cord involvement.

Postmortem examination of both cases showed striking changes in the spinal cord. There was patchy and symmetrical, but not anatomically localised, necrosis of white and grey matter. In the first case this extended from lower cervical to lumbar and sacral segments, in the second from fourth to sixth dorsal segments. Inflammatory change and glial reaction were minimal, but there was well-marked necrosis of vessel walls in the affected areas, with some adventitial fibrosis and occasional luminal thrombotic occlusion in the less acute case.

In a review of cases previously published, Mancall and Rosales listed another nine patients showing a similar clinical and pathological syndrome. They also mentioned a further three where, despite a comparable clinical picture, the pathological data were felt to be incomplete or at variance with the listed cases. All three of these had carcinoma of the stomach. Since 1964 only a further two cases (Bazzan, 1968; Ody, 1969) have been found from listings in the *Index Medicus*, bringing the total—including the dubious instances—to 16. The extreme rarity of the association of necrotising myelopathy with malignancy is apparent.

The tumours present in the reported cases include five bronchial carcinomas, four gastric carcinomas (Lubarsch, 1897, Case 1; Spiller, 1925, Case 2; Juba, 1938; Hetzel, 1960), and neoplasms of prostate, connective tissue of leg ('giant cell sarcoma'), skin (squamous carcinoma and melanoma), breast, cervix and thyroid. In most of these cases, ranging in age from 17 to 74 years, a uniform clinical picture is encountered. The patients present with weak, numb legs, sphincter dysfunction and a flaccid paraplegia sometimes extending up to the arms. The condition progresses over periods varying between two weeks and two months, necropsy revealing necrosis of the cord in the pattern described above, the lower dorsal region normally being worst affected.

The case for considering necrotising myelopathy associated with malignancy as a specific syndrome rests on two considerations: first, its special association with neoplasms and, secondly, its pathological distinctiveness. On neither ground is the case unequivocally proven.

Some of the reported cases cannot be whole-heartedly accepted. These include not only those with unusual tumours but also at least two with proven gastric carcinoma. These are summarised in Tables 14.2 and 14.3.

In Feindel's (1921) case, the tumour was removed months before the development of cord symptoms. Although incompletely described, D'Antona's (1926) case may have had spinal cord metastases. Moersch and Kernohan's (1934) case must be rejected both because of the nature of the tumour (see Table 14.2) and the complicating factor of radiotherapy to the back. The thyroid tumour in Jaffe and Freeman's (1943) case was likely to be a chance

Table 14.2

Doubtful Cases of Necrotising Myelopathy Associated with Neoplasia

	Sex	Age (years)	Type of tumour	Tumour symptoms before neurological symptoms	Neurological symptoms before tumours symptoms	Pathology	Comment
Feindel (1921)	M	23	Giant-cell sarcoma of leg	8 months	—	Necrosis of cord below mid-dorsal level	Tumour removed 6 months before development of myelopathy Myelopathy followed neo-arsphenamine treatment
D'Antona (1926)	M	41	Carcinoma of lung	—	3 weeks	Circumscribed lesion D2 Necrosis of mid and lower dorsal cord	Intramedullary metastasis?
Moersch & Kernohan (1934) Case 3	F	17	Squamous carcinoma in burn of back	Years	—	Necrosis of entire cord below thoracic segments	Back x-irradiated 2 weeks before development of myelopathy Tumour unrelated to myelopathy?
Jaffe & Freeman (1943) Case 2	F	70	Carcinoma of thyroid	—	—	Upper dorsal cord necrosis; cavitation and gliosis Moderate hyperplastic change of surface and penetrating vessels	No evidence that tumour related to neurology; likely to be chance finding Vascular changes suggest Foix–Alajouanine type of myelopathy
Bazzan (1968)	F	44	Carcinoma of cervix	4 years	—	None	Responded to vitamin therapy, with minimal residual disorder Carcinoma found at hysterectomy for menorrhagia

Table 14.3

Cases of Necrotising Myelopathy with Gastric Cancer

	Sex	Age (years)	Tumour symptoms before neurological symptoms	Neurological symptoms before tumour symptoms	Pathology	Comment
Lubarsch (1897) Case 2	F	44	—	1 year	Extensive dorsal column degeneration; anterior and lateral columns, and grey matter affected in cervical and dorsal regions	—
Spiller (1925) Case 2	M	69	2 months	—	Cord necrosis D6; vertebral metastases D3–4	Stomach tumour was x-irradiated Necrosis possibly related to vascular involvement by tumour
Juba (1938)	M	47	—	2 months	Lower dorsal cord necrotic	Vascular proliferation suggested diagnosis of Foix–Alajouanine myelopathy
Hetzel (1960)	M	58	—	2 years	High syringomyelia; extensive vascular proliferation in necrotic dorsal cord	Early symptoms due to syrinx Myelopathy of Foix–Alajouanine type

finding, while the patient of Bazzan (1968) had a minor, reversible neurological disease and a coincidental cervical cancer. Points against acceptance of some of the stomach cancer cases are given in Table 14.3. The number of totally acceptable cases other than those of Mancall and Rosales themselves is thus seen to be very small.

Necrotising myelopathy with carcinoma was thought to be a specific syndrome because the lesions differed from those of other forms of subacute myelopathy and in particular from those of the subacute necrotic myelitis of Foix and Alajouanine (1926). However, the distinction is by no means clear-cut. Foix and Alajouanine described cases with progressive amyotrophic paraplegia with sensory loss, extending upwards and causing death in from one to two years. There was necrosis in the sacral, lumbar and lower dorsal cord segments, mainly central, and a striking 'endo-méso-vascularite' with extreme hypertrophy and dilatation of extramedullary and some penetrating vessels. The absence of this vascular change in Mancall and Rosales' cases was considered a crucial differential diagnostic point. Nevertheless, published reports contain numerous instances of necrotising myelopathy *without* carcinoma, with only mild to moderate vascular hypertrophy, and in a distribution corresponding to that described by Mancall and Rosales. Some of these had evidence of multiple sclerosis, and in others there were no clear aetiological factors.

Perhaps the first of these cases was that of van Gehuchten (1927), a woman aged 34 who died in three months with necrosis of the lower dorsal cord and only moderate vascular hyperplasia. Marinesco and Draganesco (1932) reported two patients who died within five weeks. The cases showed lower cervical and mid-dorsal cord necrosis, and again only mild increase in vascularity. It was suggested that the rapid progression of the pathological process explained the less pronounced degree of vascular change, in comparison with the hypertrophy described by Foix and Alajouanine. Greenfield and Aldren Turner (1939) also believed that venous enlargement was related to chronicity.

Further support for the non-specificity of Mancall and Rosales' findings comes from Hoffman's (1955) description of three cases of necrotising myelopathy without malignancy. Two had no vascular change in a shrunken dorsal cord. A third—with a previous clinical diagnosis of neuromyelitis optica—died in three weeks and showed necrosis throughout the dorsal cord and infarction of superficial and penetrating venules.

In conclusion, it must be said that the number of cases of necrotising myelopathy associated with visceral carcinoma is very small. The evidence for this being a peculiar syndrome is still inconclusive, and the association may be a chance one, or may rest on a non-specific nutritional basis. Certainly, a very similar form of myelopathy occurs in the absence of neoplasia. There is no evidence for a special link between necrotising myelopathy and stomach cancer.

Dermatomyositis and polymyositis are familiar diseases which are far more convincingly related to neoplasia, particularly of the gastrointestinal tract. In 1959 Williams collected 590 reported cases of these disorders, of which 92 (15·6 per cent) were described as having tumours. By 1963 Mills was able to add a further 28 instances of tumour-associated dermatomyositis.

Most of these cases of dermatomyositis with neoplasm (or 'carcinomatous myopathy' in the nomenclature of Henson, Russell and Wilkinson, 1954) occur in the age range of 40 to 70 years. In one series (Arundell, Wilkinson and Haserick, 1960) more than 50 per cent of patients with dermatomyositis aged over 40 years had a malignant tumour. The most frequent, according to Williams' analysis, was carcinoma of the stomach (17 per cent of tumour cases), followed closely by carcinomas of breast (16 per cent), bronchus (15 per cent) and ovary (11 per cent). There are several reported instances of dermatomyositis developing in patients with carcinomas of gallbladder and large bowel. After exclusion of one or two improbable tumour associations listed by Williams (such as chromophobe adenoma of the pituitary), the incidence of gastrointestinal neoplasia, considered as a proportion of those cases of dermatomyositis associated with malignancy, can be reckoned to be at least 25 to 30 per cent (or about 4 per cent of all cases of dermatomyositis).

Dermatomyositis—or polymyositis if skin involvement is not apparent (Eaton, 1954)—shows similar clinical and pathological features, whether it be related to carcinoma or not. The clinical findings are so well known that their detailed description here is not appropriate. However, some reports suggest that carcinomatous cases form a homogeneous group, with a more acutely evolving rash on parts of the skin exposed to sunlight. Muscular symptoms and signs are undoubtedly the same in the two groups, involvement of girdle musculature and disturbances of deglutition being prominent.

A frequently encountered appearance, in muscle biopsies, is that of a necrotising myopathy with some phagocytosis of degenerating fibres and regenerative changes, but without evidence of an interstitial or perivascular inflammatory infiltrate (Walton and Adams, 1958; Smith, 1969; Urich and Wilkinson, 1970). This picture of extensive muscle destruction is in some respects different from the histological variety of polymyositis associated with an immune-type inflammatory reaction. However, as Urich and Wilkinson argue, the retention of 'polymyositis' as a clinical diagnostic term is valid. These authors collected 18 cases, well documented from both clinical and pathological aspects, illustrating destructive muscle disease in patients with neoplasms. Seven of the 18 tumours were gastrointestinal (four gastric—three carcinomas and one plasmacytoma—two colonic carcinomas and one gallbladder carcinoma). The proportion of gastrointestinal tumours in this series (39 per cent) is similar to that found in the clinical series already mentioned.

The lack of histological evidence for an 'auto-immune' mechanism in muscle lesions of tumour-associated dermatomyositis is interesting and rather surprising in view of the work of Grace and Dao (1959) and others, which implicates such a mechanism in the genesis of the skin component of the disease. Grace and Dao studied a patient with inoperable breast cancer, and found that she had cutaneous hypersensitivity to an aqueous extract of her tumour but not to extracts of her skin, subcutaneous tissue or muscle. Passive transfer tests were positive, indicating the presence of humoral antibodies, and it was concluded that the skin reaction was due to the interaction of tumour antigen with specific antibodies.

Syndromes believed sometimes to occur in association with gastrointestinal carcinomas

We come finally to two groups of disorders which are poorly characterised, both physically and conceptually, yet which seem to comprise the majority of reported cases of non-metastatic neurological disease in patients with cancer. Of the patients studied by Croft and Wilkinson (1965) less than a quarter suffered from the syndromes discussed up until now in this chapter. Fifty-six per cent had 'neuromuscular disorders' associated with carcinoma and 20 per cent had a mixed polyneuropathy. In most of the patients in these two groups the diagnosis was made on clinical grounds alone (proximal weakness of the lower limbs and a diminution of tendon reflexes being the important diagnostic criteria). Electrophysiological investigations were not reported, neither were biopsy studies, and it is hardly surprising that a reviewer should have difficulty in coming to positive conclusions about the aetiology and nosology of these disorders. In particular the relationship of gastric and bowel carcinoma to 'neuromuscular disorders' and polyneuropathy is far from clear.

Neuromuscular disorders. The terms 'carcinomatous neuromyopathy', 'carcinomatous myopathy' and 'neuromuscular disorders' have been widely used. They are confusing because they have been defined in varying ways, meaning different things to different authors. At times they have been used to describe conditions overlapping some of the clinicopathological entities already discussed. For instance, 'carcinomatous neuromyopathy' is often diagnosed (Croft and Wilkinson, 1963) when abnormal neurological signs in patients with malignancy are not explicable either by tumour metastases or by some other non-neoplastic neurological disorder: in other words they refer to *all* the syndromes of paraneoplastic nervous involvement. Other authors (Shy and Silverstein, 1965) have defined neuromyopathy as a clinical syndrome of symmetrical, proximal muscle weakness and wasting, associated with a decrease of the appropriate tendon reflexes. *Either* a myopathic *or* a combination of myopathic and neuropathic lesions might be found at biopsy. Brain and Henson (1958) reserve the term 'neuromyopathy' for those cases with clinical and pathological evidence of a lesion in both nerve *and* muscle, and prefer to call the cases without neural lesions 'carcinomatous myopathy'. As already noted, this may be the same as 'polymyositis'.

Brain and Henson's group of patients with 'neuromuscular disorders' broadly corresponds to Shy and Silverstein's 'neuromyopathies'. A small proportion (7·5 to 15 per cent) of these have carcinomas of stomach or rectum, but since both groups include a number of patients with dermatomyositis it is impossible to determine whether these carcinomas might be related to any proximal muscle disorders of a different kind. What seems likely, however, is that the relatively prominent position of stomach carcinoma in the 'neuromyopathy' league (Table 14.1) is due to its association with dermatomyositis rather than with any of the distinctive neurological syndromes.

Mixed polyneuropathy and carcinoma. Of 32 cases of peripheral neuropathy with carcinoma tabulated by Henson and Urich (1969), a bronchial primary tumour was present in 23, a gastric tumour in three and a colonic and pancreatic tumour in one case each. Thus in this small series, a significant proportion of cases—16 per cent—was associated with a gastrointestinal carcinoma. However, the same authors give figures for the incidence of peripheral neuropathy in unselected groups of patients with cancer. These figures include: 5·3 per cent for bronchial carcinoma (17 with neuropathy out of 316 patients), 2·8 per cent for stomach cancer (5 of 178) and 1·2 per cent for breast (3 of 250) and colonic (2 of 160) cancer. When it is recalled that about 1·5 per cent of non-cancer patients were shown to have comparable clinical abnormalities, the figures for the incidence of neuropathy in carcinoma of the breast and colon—and possibly also of the stomach—become insignificant.

Conclusions

On the available evidence, there is little to support the belief that gastrointestinal neoplasms are specifically related to any of the well-recognised neurological syndromes of carcinomatous origin. In contrast, dermatomyositis is a well-proven accompaniment of alimentary cancers, and this association *alone* seems to account for the apparently high incidence of gastric tumours in *aggregated* figures for 'carcinomatous neuromyopathies'. It follows that in a patient presenting with unexplained neurological disease, investigation of the gastrointestinal tract for occult neoplasm is likely to prove fruitless. Carcinoma of the bronchus, especially the oat-cell variety, should always be suspected in such circumstances.

References

Arundell, F. D., Wilkinson, P. D. & Haserick, J. R. (1960). Dermatomyositis and malignant neoplasms in adults: a survey of 20 years experience. *Archives of Dermatology*, **82,** 772–775.

Åström, K. E., Mancall, E. L. & Richardson, E. P. Jr (1958). Progressive multifocal leukoencephalopathy: hitherto unrecognised complication of chronic lymphatic leukaemia and Hodgkin's disease. *Brain*, **81,** 93–111.

Azzopardi, J. G. (1966). Systemic effects of neoplasia. In *Recent Advances in Pathology*, 8th edition, ed. Harrison, C. V., pp. 98–184. London: Churchill.

Balla, J. I. (1968). Cerebellar degeneration in association with carcinoma of the stomach. *British Medical Journal*, **1,** 34.

Bazzan, A. (1968). In tema di sindromi neurologiche paraneoplastiche 'la mielite trasversa o mielomalacia paraneoplastica'. *Minerva medica*, **61,** 47–54.

Brain, R. & Henson, R. A. (1958). Neurological syndromes associated with carcinoma. The carcinomatous neuromyopathies. *Lancet*, **2,** 971–974.

Brain, W. R., Daniel, P. M. & Greenfield, J. G. (1951). Subacute cortical cerebellar degeneration and its relation to carcinoma. *Journal of Neurology, Neurosurgery and Psychiatry*, **14,** 59–75.

Corsellis, J. A. N., Goldberg, G. J. & Norton, A. R. (1968). 'Limbic encephalitis' and its association with carcinoma. *Brain*, **91,** 481–496.

Croft, P. B., Henson, R. A., Urich, H. & Wilkinson, P. C. (1965). Sensory neuropathy with bronchial carcinoma: a study of four cases showing serological abnormality. *Brain*, **88,** 501–514.

Croft, P. B. & Wilkinson, M. (1963). Carcinomatous neuromyopathy. Its incidence in patients with carcinoma of the lung and carcinoma of the breast. *Lancet*, **1,** 184.

Croft, P. B. & Wilkinson, M. (1965). The incidence of carcinomatous neuromyopathy with special reference to carcinoma of the lung and the breast. In *The Remote Effects of Cancer on the Nervous System*, ed. Brain, W. R. & Norris, F. Jr, pp. 44–54. New York: Grune & Stratton.

Croft, P. B. & Wilkinson, M. (1969). The cause and prognosis in some types of carcinomatous neuromyopathy. *Brain*, **92,** 1–8.

D'Antona, S. (1926). Sulla necrosi spinale acuta nel corso dei tumori maligni, con un contributo alla conoscenza delle 'ernie spinali malaciche'. *Neurologica*, **3**, 65–90.

Denny-Brown, D. (1948). Primary sensory neuropathy with muscular changes associated with carcinoma. *Journal of Neurology, Neurosurgery and Psychiatry*, **11**, 73–87.

Dodgson, M. C. H. & Hoffman, H. L. (1953). Sensory neuropathy associated with carcinoma of the esophagus: report of a case. *Annals of Internal Medicine*, **38**, 130–134.

Eaton, L. M. (1954). The perspective of neurology in regard to polymyositis; study of 41 cases. *Neurology (Minneapolis)*, **4**, 245–263.

Feindel, R. (1921). Über akute aufsteigende Rückenmarksnekrose. *Zeitschrift für die gesamte Neurologie und Psychiatrie*, **68**, 147–159.

Foix, C. & Alajouanine, T. (1926). La myélite nécrotique subaiguë. *Revue neurologique*, **2**, 1–42.

Gehuchten, P. van (1927). Un cas de myélite nécrotique aiguë (étude clinique et anatomopathologique). *Revue neurologique*, **1**, 505–519.

Grace, J. T. & Dao, T. L. (1959). Dermatomyositis in cancer: a possible etiological mechanism. *Cancer*, **12**, 648–650.

Greenfield, J. G. (1934). Subacute spino-cerebellar degeneration occurring in elderly patients. *Brain*, **57**, 161–176.

Greenfield, J. G. & Turner, J. W. A. (1939). Acute and subacute necrotic myelitis. *Brain*, **62**, 227–257.

Henson, R. A., Hoffman, H. L. & Urich, H. (1965). Encephalomyelitis with carcinoma. *Brain*, **88**, 449–464.

Henson, R. A., Russell, D. S. & Wilkinson, M. (1954). Carcinomatous neuropathy and myopathy, a clinical and pathological study. *Brain*, **77**, 82–121.

Henson, R. A. & Urich, H. (1969). Peripheral neuropathy associated with malignant disease. In *Disease of Nerves. Part II. Handbook of Clinical Neurology*, ed. Vinken, P. J. & Bruyn, G. W., Vol. 8, pp. 131–148. Amsterdam: North Holland.

Hetzel, H. (1960). Ein fall von 'Myélite nécrotique subaiguë' (Foix-Alajouaninesche Krankheit) mit Syringobulbie und Syringomyelie. *Schweizer Archiv für Neurologie, Neurochirurgie und Psychiatrie*, **86**, 70–81.

Hoffman, H. L. (1955). Acute necrotic myelopathy. *Brain*, **78**, 377–393.

Jaffe, D. & Freeman, W. (1943). Spinal necrosis and softening of obscure origin. *Archives of Neurology and Psychiatry*, **49**, 683–707.

Juba, A. (1938). Myelitis necroticans subacuta (Foix-Alajouanine). *Deutsche Zeitschrift für Nervenheilkunde*, **148**, 17–30.

Julien, J. & Vital, C. (1969). Encéphalomyélite para-néoplastique, à propos d'une observation anatomoclinique. *Revue neurologique*, **120**, 77–88.

Lubarsch, O. (1897). Ueber Rückenmarksveränderungen bei Carcinomatösen. *Zeitschrift für klinische Medizin*, **31**, 389–415.

Mancall, E. L. & Rosales, R. K. (1964). Necrotising myelopathy associated with visceral carcinoma. *Brain*, **81**, 639–656.

Marinesco, G. & Draganesco, S. (1932). Myélite nécrotique aiguë (étude anatomoclinique de deux cas). *Annales de Médecine*, **31**, 5–20.

Mills, J. A. (1963). Connective tissue disease associated with malignant neoplastic disease. *Journal of Chronic Diseases*, **16**, 797–811.

Moersch, F. P. & Kernohan, J. W. (1934). Progressive necrosis of the spinal cord. *Archives of Neurology and Psychiatry*, **31**, 504–526.

Ody, R. (1969). Nekrotisierende Myelopathie bei metastasierendem malignen Melanom. *Archiv für Psychiatrie und Nervenkrankheiten, vereinigt mit Zeitschrift für die gesamte Neurologie und Psychiatrie*, **212**, 289–293.

Richardson, E. P. Jr (1961). Progressive multifocal leukoencephalopathy. *New England Journal of Medicine*, **265**, 815–823.

Richardson, E. P. Jr (1965). Progressive multifocal leukoencephalopathy. In *The Remote Effects of Cancer on the Nervous System*, ed. Brain, W. R. & Norris, F. Jr, pp. 6–16. New York: Grune & Stratton.

Rooke, E. D., Eaton, L. M., Lambert, E. H. & Hodgson, C. H. (1960). Myasthenia and malignant intrathoracic tumor. *Medical Clinics of North America*, **44**, 977–988.

Shy, G. M. & Silverstein, I. (1965). A study of the effects upon the motor unit by remote malignancy. *Brain*, **88**, 515–528.

Smith, B. (1969). Skeletal muscle necrosis associated with carcinoma. *Journal of Pathology*, **97**, 207–210.
Spiller, W. G. (1925). Rapidly developing paraplegia associated with carcinoma. *Archives of Neurology and Psychiatry*, **13**, 471–478.
Urich, H. & Wilkinson, M. (1970). Necrosis of muscle with carcinoma: myositis or myopathy? *Journal of Neurology, Neurosurgery and Psychiatry*, **33**, 398–407.
Walton, J. N. & Adams, R. D. (1958). *Polymyositis*, p. 241. Edinburgh: Livingstone.
Williams, R. C. Jr (1959). Dermatomyositis and malignancy: a review of the literature. *Annals of Internal Medicine*, **50**, 1174–1181.

CHAPTER FIFTEEN

Concomitant Involvement of Nervous System and Alimentary Tract in Systemic Disease

In this chapter we will look at some of the more interesting or best described diseases in which brain and gastrointestinal tract may be concurrently affected. We have had to exercise a choice in selecting diseases to be discussed under this heading. For instance, we have not dealt with the ingestion of various toxic substances capable of producing first abdominal symptoms and then a disturbance of neural function, either central or peripheral. Nor have we discussed disorders like acute intermittent porphyria which may again combine neurological and abdominal symptoms. Polyarteritis nodosa, although capable of involving both gut and nervous system, is beyond the compass of our survey. Although intestinal ulceration may be a feature of Behçet's disease (in which pronounced involvement of the nervous system may occur) the usual site of alimentary tract ulceration, in this disease, is the mouth. Despite the claims of embryology, few gastroenterologists would currently consider this territory their province, and we have left Behçet's disease to some future student of stomatological neurology.

DYSTROPHIA MYOTONICA

This disease (inherited as an autosomal dominant) affects many body systems. Although variable in its clinical manifestations and age of onset, it is usually diagnosed without difficulty because of the classical combination of distal myopathy with myotonia, cataracts, frontal baldness and hypogonadism. Other well-recognised features include involvement of the myocardium, a thickened skull vault, high serum insulin (Huff, Horton and Lebovitz, 1967) and low immunoglobulin levels (Zinneman and Rotstein, 1956; Wochner et al, 1966; Bundey, Carter and Soothill, 1970). The disease is so well known to neurologists that it is surprising that one prominent and important group of manifestations (relating to *central* nervous system involvement) is still poorly recognised. It is perhaps less paradoxical that features of the disease due to alimentary tract involvement should be better known to gastroenterologists than to neurologists. We shall try here to review briefly these two somewhat neglected aspects of a fascinating disorder.

Central nervous system involvement

The most striking manifestation of this is intellectual and social deterioration, often increasingly apparent in successive generations. Although the existence of this feature of dystrophia myotonica was denied—in characteristic dismissive fashion—by Kinnier Wilson (1954) there can be no doubt of its frequent occurrence, as many reports over the last 35 years attest. Mental changes in adults include personality disturbance and dementia, while affected children may be intellectually subnormal. Maas and Paterson (1937) found that 17 of 29 patients with the disease were of low intelligence, 11 being 'congenitally' so and six showing deterioration in adult life. Vanier (1960) and Dodge et al (1965) confirm the frequent occurrence of mental retardation in cases starting in infancy. In adults, EEG changes are common: nearly two-thirds of patients with myotonic dystrophy have recognisable abnormalities (Barwick, Osselton and Walton, 1965). Pneumoencephalography shows progressive dilatation of the cerebral ventricles in 50 per cent of cases (Refsum et al, 1967).

The pathological correlates of these clinical abnormalities have not been well worked out. In four patients with the disease, three of whom had severe intellectual impairment, Rosman and Kakulas (1966) found gross cerebral malformations and cortical dysplasias ranging from pachygyria to microscopic foci of heterotopia.

Evidence of lesions in the diencephalon and brainstem is sketchy. The change of habitus which often occurs, together with multiple endocrine dysfunction (Bauer and Aschner, 1938), has suggested the existence of a hypothalamic disturbance. Hypersomnia (Phemister and Small, 1961) and central alveolar hypoventilation (Kilburn, Eagen and Heyman, 1959) hint at diencephalic and brainstem disease, though this localisation is purely speculative in the absence of confirmatory pathology. Neuropathological evidence of brainstem involvement is limited to an unpublished case examined at the London Hospital by Professor H. Urich which showed glial alterations in pons and medulla reminiscent of those in olivopontocerebellar degeneration.

Unequivocal changes in the spinal cord have yet to be described, though there is some circumstantial evidence pointing to the existence of anterior horn cell disease. Electromyographic changes, minor alterations in muscle histology and histochemistry, and degeneration of motor nerve terminals (MacDermot, 1961; McComas, Campbell and Sica, 1971; Caccia, Negri and Parvis, 1972) have been reported and are compatible with this suggestion.

Gastrointestinal involvement

Disordered gastrointestinal motility in dystrophia myotonica frequently causes 'unexplained' abdominal pain and may lead to laparotomy and even to cholecystectomy. Wider knowledge of this fact might save a few patients from needless abdominal surgery. It is certainly our impression that the abdominal wall of patients with dystrophia myotonica bears witness to past surgical interference far more often than that of other 'neurological' patients.

The pharynx and oesophagus seem to be the most commonly involved parts of the alimentary tract, and dysphagia, nasal regurgitation and aspiration of ingested fluid are frequent symptoms (Harvey, Sherbourne and Siegel, 1965). Abnormal oesophageal peristalsis has been studied radiologically and manometrically. Pruzanski (1965) showed that 43 out of 44 patients retained contrast medium in the pharynx after swallowing; Gleeson et al (1967) also found pooling of contrast in the pharynx, inability to propel a normal-sized bolus into the upper oesophagus and poor oesophageal peristalsis. Siegel, Hendrix and Harvey (1966) reported a low resting pressure at the upper end of the oesophagus and a reduced amplitude of peristalsis throughout the length of the viscus. Patients with dystrophia myotonica were unable to initiate swallowing of water on 50 per cent of attempts, compared with 11 per cent in controls. Prolonged contraction and relaxation, as well as decreased amplitude of contraction, were seen both in upper and lower oesophagus, indicating involvement of smooth as well as striated muscle (Kelley, 1964; Harvey et al, 1965).

An atonic, dilated oesophagus (Ludman, 1962) is sometimes found, and gastric retention due to failure of peristalsis has been described (Kuiper, 1971). In the latter case, food concretions in the gastric antrum at first sight gave the radiological appearance of a carcinoma. The possibility of gastric dilatation should clearly be borne in mind when assessing upper abdominal symptoms in a patient with dystrophia myotonica.

A few case reports suggest that steatorrhoea and malabsorption may occur in this disease. These are certainly uncommon. Lups' patient (1941), a man aged 29, had a 15-year history both of myotonia and of fatty stools, and was severely anaemic. He clearly suffered from malabsorption, but might have had coincidental coeliac disease. His sister had abdominal pains and diarrhoea (without steatorrhoea), a more common state of affairs in myotonic dystrophy. Three of the 16 patients studied by Harvey et al (1965) had diarrhoea, but in only one was the faecal fat in excess of normal. Other authors (Kaufman and Heckert, 1954; Chiu and Englert, 1962; Welch, Haase and Bynum, 1964) have shown that some cases of dystrophia myotonica have steatorrhoea or D-xylose malabsorption. In a few of these cases, jejunal biopsy has failed to show a structural abnormality and any malabsorption is likely to be a consequence of impaired small bowel motility, and of altered bacterial content, rather than of changes in the absorptive surface.

Colonic smooth muscle dysfunction may produce diarrhoea or constipation. An ahaustral, dilated or hosepipe large bowel, the appearance of which may resemble ulcerative colitis on barium enema, may be seen (Bertrand, 1949; Kohn, Faires and Rodman, 1964). Prolonged contraction and slow relaxation of the muscles of the internal and external anal sphincters have also been reported (Schuster, Tow and Sherbourne, 1965).

Using intravenous cholangiography, Harvey et al (1965) showed an absent or impaired response to cholecystokinin, implying an abnormality of the smooth muscle of the gallbladder. There appears to be a high incidence of cholelithiasis in dystrophia myotonica (Chiu and Englert, 1962). If true, the relationship of gallstone formation to the disturbance of smooth muscle function might be significant, and raise broader issues.

Histopathological alterations in intestinal smooth muscle have been reported by Pruzanski and Huvos (1967). They examined two patients who had been without gastrointestinal symptoms during life. Muscle coats of stomach, small and large intestine and gallbladder were said to show a variety of changes including atrophy and focal necrosis of fibres (with possible regeneration in one case) fatty infiltration and fibrosis. Examination of the intrinsic nerves of the gastrointestinal tract by metallic impregnation of the abnormal muscle, and using electron microscopy, has yet to be carried out. It is probable, however, from clinical findings alone that the muscle of the gastrointestinal tract is the seat of a primary degenerative process in dystrophia myotonica.

AMYLOIDOSIS

Deposition of amyloid in body tissues as a primary event is uncommon. It occurs in a metabolic disorder which may be inherited (usually as an autosomal dominant) or it may occur sporadically. Amyloid deposits are also found in association with ageing, myelomatosis, and certain neoplasms, and 'secondary' amyloidosis is an important complication in some patients with chronic infections and collagen disorders.

Amyloid has an immunoglobulin origin. One variety at least is partly derived from the variable part of the immunoglobulin light chain. Experimental amyloidosis in laboratory animals, induced by injection of casein (Kuczynski, 1922), has been ascribed by some workers (Teilum, 1964; Briccetti, Cathcart and Cohen, 1972) to a defective immune response to chronic antigenic stimulation. Such a mechanism, however, has yet to be convincingly shown in either the animal or the human disease.

Whatever the stimulus to its production, amyloid has a uniform histological and ultrastructural appearance. Essentially it is a fibrous glycoprotein which accumulates extracellularly in connective tissue. It is eosinophilic. When stained with a variety of dyes and viewed through the light microscope, using a crossed polariser and analyser, amyloid shows a whorled birefringence, a feature which suggests a structural periodicity. Electron micrographs reveal amyloid to be composed mainly of long, thin, non-branching fibrils. Each fibril is made of one to four filaments 7·0 to 7·5 nm wide, each of which in turn is formed from protofibrils, themselves built up of units about 3·5 nm in diameter. Chemically, the fibrils are found to be largely protein, with 2 to 5 per cent of carbohydrate. They are non-immunogenic and contain no antigen–antibody complexes or immunoglobulin. A second constituent of amyloid, physically and ultrastructurally distinct from the main component, is a non-fibrillar particulate immunogenic glycoprotein (Cohen, 1972).

Involvement of the nervous system is a feature of primary amyloidosis (and more particularly of its hereditary variants). So is involvement of the gastrointestinal tract severe enough to cause symptoms. Secondary amyloidosis does not produce significant nervous or prominent gastrointestinal symptoms. The types of amyloid disease that fall within the scope of this chapter are all primary. In so far as the genetically determined forms of the disease are almost certainly due to some as yet undetermined 'inborn error of metabolism', the term 'primary' should be used with caution. The whole subject of the hereditery amyloidoses is well reviewed by Mahloudji et al (1969).

Both sporadic and hereditary forms of 'primary' amyloidosis may come to the attention of neurologist or gastroenterologist. It should be remembered, however, that not all varieties of hereditary amyloidosis involve the nervous system. Eight clinical forms of hereditary amyloid disease have been recognised and differentiated from one another on grounds of mode of inheritance, age of onset, rate of progression, organ predominantly affected, and usual mode of death. The first five are of no immediate relevance here, but are mentioned to stress the genetic and clinical heterogeneity of 'familial primary amyloidosis'. They are:

(a) amyloid nephropathy (Ostertag, 1932; Maxwell and Kimbell, 1936) (autosomal dominant inheritance);
(b) familial Mediterranean fever (Heller, Sohar and Sherf, 1958) (autosomal recessive inheritance);
(c) fever, urticaria, perceptive deafness and nephropathy (Muckle and Wells, 1962) (autosomal dominant inheritance);
(d) cold hypersensitivity and renal failure (McKusick and Goodman, 1962) (autosomal dominant inheritance);

Table 15.1

A Comparison of some Findings in Four Types of Amyloidosis Affecting Nerves and Gastrointestinal Tract

	Hereditary type I ('Portuguese')	Hereditary type II ('Indiana')	Hereditary type III ('Iowa')	Sporadic primary
Age at onset (years)	20–50	35–50	20–40	30–60
Initial neurological involvement	Feet	Hands	Feet	Hands or feet
Subsequent neurological involvement	Lower > upper limbs	Upper limbs (rarely feet)	Lower > upper limbs	Lower and upper limbs
Gastrointestinal involvement	Frequent	Rare	Frequent	Frequent
Other autonomic involvement	Frequent	Rare	Frequent	Frequent
Renal involvement	Rare	Never	Frequent	Frequent
Duration (years)	7–12	14–40+	1–26	1–5
Cause of death	Cachexia, intercurrent infection	Unrelated	Renal failure	Often renal, cardiac or hepatic failure
Mode of inheritance	Autosomal dominant	Autosomal dominant	Autosomal dominant	-

(e) amyloid cardiomyopathy (Frederiksen et al, 1962) (mode of inheritance uncertain).

In addition, there are three varieties of hereditary amyloidosis with neurological *and* gastroenterological involvement, the latter being conspicuous in two of the forms and unusual in the other:

(f) type I amyloid neuropathy ('Portuguese type') (Andrade, 1951, 1952; Kantarjian and DeJong, 1953; Araki et al, 1968);
(g) type II amyloid neuropathy ('Indiana type') (Rukavina et al, 1956; Schlesinger, Duggins and Masucci, 1962; Mahloudji et al, 1969);
(h) type III amyloid neuropathy ('Iowa type') (van Allen, Frohlich and Davis, 1969).

Some of the features of the three hereditary neuropathic types listed above, as well as of sporadic primary amyloidosis, are set out in Table 15.1. These four distinct varieties of amyloid disease capable of involving the gut and nervous system will now briefly be discussed. An Icelandic family with cerebral haemorrhage and possible amyloid deposition in cerebral arteries (Gudmundsson et al, 1972) is too poorly documented pathologically to be added to these varieties.

Type I amyloid neuropathy ('Portuguese type')

Andrade's description (1951, 1952) of 'a peculiar form of peripheral neuropathy' was the first clear account of familial amyloid involvement of peripheral nerves, though primary amyloidosis affecting neural tissue had been described previously in isolated cases (De Navasquez and Treble, 1938) and possible in one sibship (De Bruyn and Stern, 1929). The patients studied by Andrade lived in or near the Oporto district. The disorder has been referred to as the Portuguese type of amyloidosis, though very similarly affected families, not of Portuguese origin, have since been described from the United States (Kantarjian and DeJong, 1953; Shulman and Bartter, 1956), Germany (Delank et al, 1965), Japan (Araki et al, 1968) and Sweden (Andersson, 1970).

The main clinical feature is a progressive peripheral neuropathy beginning in the feet and extending proximally, the hands occasionally being involved. The limb disorder is associated with alimentary symptoms, disturbances of sphincter control and impotence. The neuropathy is predominantly sensory and may lead to trophic changes and perforating ulcers of the feet. Thermal sense and pain sense are lost early, tactile sense and position sense later. Weakness, which develops late, produces a severe 'steppage' disturbance of gait. The patient ultimately becomes bedridden. Fasciculation is often present but marked muscle wasting is rare. Severe visual impairment may result from linear vitreous opacities, which have been likened to a 'glass wool network' (Kaufman and Thomas, 1959). The irides may also be involved and show irregular outlines and fringed edges. Pupillary contractility may be grossly reduced.

Gastrointestinal complaints range from vague dyspeptic symptoms to prolonged debilitating diarrhoea. Vomiting, violent colic and persistent constipation may also be prominent features. Bouts of alternating constipation and diarrhoea are common in patients with 'Portuguese' amyloidosis, though in the later stages diarrhoea is unremitting. Malabsorption has been reported by some authors (Ribeiro do Rosario, 1961; Ribeiro do Rosario et al, 1963) though demonstrable steatorrhoea is rare.

These symptoms are accompanied by loss of weight and appetite and by obvious features of autonomic neuropathy. Impotence is an important presenting complaint, and disorders of vesical and rectal control are common. The Japanese patients are recorded as having no sensation of bladder fullness or of defaecation. Anhidrosis has been described in some cases. The majority of patients show orthostatic hypotension at the time of first examination, and dizziness and fainting spells occur frequently. Uraemia is significantly absent, although renal involvement is common at necropsy.

This severe disease usually kills the bedridden, debilitated patient within a decade, intercurrent infection developing terminally. At necropsy most organs are involved. The kidney, peripheral nerves, pancreas and heart are the most frequently affected, and liver and spleen the least involved. The cerebral and spinal pia mater may be infiltrated. In peripheral nerves deposits are found between nerve fibres, in the perineurium and in the vasa nervorum. There may be associated demyelination and Schwann cell proliferation. Wallerian degeneration is sometimes seen at a late stage. Large amounts of amyloid are present in the connective tissue of the gastric lamina propria and muscularis and a similar but less severe pattern of deposition is found in the intestines. Intramural nerve plexuses are similarly affected. The gastrointestinal features of this disorder are likely to be the result of such infiltration, although the contributory effect of destruction of exocrine pancreatic tissue should also be considered.

The mode of inheritance of this disorder is autosomal dominant.

Type II amyloid neuropathy ('Indiana type')

A family of Swiss origin, living in Indiana, was found by Rukavina et al (1956) to have a different type of hereditary amyloid neuropathy. It started later and lasted longer, the patients generally dying of unrelated causes. This type of amyloid neuropathy presented as a carpal tunnel syndrome, neuropathic features in the lower limbs being restricted to distal sensory impairment and hyporeflexia. Punctate vitreous opacities were present in some cases. Gastrointestinal involvement and features of autonomic neuropathy were not observed.

In 1969 Mahloudji et al reported a large sibship with an identical disorder from Maryland. This kindred included 11 apparently unrelated families examined in a survey of hereditary neurological disease and eventually traced back to a German couple, married about 1775. At least 146 individuals in seven generations were believed to have been affected. Their neurological disorder had been variously labelled Charcot–Marie–Tooth disease, syringomyelia, carpal tunnel syndrome and polyneuritis. It presented with a picture of median nerve compression in the carpal tunnel, followed by evidence of sensory involvement in other nerves of the upper limbs. Eventually the upper limb reflexes disappeared. Some patients, usually male, had painful paraesthesiae of feet and legs. Men, as a whole, were more severely affected than women. Foot drop sometimes developed. In contrast to Andrade's syndrome, ulceration of the feet was very rare, while trophic lesions of the hands were not uncommon. Vitreous opacities were well documented by Kaufman (1958) in this type of amyloid neuropathy. They were likened to yellow pencil shavings in one of the patients reported by Schlesinger et al (1962). Occasional symptoms of autonomic neuropathy were present, and included impaired sphincter control in two patients and impotence in one.

Gastrointestinal features, encountered in several cases, consisted of mild dyspepsia and chronic constipation. Only one patient had severe watery diarrhoea. Amyloid deposition in the intestinal wall was found at necropsy in one case without abdominal symptoms and might possibly have been the cause of the alimentary disturbances in this sibship.

The mode of inheritance was autosomal dominant.

Type III amyloid neuropathy ('Iowa type')

Only one family suffering from a syndrome of amyloidosis with neuropathy, nephropathy and peptic ulcer has so far been reported (van Allen et al, 1969). The average survival after the onset of symptoms ranged from 12 to 17 years, in different generations. Death was usually due to amyloid renal disease. The initial manifestations appeared in the third and fourth decades.

A very slowly progressive sensorimotor neuropathy was observed, the lower extremities being affected more than the upper. The involvement was sometimes as severe as in the Portuguese type of amyloidosis. Visual loss was present in some cases, lenticular rather than vitreous opacities being the cause. Anhidrosis and impotence suggested associated autonomic neuropathy.

In almost every case duodenal ulceration had occurred at some time during the patient's illness. Some patients had severe chronic dyspepsia and vomiting, while others developed severe gastrointestinal haemorrhage, pyloric stenosis, or perforation of an ulcer. One patient had died from peritonitis following such an event. Several patients had undergone gastrectomy.

Amyloid infiltration of the vagus was seen in a biopsy specimen, but in other biopsy and autopsy material insignificant amounts of amyloid were found in relation to the area of peptic ulceration. The cause of this ulceration remains obscure. However, both neuropathy (somatic and autonomic) and nephropathy were shown to be due to extensive amyloid deposition.

The mode of inheritance was autosomal dominant.

Sporadic primary amyloidosis

When there is a positive family history and the patient presents one of the disease patterns just described a clinical diagnosis of primary amyloidosis should be relatively easy to make, and then to confirm by biopsy. Greater difficulty is encountered in sporadic cases, which may present bizarre symptoms and elude diagnosis in life. Prominent among the clinical features of such cases are severe diarrhoea, evidence of autonomic neuropathy, hoarseness and electrocardiographic abnormalities.

The case described by French et al (1965) is representative of this group, illustrating the various problems of diagnosis and the evolution of neurological and gastroenterological signs. A 42-year-old man presented with pain in the feet and legs, associated with sensory impairment and recurrent ulceration of the toes. Four years later he developed profuse watery diarrhoea, urinary incontinence and impotence, and his polyneuritis began to affect his upper limbs. Macrocytic anaemia was found and malabsorption demonstrated. Over the next two years his neuropathy and diarrhoea worsened, and he became bedridden. Postural hypotension was an additional problem. The possibility of amyloidosis was considered in life, but nerve and gastric biopsies were negative. Death from bronchopneumonia occurred nine years after the first symptoms. At necropsy deposits of amyloid in vessels and nerves were found in many organs. There was extensive involvement of autonomic nerves (including myenteric and submucosal plexuses). In the absence of amyloid infiltration of bowel mucosa or muscle coats, such nervous infiltration might well have been a cause of his diarrhoea.

The prevalence of gastroenterological symptoms in sporadic primary amyloidosis is difficult to assess, early accounts of such patients (Chambers, Medd and Spencer, 1958) sometimes aggregating sporadic and familial cases in their discussion of this problem, and others (Barth et al, 1969) being so slanted towards the immunochemical and metabolic aspects as to leave one in some doubt as to basic clinical facts. Of the three patients with sporadic primary amyloidosis involving the nervous system reported by Chambers et al (1958), two had severe diarrhoea. Munsat and Poussaint (1962) reported gastrointestinal symptoms in 13 of 19 patients with amyloid neuropathy. The abdominal symptoms were initially of a rather vague nature but were followed by severe constipation or diarrhoea. Other abdominal symptoms are less frequent. These include vomiting, dyspepsia, and a picture of acute abdomen (Barth et al, 1969) due to haemorrhage into abdominal lymph nodes.

Sporadic primary amyloidosis may present as a neuropathy (Chambers et al, 1958; Munsat and Poussaint, 1962). The neuropathy is predominantly sensory, and while frequently taking the form of a carpal tunnel syndrome it may begin in the lower limbs, as in the case already described, or it may be generalised from the onset (Munsat and Poussaint, 1962). The neurological aspects may be quite striking. The patients may present with lightning pains in the legs, suggestive of tabes, and the pupillary signs (irregularity, poor response to light) may lead to serious diagnostic errors, particularly as motor signs (such as weakness and wasting) may be delayed in their appearance. The CSF protein may be raised and the colloidal gold curve abnormal, further adding to the diagnostic difficulties. The nerves may be enlarged. Pain and thermal sensation are affected early and sensory symptoms may appear with great suddenness. The tendon reflexes are often long preserved (Chambers et al, 1958), this presumably representing the rather late involvement of large diameter, faster conducting afferent fibres. The combination of distal analgesia of stocking type with retained reflexes may lead to misdiagnoses of hysteria or (if there is ulceration) of dermatitis artefacta (Chambers et al, 1958). The main differential diagnosis is from tabes, hereditary sensory radicular neuropathy, hypertrophic polyneuritis and leprosy. Nerve biopsy may be very informative. The association of hoarseness, abnormal ECG and peripheral neuropathy (Sullivan et al, 1955), or of renal failure, cardiac failure and peripheral neuropathy, have been stressed as highly suggestive of sporadic primary amyloidosis.

Infiltration of muscles, with and without gastroenterological accompaniment may occur and present with swelling, induration and pain on exercise, a diagnostic problem which is solved by biopsy. Macroglossia occurs in one-third to half of cases and may be a helpful clue. It is not a feature of familial primary amyloidosis (Rukavina et al, 1956). Chambers et al (1958) stress the significance of some little known signs or symptoms that might suggest that a severe peripheral neuropathy might be due to primary amyloidosis. Among such features are hoarseness (at times due to amyloidosis of the vocal cords), symmetrical swelling of the submandibular region (suggestive of enlargement of the root of the tongue), and generalised pigmentation. Amyloid purpura is frequently noted about the head and neck (Barth et al, 1969) and is probably due to traumatic rupture of thickened, inelastic small vessels. Many cases show increased numbers of plasma cells in the marrow, though there is no evidence of myelomatosis and in fact immunoglobulin synthesis is decreased. Most patients die from involvement of kidneys, heart or liver within a few years (Chambers et al, 1958; Barth et al, 1969).

Biopsy of liver, tongue, lymph node or other organs and examination by modern methods should enable a diagnosis of amyloid disease to be made in most of these sporadic cases.

PSEUDOXANTHOMA ELASTICUM

Patients with pseudoxanthoma elasticum (PXE), a hereditary disease of connective tissue, may on occasion come under the care of either gastroenterologist or neurologist. PXE is a rare disease, having an estimated prevalence in Great Britain of between one and six per million (Berlyne, Bulmer and Platt, 1961). The condition is inherited as an autosomal recessive trait. The nature of the basic defect is uncertain (McKusick, 1966) but the essential pathological change is the deposition of abnormal, partly fibrillar material in the deeper parts of the dermis and in the walls of muscular arteries. This material has some of the tinctorial features of elastic (e.g. orceinophilia) but under the electron microscope it has the appearances, including periodicity, of normal collagen (Tunbridge et al, 1952). Whether it is derived from true elastic fibres or from a degenerative process occurring in collagen and akin to solar or senile elastosis is disputed. Fragmentation and calcification of the abnormal fibres occurs. This leads to a marked reduction of elasticity in affected skin and blood vessels, which may also develop medial fibrosis.

A tendency to spontaneous arterial haemorrhage results from increased rigidity, and may lead to luminal narrowing. Most of the major organs may be affected. Disease of the cardiovascular system includes coronary insufficiency, myocardial infarction, hypertension and intermittent claudication. The radial pulses may not be palpable. The most important gastrointestinal effect of PXE is haemorrhage, which is common and may be fatal.

Haemorrhage usually comes from small gastric lesions, such as areas of superficial erosion. These are presumed to have a partly ischaemic origin.

Only occasionally is an obvious abnormality, such as peptic ulcer or hiatus hernia, revealed by contrast radiography. Bleeding is not always from the stomach, and massive haemorrhage from the jejunum has been described (Sames, 1961). Children may be affected (McKusick, 1966) and pregnancy may predispose patients with PXE to gastrointestinal bleeding.

The skin lesions, which the patient has sometimes known to be present from childhood, are the most obvious diagnostic clue. Typically, areas with lax, redundant, inelastic folds, covered with small yellowish plaques and resembling the skin of a plucked chicken, are seen on the neck and abdominal wall and in the axillae, antecubital fossae and groins. Facial creases may be exaggerated. Skin biopsy shows a picture of abnormal, calcified, elastic-staining granular or fibrillar material in the middle and deep parts of the dermis, usually associated with a foreign-body type giant-cell inflammatory reaction.

The eye lesions in PXE are also characteristic. Ocular fundi show grey or reddish, pigmentless angioid streaks, often orientated like vessels but several times wider than veins. They lie deep to the retinal vessels and probably represent cracks in Bruch's membrane resulting from elastic degeneration. A non-specific choroidoretinitis may also be found. Extensive retinal scarring may develop, and together with intraocular haemorrhage may lead to blindness.

Clinical involvement of the central nervous system, distinct from the eye, is relatively uncommon, but a number of patients have had severe or fatal neurological disease in consequence of the combined effects of cerebral arterial degeneration and hypertension. These are summarised in Table 15.2. Several other cases, including that of Benedict and Montgomery (1935), others collected by Témime (1940), and Case 9 of Carlborg et al (1959) have had PXE and what was probably fortuitously associated nervous disease, such as epilepsy or a glioma. There are also reports of patients (such as the 13-year-old child—Case 3—described by McKusick in 1966) who were neurologically asymptomatic in life but had demonstrable lesions of the cerebral arteries at autopsy. Berry aneurysm in association with PXE was reported by Dixon (1951). Scheie and Hogan (1957) described a patient with bilateral calcified internal carotid aneurysms. Premature calcification of the choroid plexus was commented on by the same authors. Calcification of the pineal and falx in a young woman aged 31 was described by Nellen and Jacobson (1956). The carotid syphon was calcified in a 30-year-old patient reported by Goodman et al (1963) and in a patient reported by Zentmayer (1946). Many authors have stressed the tendency to premature calcification of peripheral arteries and other structures in PXE.

The need to examine every patient with haematemesis or melaena (and every patient—and in particular every young patient—with a 'stroke') for the characteristic skin and ocular lesions of PXE has often been emphasised. Correct diagnosis in the casualty department (Berlyne, 1960) or outpatient clinic may save patients with PXE, bleeding from the gastrointestinal tract, from inappropriate surgery, though surgery may be the only means of stopping disastrous blood loss. The occurrence of gastrointestinal bleeding in a young patient who has had a stroke, or of a stroke in a young patient with a previous

Table 15.2

Involvement of the Nervous System in Pseudoxanthoma Elasticum

Author	Sex	Age	Neurological findings	Autopsy	Neuropathological findings
Urbach & Nékám (1936) Urbach & Wolfram (1937)	M	47	3 years headache, speech disturbance; Korsakoff psychosis; death after right hemiplegia	Yes	Multiple cerebral and pontine infarcts; arteriosclerotic vascular changes
Prick (1937)	F	48	Left hemiparesis; death several days later from massive pontine lesion	Yes	Pontine infarct; hyalinisation of pontine vessels, which had normal elastic
Carlborg et al (1959) Case 10	F	59	Coma; right sided motor signs; death in a few hours	Yes	Plum-sized cerebellar haemorrhage; normal adjacent vessels
van Bogaert (1961)	F	21	Acute onset of headache and massive brainstem lesion, with subarachnoid bleeding; death 2 days later	?	
van Bogaert (1961)	F	17	Three acute brainstem episodes over 12 days; death	No	
Messis & Budzilovitch (1970)	M	41	Psychosis in last few weeks of life	Yes	Calcification of cerebral arteries and arterioles; softenings in thalamus and cerebral white matter
Rios-Montenegro et al (1972)	M	20	Right proptosis due to carotico-cavernous fistula; alive		

history of gastrointestinal bleeding, should lead one to suspect PXE. The detection of absent peripheral pulses, angioid streaks, characteristic skin lesions or premature arterial calcification would be strong corroborative evidence of the disease.

ABETALIPOPROTEINAEMIA (BASSEN–KORNZWEIG SYNDROME)

In 1950 Bassen and Kornzweig reported the case of an 18-year-old girl, born of parents who were first cousins, with a hitherto unreported syndrome of retinitis pigmentosa, central nervous disease resembling Friedreich's ataxia, and peculiar crenated red cells in the peripheral blood. Walking had been delayed until she was two years old, and steatorrhoea had been present up to the age of six. Two years later Singer, Fisher and Perlstein described a patient with the same condition. This was a 13-year-old boy, also of consanguineous parents, with 'coeliac disease' in early childhood, progressive ataxic neuropathy, and a similar malformation of red cells, for which the name 'acanthrocytosis' was coined. The third case (Kornzweig and Bassen, 1957) was the younger brother of the first, and the fourth a Belgian girl reported by Druez (1959), who having had the dubious benefit of a classical education corrected 'acanthrocytosis' to 'acanthocytosis' (Greek *akantha*, a thistle). By 1968 28 patients affected with this rare condition had been documented (Fredrickson, Gotto and Levy, 1972).

The Bassen–Kornzweig syndrome is characterised biochemically by the absence of betalipoprotein in the blood. The various plasma lipoproteins (chylomicrons, prebeta-, beta- and alpha-lipoproteins) are absent or deficient in three genetically determined disorders of lipid transport (the other two being familial hypobetalipoproteinaemia and Tangier disease). All three disorders are of neurological interest, but only abetalipoproteinaemia is associated with clinical gastrointestinal disease and therefore falls within the scope of our survey.

Biochemical disorder

In the Bassen–Kornzweig syndrome betalipoprotein is totally absent from the blood. It was at one time believed that small amounts might indeed be present, ultracentrifugation of plasma producing a lipoprotein fraction with the same density as betalipoprotein; this, however, turned out to have a different chemical composition. The likely metabolic defect is a failure of synthesis, probably in the liver, of the protein moiety (apoprotein) which has a molecular weight of 500 000, and is made up of subunits of molecular weight between 26 000 and 80 000 (Fredrickson et al, 1972). Biochemical diagnosis begins with the finding of a low serum cholesterol and is confirmed by a variety of protein separation and identification techniques, notably immunoelectrophoresis. These define the absence of betalipoprotein.

Clinical features

Clinical manifestations appear early. Affected children seem normal at birth but soon develop steatorrhoea and abdominal distension. They fail to grow and to gain weight normally in infancy. Between the ages of 5 and 10 years a typical retinitis pigmentosa and an ataxic neurological disorder appear. There is progressive disability and death may occur in childhood, though some patients survive to middle life.

Intestinal. Steatorrhoea is prominent in early infancy, in fact *before* gluten is added to the diet. In several cases it has lessened or disappeared by the age of six, perhaps because of the reduction of fat intake. Pancreatic and intestinal enzymes and bile salts are present in the bowel in normal amounts and fat is handled normally in the lumen of the small bowel. Up to 80 per cent of an ingested fat load may be absorbed into the intestinal mucosa, but it cannot be removed from this site because of a defective transport mechanism. No chylomicrons enter the lymphatic system. This failure of transmucosal transport produces steatorrhoea and also results in a pathognomonic abnormality on jejunal biopsy. This shows a mucosa of normal thickness, with normal shaped and sized villi but (if the diet has contained fat in the previous 14 days) with many lipid droplets. These give a characteristic foamy, vacuolated appearance to the epithelial cells, especially at the tips of the villi.

Haematological. Acanthocytes, which are erythrocytes with spiky or tentacular processes, are seen in wet preparations of fresh peripheral blood. It should be noted that acanthocytosis occurs in other diseases without lipoprotein abnormalities, some of which have neurological features (Critchley, Clark and Wikler, 1968; Levine, Estes and Looney, 1968).

Retinal. Retinitis pigmentosa developed between the ages of 18 months and 6 years in one patient (Salt et al, 1960; Wolff, Lloyd and Tonks, 1964) and between 13 and 19 years in another (Singer et al, 1952; Jampel and Falls, 1958). The earliest ophthalmoscopic change is the appearance of pigment granules in the macular region. Pigment later appears at the periphery of the fundi. By the time pigmentary retinopathy has become well developed, impaired visual acuity, scotomata, constricted visual fields and night blindness are likely to be present.

Neurological. As has already been noted, the neurological component of the Bassen–Kornzweig syndrome is slowly progressive and bears some resemblance to Friedreich's ataxia. In 10 cases reviewed by Schwartz et al 1963) neurological features, in order of decreasing frequency, included areflexia, proprioceptive loss, ataxia of gait, trunk and limbs, muscle weakness external ophthalmoplegia, extensor plantar responses and cutaneous sensory loss. Abnormal neurological signs were first detected in this group of patients, between the ages of 2 and 17 years. Motor abnormalities have, however, been found as early as 20 months (Becroft, Costello and Scott, 1965). Deformities—pes cavus and kyphoscoliosis—often occur and are presumably a sequel of the chronic disturbance of motor function. The progression of the disease is relentless. Most patients are unable to stand by the time they reach the age of 30.

Neuropathology

These symptoms and signs point to lesions of the long tracts, brainstem and cerebellum, and possibly of peripheral nerves. The nature of such lesions is poorly defined pathologically for no adequate description of the brain, cord and nerves in the Bassen–Kornzweig syndrome has yet been published. All that is available is minimal information about two autopsies and one sural nerve biopsy.

The patient described by Sobrevilla, Goodman and Kane (1964) was a 36-year-old woman. An abnormal gait was recognised in early childhood; bilateral pes cavus had been present since the age of 15, and in the last 11 years she had developed weak, areflexic limbs, distal proprioceptive deficit and extensor plantar responses. At the age of 30, visual impairment and macular degeneration were noted, and deposits of brown pigment were subsequently observed in each macular region. Visual loss and difficulty with walking were severe by the time she died (of heart disease). In life, the diagnosis was suggested by the presence of acanthocytosis and a low serum cholesterol. Autopsy revealed marked pallor of myelin staining in the dorsal columns and some demyelination in the spinocerebellar tracts. Focal loss of myelin was also seen in sections of peripheral nerves. The cerebellum was said to show decreased numbers of Purkinje cells and to contain demyelinated foci, but the documentation of these statements was very sketchy.

A second autopsied case is the 10-year-old boy reported by Dische and Porro (1970). Steatorrhoea was present from early infancy and a neurological picture of broad-based gait, coarse intention tremor, slurred speech, impaired position and vibration sense and areflexia began to develop two years before he died, also from cardiac failure. At post-mortem examination, evidence of a cardiomyopathy was present. The cerebrum was normal (apart from prominent lipofuscin deposits in cortical neurones). The cerebellum showed no loss of cells or abnormality of white matter. However, as in the first autopsied case, marked demyelination of the dorsal columns, with gliosis, was found, and there were similar but less severe changes in the spinocerebellar tracts. Anterior horn cells, like cortical neurones, showed an increased amount of lipochrome pigment, possibly a significant finding (see below). Peripheral nerves again contained demyelinated areas, an observation also made on a sural nerve biopsy by Schwartz et al (1963). No significant muscle lesions were found in these cases.

The neuropathology of the Bassen–Kornzweig syndrome is thus too poorly worked out for an involved discussion to be worthwhile. One point may perhaps be made. It has often been noted that the neurological part of this syndrome clinically resembles Friedreich's ataxia. Inasmuch as the most obvious nervous lesions in abetalipoproteinaemia, as in Friedreich's ataxia, are in the long ascending tracts of the spinal cord, there is pathological support for this view. However, until an autopsy report with an adequate description of cerebellum, brainstem, dorsal roots and dorsal root ganglia is published, a valid comparison between the two conditions cannot be made.

Aetiology

The spinocerebellar degeneration in the Bassen–Kornzweig syndrome (as in Friedreich's ataxia) is probably 'abiotrophic' (Gowers, 1902), and future research may conceivably demonstrate a specific neuronal enzymic defect, presumably resulting from the same abnormal gene which is responsible for deficient synthesis of betalipoprotein in the liver. Nervous, biochemical, haematological and intestinal changes are probably separate manifestations of a multisystem disease, and there is probably no direct relationship between fat and vitamin malabsorption on the one hand and the central nervous lesions on the other.

The role of vitamin E. Attempts have nevertheless been made to link the neurological features of the syndrome to vitamin E deficiency. The argument rests on the finding of unrecordable vitamin E levels in the blood of patients with Bassen–Kornzweig syndrome (Kayden, Silber and Kossmann, 1965), the occurrence of nervous disease in rats deprived of dietary vitamin E, and the existence of microscopic nervous lesions in infants with abnormal fat absorption and presumed low vitamin E levels. Our currently inadequate knowledge of the nature of the neurological component of the Bassen–Kornzweig syndrome makes the argument worth recapitulating, even though it is hard to envisage how a simple dietary deficiency of this sort could produce such an anatomically restricted form of system degeneration.

In experimental animals, it is well known that vitamin E deficiency may produce both a myopathy (which will not be discussed further) and degeneration in the central nervous system. Acutely developing muscular paralysis in rats whose mothers had been deprived of the vitamin was reported as long ago as 1928 by Evans and Burr. In 1935 Ringsted first described a nervous disorder resulting from chronic vitamin E deficiency in adult rats. Clinical and pathological features were comprehensively reviewed by Einarson and Ringsted (1938), and many confirmatory reports have appeared (Luttrell and Mason, 1949; Malamud, Nelson and Evans, 1949). The essential signs which evolve over 6 to 15 months, are a progressive ataxic paraparesis with marked muscle wasting, hypalgesia, and urinary incontinence. The underlying pathology is a combined neural and muscular one, atrophy of spinal origin supervening on an initial myopathic process. The earliest central nervous lesions are degeneration of posterior spinal roots and posterior columns, with demyelination, loss of axons and gliosis. The neurones of the anterior spinal horns subsequently show chromatolysis, become filled with lipochrome pigment, and eventually disappear, leaving a glial residue. Some pyramidal tract degeneration may be present. Einarson (1952) finds the overall morbid anatomical picture reminiscent 'of the combined features of tabes dorsalis, muscular dystrophy and muscular atrophy of spinal origin'.

Pentschew and Schwarz (1962) and Lampert, Blumberg and Pentschew (1964) found microscopic eosinophilic bodies in the gracile and cuneate nuclei of rats deprived of dietary vitamin E for many months. These bodies appear before obvious dorsal column degeneration and are thought to represent the earliest effect of degeneration occurring distally in long fibres. Similar bodies have been seen in children with cystic fibrosis (Sung, 1964) and biliary atresia (Sung and Stadlan, 1966), and it has been argued that since vitamin E deficiency is present in these states (Nitowsky, Gordon and Tildon, 1956) distal neuronal degeneration of this type is related to avitaminosis E. Unfortunately, eosinophilic bodies have no such specificity: they occur in a variety of toxic or metabolic nervous diseases where there is no evidence whatsoever of vitamin E deficiency. They are seen for instance in a spontaneous disease of childhood known as infantile neuroaxonal dystrophy

(Seitelberger, 1957; Cowen and Olmstead, 1963), and in rats poisoned with parabromophenylacetylurea (Blakemore and Cavanagh, 1969). In all probability they result from attempted terminal regeneration of the central axon of any neurone whose metabolism has been impaired, irrespective of cause.

It is interesting that eosinophilic axonal bodies have been seen in the dorsal horns of the spinal cord in Friedreich's ataxia (Blakemore and Cavanagh, 1969). A tenuous link between the Bassen–Kornzweig syndrome and the neurological effects of hypovitaminosis E is thus provided. The link is indeed tenuous, since the neuronal and axonal lesions in the cords of vitamin-E-deficient rats are far more widespread than in the human diseases. Moreover, attempts to induce a similar neurological syndrome in dietarily deprived primates have failed. Einarson and Telford (1960) maintained young rhesus monkeys on vitamin-E-deficient diets for up to three years: while a florid muscle disorder was produced, abnormality in the central nervous system was restricted to pigment deposition and chromatolysis in neurones, with little evidence of cell death and none of tract degeneration. In the absence of the protective antioxidant effect of vitamin E, it is conceivable that the accumulated intraneuronal pigment under these circumstances as well as in the rat and in one of the autopsied cases of Bassen–Kornzweig syndrome (Dische and Porro, 1970) is an end-product of excessive lipid peroxidation (Tappel, 1962). It is hard, however, to reconcile the lack of tract lesions in Einarson and Telford's vitamin-deficient monkeys either with the cord lesions in rats or with the dorsal column and spinocerebellar degeneration seen in the human syndrome.

Lipochrome deposition apart, there is some circumstantial evidence that vitamin E deficiency may play a part in the pathogenesis of some of the lesions of the Bassen–Kornzweig syndrome. Kayden et al (1965) have shown that the increased susceptibility of acanthocytes to autohaemolysis when exposed to hydrogen peroxide was reversed by the vitamin, while Molenaar et al (1968) have given vitamin E to two patients with low blood levels, and have shown that poorly defined intracellular membranes in jejunal epithelium gain a normal appearance after such treatment.

References

Dystrophia myotonica

Barwick, D. D., Osselton, J. W. & Walton, J. N. (1965). Electroencephalographic studies in hereditary myopathy. *Journal of Neurology, Neurosurgery and Psychiatry*, **28,** 109–114.

Bauer, J. & Aschner, B. (1938). Beziehungen zwischen Endokrinologie und Neurologie. *Confinia neurologica*, **1,** 318–343.

Bertrand, L. (1949). Le mégacolon dans la maladie de Steinert. *Revue neurologique*, **81,** 480–486.

Bundey, S., Carter, C. D. & Soothill, J. F. (1970). Early recognition of heterozygotes for the gene for dystrophia myotonica. *Journal of Neurology, Neurosurgery and Psychiatry*, **33,** 279–293.

Caccia, M. R., Negri, S. & Parvis, V. P. (1972). Myotonic dystrophy with neural involvement. *Journal of the Neurological Sciences*, **16,** 253–269.

Chiu, V. S. W. & Englert, E. Jr (1962). Gastrointestinal disturbances in myotonia dystrophica. *Gastroenterology*, **42,** 745–746.

Dodge, P. R., Gamstorp, I., Byers, R. K. & Russell, P. (1965). Myotonic dystrophy in infancy and childhood. *Pediatrics*, **35,** 3–19.

Gleeson, J. A., Swann, J. C., Hughes, D. T. D. & Lee, F. I. (1967). Dystrophia myotonica—a radiological survey. *British Journal of Radiology*, **40**, 96–100.

Harvey, J. C., Sherbourne, D. H. & Siegel, C. I. (1965). Smooth muscle involvement in myotonic dystrophy. *American Journal of Medicine*, **39**, 81–90.

Huff, T. A., Horton, E. S. & Lebovitz, H. E. (1967). Abnormal insulin secretion in myotonic dystrophy. *New England Journal of Medicine*, **277**, 837–841.

Kaufman, K. K. & Heckert, E. W. (1954). Dystrophia myotonica with associated sprue-like symptoms. *American Journal of Medicine*, **16**, 614–616.

Kelley, M. L. (1964). Dysphagia and motor failure of the esophagus in myotonia dystrophica. *Neurology (Minneapolis)*, **14**, 955–960.

Kilburn, K. H., Eagen, J. T. & Heyman, A. (1959). Cardiopulmonary insufficiency associated with myotonic dystrophy. *American Journal of Medicine*, **26**, 929–935.

Kohn, N. N., Faires, J. S. & Rodman, J. (1964). Unusual manifestations due to involvement of involuntary muscle in dystrophia myotonica. *New England Journal of Medicine*, **271**, 1179–1183.

Kuiper, D. H. (1971). Gastric bezoar in a patient with myotonic dystrophy. A review of the gastrointestinal complications of myotonic dystrophy. *American Journal of Digestive Diseases*, **16**, 529–534.

Ludman, H. (1962). Dysphagia in dystrophia myotonica. *Journal of Laryngology and Otology*, **76**, 234–236.

Lups, S. (1941). Dystrophia myotonica mit Steatorrhoe. *Acta medica scandinavica*, **106**, 557–578.

McComas, A. J., Campbell, M. J. & Sica, R. E. P. (1971). Electrophysiological study of dystrophia myotonica. *Journal of Neurology, Neurosurgery and Psychiatry*, **34**, 132–139.

MacDermot, V. (1961). The histology of the neuromuscular junction in dystrophia myotonica. *Brain*, **84**, 75–84.

Maas, O. & Paterson, A. S. (1937). Mental changes in families affected by dystrophia myotonica. *Lancet*, **1**, 21–23.

Phemister, J. C. & Small, J. M. (1961). Hypersomnia in dystrophia myotonica. *Journal of Neurology, Neurosurgery and Psychiatry*, **24**, 173–175.

Pruzanski, W. (1965). Myotonic dystrophy—a multisystem disease. Report of 67 cases and a review of the literature. *Psychiatria et Neurologia*, **149**, 302–322.

Pruzanski, W. & Huvos, A. G. (1967). Smooth muscle involvement in primary muscle disease. I. Myotonic dystrophy. *Archives of Pathology*, **83**, 229–233.

Refsum, S., Lønnum, A., Sjaastad, O. & Engeset, A. (1967). Dystrophia myotonica. Repeated pneumoencephalographic studies in ten patients. *Neurology (Minneapolis)*, **17**, 345–348.

Rosman, N. P. & Kakulas, B. A. (1966). Mental deficiency associated with muscular dystrophy. A neuropathological study. *Brain*, **89**, 769–787.

Schuster, M. M., Tow, D. E. & Sherbourne, M. E. (1965). Anal sphincter abnormalities characteristic of myotonic dystrophy. *Gastroenterology*, **49**, 641–648.

Siegel, C. I., Hendrix, T. R. & Harvey, J. C. (1966). The swallowing disorder in myotonia dystrophica. *Gastroenterology*, **50**, 541–550.

Vanier, T. M. (1960). Dystrophia myotonica in childhood. *British Medical Journal*, **2**, 1284–1288.

Welch, J. D., Haase, G. R. & Bynum, T. E. (1964). Myotonic muscular dystrophy. Systemic manifestations. *Archives of Internal Medicine*, **114**, 669–679.

Wilson, S. A. K. (1954). *Neurology*, 2nd edition, p. 1172. London: Butterworth.

Wochner, R. D., Drews, G., Strober, W. & Waldmann, T. A. (1966). Accelerated breakdown of immunoglobulin G (IgG) in myotonic dystrophy. A hereditary error of immunoglobulin catabolism. *Journal of Clinical Investigation*, **45**, 321–329.

Zinneman, H. H. & Rotstein, J. (1956). A study of gamma globulins in dystrophia myotonica. *Journal of Laboratory and Clinical Medicine*, **47**, 907–916.

Amyloidosis

Andersson, R. (1970). Hereditary amyloidosis with polyneuropathy. *Acta medica scandinavica*, **188**, 85–94.

Andrade, C. (1951). Note préliminaire sur une forme particulière de neuropathie périphérique. *Revue neurologique*, **85**, 302–306.

Andrade, C. (1952). A peculiar form of peripheral neuropathy. *Brain*, **75**, 408–427.

Araki, S., Mawatari, S., Ohta, M., Nakajima, A. & Kuroiwa, Y. (1968). Polyneuritic amyloidosis in a Japanese family. *Archives of Neurology*, **18**, 593–602.

Barth, W. F., Willerson, J. T., Waldmann, J. A. & Decker, J. L. (1969). Primary amyloidosis. Clinical, immunochemical and immunoglobulin metabolism studies in fifteen patients. *American Journal of Medicine*, **47**, 259–273.

Briccetti, A. B., Cathcart, E. S. & Cohen, A. S. (1972). Casein-induced experimental amyloidosis. 2. Lymphocyte transformation in preamyloidotic and amyloidotic guinea pigs. *Acta pathologica et microbiologica scandinavica, Section A*, **80**, Supplementum 233, 162–166.

Chambers, R. A., Medd, W. E. & Spencer, H. (1958). Primary amyloidosis, with special reference to involvement of the nervous system. *Quarterly Journal of Medicine*, **27**, 207–226.

Cohen, A. S. (1972). Inherited systemic amyloidosis. In *The Metabolic Basis of Inherited Disease*, 3rd edition, ed. Stanbury, J. B., Wyngaarden, J. B. & Fredrickson, D. S. New York: McGraw-Hill.

De Bruyn, R. S. & Stern, R. O. (1929). A case of the progressive hypertrophic polyneuritis of Dejerine and Sottas, with pathological examination. *Brain*, **52**, 84–107.

Delank, H. W., Koch, G., Könn, G., Missmahl, H. P. & Suwelack, K. (1965). Familiäre Amyloid-polyneuropathie typus Wohlwill-Corino Andrade. *Ärztliche Forschung*, **19**, 401–416.

De Navasquez, S. & Treble, H. A. (1938). A case of primary generalized amyloid disease with involvement of the nerves. *Brain*, **61**, 116–128.

Frederiksen, T., Gøtzsche, H., Harboe, N., Kiær, W. & Mellemgaard, K. (1962). Familial primary amyloidosis with severe amyloid heart disease. *American Journal of Medicine*, **33**, 328–348.

French, J. M., Hall, G., Parish, D. J. & Smith, W. T. (1965). Peripheral and autonomic nerve involvement in primary amyloidosis associated with uncontrollable diarrhoea and steatorrhoea. *American Journal of Medicine*, **39**, 277–284.

Gudmundsson, G., Hallgrímson, J., Jónasson, T. A. & Bjarnason, O. (1972). Hereditary cerebral haemorrhage with amyloidosis. *Brain*, **95**, 387–404.

Heller, H., Sohar, E. & Sherf, L. (1958). Familial Mediterranean fever. *Archives of Internal Medicine*, **102**, 50–71.

Kantarjian, A. D. & DeJong, R. N. (1953). Familial primary amyloidosis with nervous system involvement. *Neurology (Minneapolis)*, **3**, 399–409.

Kaufman, H. E. (1958). Primary familial amyloidosis. *Archives of Ophthalmology*, **60**, 1036–1043.

Kaufman, H. E. & Thomas, L. B. (1959). Vitreous opacities diagnostic of familial primary amyloidosis. *New England Journal of Medicine*, **261**, 1267–1271.

Kuczynski, M. H. (1922). Edwin Goldmanns Untersuchungen über celluläre Vorgänge im Gefolge des Verdauungsprozesses auf Grund nachgelassener Präparate dargestellt und durch neue Versuche ergänzt. *Virchows Archiv für pathologische Anatomie und Physiologie und für klinische Medizin*, **239**, 185–302.

McKusick, V. A. & Goodman, R. M. (1962). Pinnal calcification. Observations in systemic diseases not associated with disordered calcium metabolism. *Journal of the American Medical Association*, **179**, 230–232.

Mahloudji, M., Teasdall, R. D., Adamkiewicz, J. J., Hartmann, W. H., Lambird, P. A. & McKusick, V. A. (1969). The genetic amyloidoses: with particular reference to hereditary neuropathic amyloidosis, Type II (Indiana or Rukavina Type). *Medicine (Baltimore)*, **48**, 1–37.

Maxwell, E. S. & Kimbell, I. (1936). Familial amyloidosis, with case reports. *Medical Bulletin of the Veterans' Administration*, **12**, 365–369.

Muckle, T. J. & Wells, M. (1962). Urticaria, deafness and amyloidosis: a new heredofamilial syndrome. *Quarterly Journal of Medicine*, **31**, 235–248.

Munsat, T. L. & Poussaint, A. F. (1962). Clinical manifestations and diagnosis of amyloid polyneuropathy. Report of three cases. *Neurology (Minneapolis)*, **12**, 413–422.

Ostertag, B. (1932). Demonstration einer eigenartigen familiären 'Para-amyloidose'. *Zentralblatt für allgemeine Pathologie und pathologische Anatomie*, **56**, 253–254.

Ribeiro do Rosario, M. (1961). Aspects cliniques et pathophysiologiques des troubles digestifs de l'amylose primaire, type portugais. *Acta gastro-enterologica belgica*, **24**, 391–399.

Ribeiro do Rosario, M., Antunes, L., Barros, F., Pinto, R. & Baptista, A. (1963). Études sur la paramyloidose portugaise à forme polyneuritique (type C Andrade) II. Le syndrome digestif. *Acta neuropathologica*, Supplement 2, 19–28.

Rukavina, J. G., Block, W. D., Jackson, C. E., Falls, H. F., Carey, J. H. & Curtis, A. C. (1956). Primary systemic amyloidosis: a review and an experimental, genetic and clinical study of 29 cases with particular emphasis on the familial form. *Medicine (Baltimore)*, **35**, 239–334.

Schlesinger, A. S., Duggins, V. A. & Masucci, E. F. (1962). Peripheral neuropathy in familial primary amyloidosis. *Brain*, **85**, 357–370.

Shulman, L. E. & Bartter, F. C. (1956). Familial primary amyloidosis. *Bulletin of the Johns Hopkins Hospital*, **98**, 238–239.

Sullivan, J. F., Twitchell, T. E., Gherardi, G. J. & Vanderlaan, W. P. (1955). Amyloid polyneuropathy. *Neurology (Minneapolis)*, **5**, 847–855.

Teilum, G. (1964). Pathogenesis of amyloidosis. The two-phase cellular theory of local secretion. *Acta pathologica et microbiologica scandinavica*, **61**, 21–45.

van Allen, M. W., Frohlich, J. A. & Davis, J. R. (1969). Inherited predisposition to generalised amyloidosis. *Neurology (Minneapolis)*, **19**, 10–25.

Pseudoxanthoma elasticum

Benedict, W. L. & Montgomery, H. (1935). Pseudoxanthoma elasticum and angioid streaks. *American Journal of Ophthalmology*, **18**, 205–212.

Berlyne, G. M. (1960). Pseudoxanthoma elasticum. *Lancet*, **1**, 77–80.

Berlyne, G. M., Bulmer, H. G. & Platt, R. (1961). The genetics of pseudoxanthoma elasticum. *Quarterly Journal of Medicine*, **30**, 201–212.

Carlborg, V., Ejrup, B., Grönblad, E. & Lund, F. (1959). Vascular studies in pseudoxanthoma elasticum and angioid streaks. *Acta medica scandinavica*, **166**, Supplementum 350, 1–84.

Dixon, J. M. (1951). Angioid streaks and pseudoxanthoma elasticum with aneurysm of the internal carotid artery. *American Journal of Ophthalmology*, **34**, 1322–1323.

Goodman, R. M., Smith, E. W., Paton, D., Bergman, R. A., Siegel, C. L., Otteson, O. E., Shelley, W. M., Pusch, A. L. & McKusick, V. A. (1963). Pseudoxanthoma elasticum: a clinical and histopathological study. *Medicine (Baltimore)*, **42**, 297–334.

McKusick, V. A. (1966). Pseudoxanthoma elasticum. In *Heritable Disorders of Connective Tissue*, 3rd edition, pp. 286–324. St Louis: Mosby.

Messis, C. P. & Budzilovitch, G. N. (1970). Pseudoxanthoma elasticum. Report of an autopsied case with cerebral involvement. *Neurology (Minneapolis)*, **20**, 703–709.

Nellen, M. & Jacobson, M. (1956). Pseudoxanthoma elasticum (Grönblad-Strandberg disease) with coronary artery calcification. *South African Medical Journal*, **32**, 649–651.

Prick, J. J. G. (1937). Pontine pseudobulbaire Paralyse bij Pseudoxanthoma Elasticum. *Nederlandsch tijdschrift voor geneeskunde*, **81**, 3093–3096.

Rios-Montenegro, E. N., Behrens, M. M. & Hayt, W. F. (1972). Pseudoxanthoma elasticum. Association with bilateral carotid rete mirabilis and unilateral carotid—cavernous sinus fistula. *Archives of Neurology*, **26**, 151–155.

Sames, C. P. (1961). Pseudoxanthoma elasticum: severe melaena from the jejunum treated by resection. *Proceedings of the Royal Society of Medicine*, **54**, 519.

Scheie, H. G. & Hogan, T. F. (1957). Angioid streaks and generalised arterial disease. *Archives of Ophthalmology*, **57**, 855–868.

Témime, P. (1940). *Contribution à l'étude de l'élastorrhexie systématisée*. Paris: Jouve, Imprimerie de la Faculté de Médecine.

Tunbridge, R. E., Tattersall, R. N., Hall, D. A., Astbury, W. T. & Reed, R. (1952). The fibrous structure of normal and abnormal human skin. *Clinical Science*, **11**, 315–331.

Urbach, E. & Nékám, L., Jr. (1936). Pathogenese des Groenblad-Strandbergschen Syndroms (Pseudoxanthoma elasticum + Angioid streaks). *Klinische Wochenschrift*, **15**, 850–857.

Urbach, E. & Wolfram, S. (1937). Veränderungen des elastischen Gewebes bei einem autoptisch untersuchten Falle von Groenblad-Strandbergschem Syndrom. *Archiv für Dermatologie und Syphilis*, **176**, 167–175.

van Bogaert, L. (1961). Neuropathologie générale des phacomatoses et de quelques dystrophies neuro-cutanées moins bien connues, chez l'enfant. *18e Congrès de l'Association des Pédiatres de Langue française, Genève*, 1961, **2**, 349–386. Bâle & New York: Karger.

Zentmayer, W. (1946). Angioid streaks of the fundus oculi observed over a period of thirty-six years; report of a case. *Archives of Ophthalmology*, **35**, 541–545.

Abetalipoproteinaemia

Bassen, F. A. & Kornzweig, A. L. (1950). Malformation of the erythrocytes in a case of atypical retinitis pigmentosa. *Blood*, **5**, 381–387.

Becroft, D. M. D., Costello, J. M. & Scott, P. J. (1965). A-β-lipoproteinaemia (Bassen-Kornzweig syndrome). *Archives of Disease in Childhood*, **40**, 40–52.

Blakemore, W. F. & Cavanagh, J. B. (1969). 'Neuroaxonal dystrophy' occurring in an experimental 'dying back' process in the rat. *Brain*, **92**, 789–804.

Cowen, D. & Olmstead, E. V. (1963). Infantile neuroaxonal dystrophy. *Journal of Neuropathology and Experimental Neurology*, **22**, 175–236.

Critchley, E. M. P., Clark, D. B. & Wikler, A. (1968). Acanthocytosis and neurologic disorder without abetalipoproteinemia. *Archives of Neurology*, **18**, 134–140.

Dische, M. R. & Porro, R. S. (1970). The cardiac lesions in Bassen–Kornzweig syndrome. *American Journal of Medicine*, **49**, 568–571.

Druez, G. (1959). Un nouveau cas d'acanthocytose: dysmorphie érythrocytaire congénitale avec rétinite, troubles nerveux et stigmates dégénératifs. *Revue d'Hématologie*, **14**, 3–11.

Einarson, L. (1952). Criticizing review of the concepts of the neuromuscular lesions in experimental vitamin E deficiency, preferably in adult rats. *Acta psychiatrica neurologica scandinavica*, Supplentum 78, 1–76.

Einarson, L. & Ringsted, A. (1938). *Effect of chronic vitamin E deficiency on the nervous system and the skeletal musculature in adult rats: a neurotropic factor in wheat germ oil.* Copenhagen: Munksgaard; London: Oxford.

Einarson, L. & Telford, I. R. (1960). Structural changes in the nervous system of monkeys deprived of vitamin E. *Anatomiske Skrifter*, **3**, 1–28.

Evans, H. M. & Burr, G. D. (1928). Development of paralysis in the suckling young of mothers deprived of vitamin E. *Journal of Biological Chemistry*, **76**, 273–297.

Fredrickson, D. S., Gotto, A. M. & Levy, R. I. (1972). Familial lipoprotein deficiency (abetalipoproteinemia, hypobetalipoproteinemia, and Tangier disease). In *The Metabolic Basis of Inherited Disease*, 3rd edition, ed. Stanbury, J. B., Wyngaarden, J. B. & Fredrickson, D. S. New York: McGraw-Hill.

Gowers, W. R. (1902). A lecture on abiotrophy. *Lancet*, **1**, 1003–1007.

Jampel, R. S. & Falls, H. F. (1958). Atypical retinitis pigmentosa, acanthrocytosis and heredodegenerative neuromuscular disease. *Archives of Ophthalmology*, **59**, 818–820.

Kayden, H. J., Silber, R. & Kossmann, C. E. (1965). The role of vitamin E deficiency in the abnormal autohemolysis of acanthocytosis. *Transactions of the Association of American Physicians*, **78**, 334–342.

Kornzweig, A. L. & Bassen, F. A. (1957). Retinitis pigmentosa, acanthrocytosis and heredodegenerative neuromuscular disease. *Archives of Ophthalmology*, **58**, 183–187.

Lampert, P. W., Blumberg, J. M. & Pentschew, A. (1964). An electron microscopic study of dystrophic axons in the gracile and cuneate nuclei of vitamin E deficient rats. *Journal of Neuropathology and Experimental Neurology*, **23**, 60–77.

Levine, I. M., Estes, J. W. & Looney, J. M. (1968). Hereditary neurological disease with acanthocytosis. A new syndrome. *Archives of Neurology*, **19**, 402–409.

Luttrell, C. N. & Mason, K. E. (1949). Vitamin E deficiency, dietary fat, and spinal cord lesions in rat. *Annals of the New York Academy of Sciences*, **52**, 113–120.

Malamud, N., Nelson, M. M. & Evans, H. M. (1949). Effect of chronic vitamin E deficiency on nervous system in rats. *Annals of the New York Academy of Sciences*, **52**, 135–138.

Molenaar, I., Hommes, F. A., Braams, W. G. & Polman, H. A. (1968). Effect of vitamin E on membranes of the intestinal cell. *Proceedings of the National Academy of Sciences of the U.S.A.*, **61**, 982–988.

Nitowsky, H. M., Gordon, H. H. & Tildon, J. T. (1956). Studies of tocopherol deficiency in infants and children. IV. The effect of alpha tocopherol on creatinuria in patients with cystic fibrosis of pancreas and biliary atresia. *Bulletin of the Johns Hopkins Hospital*, **98**, 361–371.

Pentschew, A. & Schwarz, K. (1962). Systemic axonal dystrophy in vitamin E deficient adult rats. *Acta neuropathologica*, **1**, 313–334.

Ringsted, A. (1935). A preliminary note on the appearance of paresis in adult rats suffering from chronic avitaminosis E. *Biochemical Journal*, **29**, 788–795.

Salt, H. B., Wolff, O. H., Lloyd, J. K., Fosbrooke, A. S., Cameron, A. H. & Hubble, D. V. (1960). On having no betalipoprotein: a syndrome comprising a-beta-lipoproteinaemia, acanthocytosis, and steatorrhoea. *Lancet*, **2**, 325–329.

Schwartz, J. F., Rowland, L. F., Eder, H., Monks, P. A., Osserman, E. F., Hirschberg, E. & Anderson, H. (1963). Bassen–Kornzweig syndrome: deficiency of serum β-lipoprotein. A neuromuscular disorder resembling Friedreich's ataxia, associated with steatorrhea, acanthocytosis, retinitis pigmentosa and a disorder of lipid metabolism. *Archives of Neurology*, **8**, 438–454.

Seitelberger, F. (1957). Zur Morphologie und Histochemie der degenerativen Axonveranderungen im Zentralnervensystem. *IIIe Congrès International de Neuropathologie, Bruxelles. Rapports et Discussions*, pp. 127–147.

Singer, K., Fisher, B. & Perlstein, M. A. (1952). Acanthrocytosis: a genetic erythrocytic malformation. *Blood*, **7**, 577–591.

Sobrevilla, L. A., Goodman, M. L. & Kane, C. H. (1964). Demyelinating central nervous disease, macular atrophy and acanthrocytosis (Bassen–Kornzweig syndrome). *American Journal of Medicine*, **37**, 821–828.

Sung, J. H. (1964). Neuroaxonal dystrophy in mucoviscidosis. *Journal of Neuropathology and Experimental Neurology*, **23**, 567–583.

Sung, J. H. & Stadlan, E. M. (1966). Neuroaxonal dystrophy in congenital biliary atresia. *Journal of Neuropathology and Experimental Neurology*, **25**, 341–361.

Tappel, A. L. (1962). Vitamin E as the biological lipid antioxidant. *Vitamins and Hormones*, **20**, 493–510.

Wolff, O. H., Lloyd, J. K. & Tonks, E. L. (1964). A-beta-lipoproteinaemia with special reference to the visual defect. *Experimental Eye Research*, **3**, 439–442.

CHAPTER SIXTEEN

The Gastrointestinal Tract in Neurological Disease

Most of our monograph has been concerned with the impact on the nervous system of disorders of gastrointestinal structure and function. In our last chapter we take a look at the other side of the coin: the production of gastroenterological disease by neurological disorders.

The clinical neurologist divides abnormalities of motor function into those caused by primary muscle disease, those caused by a lower motor neurone lesion and those caused by lesions of the upper motor neurone, but it is not convenient to envisage disorders of alimentary motility in an analogous way. Post-ganglionic autonomic fibres arise either from *sympathetic* paravertebral ganglion cells or from *parasympathetic* ganglion cells, close to or within the bowel wall. The complex anatomy of these systems precludes a simple, arbitrary grouping of disorders of intestinal motor function comparable to that used for abnormalities in the innervation of striated muscle. Hence instead of using terms like 'lower motor neurone' or 'upper motor neurone' disorders, we will here consider alterations of gastrointestinal function as due to abnormalities of *intrinsic* and of *extrinsic* bowel innervation. In addition, alimentary smooth muscle may itself be the seat of primary disease. This is seen in association with some primary diseases of voluntary muscle.

SMOOTH MUSCLE INVOLVEMENT IN DISEASES OF VOLUNTARY MUSCLE

Acute gastric dilatation in patients with Duchenne, limb-girdle or facio-scapulo-humeral dystrophy has been described by Crowe (1961), Robin and Falewski (1963), and earlier by Berblinger and Dukens (1929) and Bevans (1945). Despite the rarity of published cases, Robin and Falewski (1963) asserted that 'acute gastric dilatation, far from being uncommon, is an almost diagnostic manifestation of muscular dystrophy'. In their experience, gained in a crippled children's hospital in Jerusalem, nearly all patients with dystrophy had suffered from repeated attacks of gastric dilatation. These began with malaise, and abdominal pain, tenderness and distension. Vomiting followed after a few hours. This was effortless and profuse, often of a 'coffee ground' appearance at first, and then clear and watery. Dehydration developed with choleraic speed. Some of the reported cases responded to the traditional 'suck-and-drip' method, but in others the outcome was fatal, either from fluid loss or from gastric perforation and peritonitis (Bevans, 1945, Case 4).

Robin and Falewski (1963) discussed the possibility that dystrophic change in the smooth muscle of the stomach wall might be responsible for acute gastric dilatation, but were unable to produce evidence to this effect. There are several papers which purport to show 'degeneration', 'fatty infiltration' or 'loss' of muscle fibres in the gastrointestinal tract in patients with muscular dystrophies, but the changes described seem to us to be either artefactual, insignificant or present in controls. Other reports reveal inadequate knowledge of muscle pathology (Bunting, 1908; Bevans, 1945; Huvos and Pruzanski, 1967). While it may well be that in the Duchenne, limb-girdle and facio-scapulo-humeral dystrophies there are degenerative changes in alimentary smooth muscle, such changes have yet to be convincingly documented.

Apart from acute gastric dilatation, there is little clinical evidence of involvement of the gastrointestinal tract in these conditions. Patterson and Rios (1959) showed impaired gastrointestinal motility in a 28-year-old patient with a myopathy of obscure nature. This had led to severe malnutrition, and was claimed to be related to atrophy of the circular muscle coat of the intestinal wall. A similar mechanism was proposed (though not confirmed histologically) by Patterson, Ong and Drake (1964) to explain impaired D-xylose absorption, in the absence of steatorrhoea, in a group of patients with muscular dystrophy. This finding has not been reported by other workers and standard accounts of the dystrophies understandably make no mention of intestinal involvement.

SMOOTH MUSCLE INVOLVEMENT IN EXTRINSIC NERVOUS DISEASE

In a book on the neurology of gastrointestinal disease space should be found for a few words on what might be termed 'the gastroenterology of neurological disease'. Description of the alimentary symptoms that may be encountered by neurologists in their clinical practice is beyond our brief. There is no point, for instance, in our dealing here with the semeiology and treatment of tabetic crises, with constipation in multiple sclerosis, vomiting from raised intracranial pressure, or with the symptoms resulting from general debility and weak abdominal muscles. Lesions of peripheral and central autonomic pathways producing gastrointestinal dysfunction are catalogued elsewhere (e.g. Hillemand, 1955; Appenzeller, 1969), though it is noteworthy how relatively little attention has been paid by neurologists to this aspect of autonomic disease compared with disturbances of vasomotor or bladder function.

Some quite important effects of denervation of the alimentary tract have received less attention than (in our opinion) they deserve. There are, for instance, very few clinical or experimental studies on changes in the motility of the bowel following lesions of the spinal cord (Connell, Frankel and Guttmann, 1963). We do not propose to discuss the complete spectrum of gastrointestinal disease resulting from damage to extrinsic nerve pathways. Instead we will confine ourselves to some common—but under-recognised—symptoms occurring in two common neurological diseases and probably due to cranial parasympathetic lesions. In addition, we will discuss the problem of diarrhoea in patients with diabetes, a syndrome held to be due to autonomic neuropathy.

Motor neurone disease

It has long been known that gastrointestinal smooth muscle may be involved in motor neurone disease (Léri, 1902), but it is only in recent years, with the use of intraluminal pressure recording, fluoroscopy and cineradiography that such involvement has been well documented. The patients so affected are those with bulbar and pseudobulbar symptomatology, rather than those with progressive muscular atrophy. Their dysphagia may result from disorders of pharyngeal function and of oesophageal motility. These patients may also develop dilatation of the stomach and first part of the duodenum, which may produce symptoms but is more often clinically silent.

Disorders of the pharynx in amyotrophic lateral sclerosis have been studied cineradiographically by Bosma and Brodie (1969) and we will say nothing more about them. Oesophageal motility was examined in 19 patients with bulbar involvement by Smith, Mulder and Code (1957). Diminished peristaltic pressures or incoordinated peristaltic activity were found. Fischer et al (1965) confirmed these findings, and showed additionally that some patients had diffuse oesophageal spasm or absent lower oesophageal sphincter activity.

Gross dilatation of oesophagus, stomach and first part of duodenum was described by Boudin et al (1954) in a clinical and radiological study from the Salpêtrière. Ten out of 12 patients with bulbar features were thus affected; usually there were no accompanying abdominal symptoms. Reduced oesophageal motility and gastric stasis were also observed. Boudin and his colleagues made an analogy between these findings and the occurrence of gastric paralysis after vagotomy (Walters and Belding, 1951), in diphtheria and in poliomyelitis, where neuronal destruction can be found in the dorsal nucleus of the vagus and nucleus ambiguus. In three of their patients they were able to confirm the existence of nerve cell damage in the dorsal motor vagal nucleus, an observation also made—about the same time—by Lawyer and Netsky (1953), thereby providing a logical anatomical basis for gastric and oesophageal dysfunction in motor neurone disease. A further case of gastric dilatation in amyotrophic lateral sclerosis has been published by Bariety et al (1961); however, this complication remains virtually undocumented in the English-language literature.

Parkinson's disease

Gastrointestinal symptoms—in particular constipation—are common in Parkinson's disease (Pallis, 1971). We shall here confine ourselves to disorders of deglutition and oesophageal function, which are less well recognised. The Parkinsonian patient with rapid weight loss and dysphagia may present a difficult diagnostic problem. Carcinoma of the stomach or oesophagus is not usually the underlying cause. Fruitless and unnecessary investigation for what are basically neurogenic symptoms is still too often undertaken.

Mild degrees of dysphagia are common in all varieties of Parkinsonism. Radiological studies (Grossiord et al, 1956) have shown delay in the initiation of swallowing, irregular movement of the epiglottis, and stasis of contrast medium in pyriform fossa and valleculae. *Oesophageal motility* may be abnormal, even in patients without dysphagia (Fischer et al, 1965). Intraluminal pressure measurements show defective peristalsis, while non-peristaltic segmental oesophageal spasm may be present on barium swallow examination (Eadie and Tyrer, 1965). These abnormalities can be related to a disturbance of vagal innervation, the dorsal nucleus of the vagus often showing neuronal loss or damage in Parkinson's disease (Eadie, 1963).

'Diabetic diarrhoea'

'Diabetic diarrhoea' is a poorly understood disorder of intestinal function, encountered in inadequately controlled diabetics, and widely held, on somewhat flimsy evidence, to be due to an autonomic neuropathy. The *objective* basis for this belief is, perhaps unavoidably, rather shaky. There is, however, a certain amount of *circumstantial* evidence, which we shall now review.

Clinical features and associations. Although there had been a few earlier reports, Rundles (1945) was the first to draw attention to the frequency of gastrointestinal disorder in patients with diabetic neuropathy. Of 125 patients with unequivocal diabetic neuropathy 76 (61·8 per cent) had 'striking abnormalities' of alimentary function 'in the form of severe constipation, chronic diarrhea, anorexia and nausea'. Many of these patients suffered from impotence and urinary difficulties, and several from orthostatic hypotension.

Diabetics without neuropathy were no more prone to develop gastrointestinal symptoms than were a comparable group of non-diabetics. The usual causes of these symptoms had been carefully excluded by customary diagnostic methods, such as radiological examination, sigmoidoscopy, stool examination, etc. Twenty-seven patients had a severe, chronic diarrhoea, often alternating with constipation. In some patients the diarrhoea was predominantly nocturnal, often being associated with faecal incontinence. The author attributed 'diabetic diarrhoea' to 'autonomic nerve disease'. Two fatal cases of diabetic neuropathy with prominent gastrointestinal symptoms were reported to have shown 'degenerative changes in the nerve trunks of the oesophageal plexus and about the celiac ganglia' but no further details were given.

Sheridan and Bailey (1946) reported 40 patients with severe diabetes and intermittent nocturnal diarrhoea. Most had also suffered from nocturnal faecal incontinence. These patients were seldom troubled by diarrhoea during the daytime but might have 8, 10 or more stools at night. The stools were watery, and quite unlike those found in steatorrhoea. The diarrhoea was strikingly intermittent, remissions lasting days or weeks being followed by relapses of similar duration. Diabetic neuropathy had preceded the onset of diarrhoea in 58 per cent of the 40 cases reported. The authors concluded, without pathological evidence, that the condition might be due to a 'disturbance of sympathetic innervation'.

In a radiological study of 30 patients with diabetic neuropathy and prominent gastrointestinal symptoms Hodges, Rundle and Hanelin (1947) found that 'some degree of gastric retention, prolonged barium transit time through the intestinal tract, and segmentation of the barium column' were fairly constant features. In many of the patients the radiological evidence of disturbed gastrointestinal function 'was less conspicuous than the clinical symptomatology would lead one to expect'. 'Abnormalities of the same type and degree occurred in those suffering from severe constipation as in those with chronic diarrhea. There were no features by which patients with nocturnal diarrhea could be separated from those with daytime diarrhea'. The authors claimed that this relative paucity of radiological signs in patients with presumed autonomic neuropathy of diabetic origin was not really very surprising. They showed that patients who had been submitted to extensive bilateral thoraco-lumbar surgical sympathectomy (for the treatment of arterial hypertension) only exhibited 'a slight slowing of transit time'.

In 1957, Malins and French reviewed the whole subject. They reported 28 cases of diabetes mellitus, complicated by chronic diarrhoea. In 10 of the 28 cases the diarrhoea was only troublesome at night. In none of the patients was the diabetes considered well controlled. Detailed studies confirmed the presence of normal pancreatic secretion. Malabsorption did not appear to be present. Seven of the patients had no evidence of neuropathy. Of the remainder, 14 had autonomic neuropathy (as evidenced by impotence, sweating disorders and/or orthostatic hypotension) in addition to more classical signs of neuropathy such as areflexia or patchy anaesthesia. Fourteen of the patients had had barium meals with follow-through films over a period of 24 hours. Five showed some delay in gastric emptying. 'Transit through the small and large intestine was generally rapid, and in no case slow.' The authors postulated 'a mechanism of small and large-intestinal hurry, due to autonomic nerve degeneration'. Chlortetracycline proved effective in controlling the diarrhoea in many cases, suggesting that a disturbance of intestinal flora might in some way be involved. Postmortem examination of the lumbar sympathetic and presacral nerves in a single case showed no abnormality.

The relation of diabetic steatorrhoea to other causes of diarrhoea in diabetics is fully reviewed by Wruble and Kalser (1964). The authors considered diabetic steatorrhoea to be a distinct entity, encountered mainly in male patients with poorly controlled diabetes of early onset, 'almost universally' associated with autonomic neuropathy, and distinguishable (by absorption studies and jejunal biopsy) from coeliac disease occurring in diabetics.

Neurophysiological evidence. We are aware of only a single neurophysiological study in 'diabetic diarrhoea'. Whalen and Soergel (reported by Hensley and Soergel, 1968) recorded the jejunal motor activity of eight patients with diabetes and chronic diarrhoea by balloon kymography. Compared with a group of 12 normal subjects jejunal motor tone and activity were normal in the fasting state. The minimum dose of adrenaline and noradrenaline, given intravenously, which temporarily abolished jejunal motor activity was identical in patients and in controls. Similarly, there was no difference in the jejunal motor response to graded doses of subcutaneously administered methacholine chloride between the two groups. These findings were taken to imply that there was no denervation hypersensitivity of the bowel in diabetic patients with diarrhoea. The inference, unstated by the authors, is that if there was a lesion of the autonomic nervous system in such cases, it would have to involve the preganglionic fibres.

Neuropathological basis. The neuropathological substratum of diabetic diarrhoea is poorly documented. Berge, Sprague and Bennett (1956) failed to find any significant pathological changes in intramural plexuses in eight autopsied cases of diabetic diarrhoea. Hensley and Soergel (1968) reported a much fuller examination of the autonomic nervous system in three patients who had suffered from diabetic diarrhoea. Each had shown evidence of motor, sensory and visceral neuropathy during life. The findings in two control groups—one consisting of nine diabetics without diarrhoea, the other of 18 non-diabetic patients—were also described.

The cell bodies of the intermediolateral columns showed no morphological differences in the three groups. The greater splanchnic nerves and the cervical portions of the vagus were normal in the patients with diabetic diarrhoea, as were the myenteric and submucosal plexuses of the small and large intestine. The only detectable histological changes were localised to the neurones of the prevertebral and paravertebral ganglia. Two types of 'abnormality' were detected: 'giant sympathetic neurones' and 'dendritic swelling'. Both changes (though mainly the latter) were found in the patients with diabetic diarrhoea. Similar changes were also found, in varying proportions, in the control groups.

It must be concluded that a firm pathological basis for this syndrome has not as yet been established. Moreover, it is difficult to conceive of an *intermittent* disturbance of function, such as is alleged to characterise diabetic diarrhoea, arising on the basis of a degeneration of a specific group (or specific groups) of neurones.

GASTROINTESTINAL DISEASE DUE TO LESIONS OF INTRINSIC BOWEL INNERVATION

In the concluding pages of this monograph we must give a brief account of some diseases which lie beyond the province of neurology yet are due *entirely* to lesions of nerves. These comprise a number of gastroenterological conditions, never seen by clinical neurologists, in which the disturbance of function is due to a local abnormality of innervation.

For many years, the morbid anatomy of the intrinsic innervation of hollow viscera in man had only been studied in the most desultory fashion. The reasons were obvious. Very few neuropathologists had devoted their careers to the study of the autonomic nervous system, of which Auerbach's and Meissner's plexuses are a small but important part. Moreover, many of the pathological variations described (e.g. de Castro, 1932) were of dubious significance, to say the least. At the same time, gcneral pathologists, who both eviscerate cadavers and examine microscopic sections of bowel in their daily work, often lack the special interest and expertise needed for a systematic examination of these plexuses. It has been left to Barbara Smith (1972) to collect and analyse published data on the neuropathology of the alimentary tract. She has applied new techniques to demonstrate the myenteric plexus and other nerves in normal and abnormal viscera. Her monograph should be consulted for further information about most of the topics dealt with here, as well as for information about the normal neuroanatomy of the oesophagus, stomach and intestine.

We will now discuss Chagas' disease, achalasia of the cardia, infantile pyloric stenosis, congenital megacolon, and ganglioneuromatous involvement of the intestines.

Chagas' disease

If the reader of this book has been saddened by the fact that the medical energy expended on a disease often seems to be inversely proportional to its prevalence, we hope he will be consoled by the subject of the next few paragraphs. Chagas' disease must be by far the commonest disorder falling within the scope of this book (and therefore the most important in terms of human ill-health). Yet we cannot help feeling that many of those reading these pages will never have seen a case and are likely to have only the vaguest knowledge concerning its features. The reason, of course, is geographical. The disease is predominantly one of tropical South America; Brazil is the source of most reports, though adjacent Latin American countries, Central America and even the southernmost United States probably harbour numerous undocumented cases. The World Health Organisation Study Group's (1960) conservative estimate of the total number of affected individuals was seven million. This illustrates the size of the problem.

In 1909 Chagas first described a previously unknown flagellate in the hindgut of the *Reduviid* bug *Panstrongylus megistus* caught in central Brazil. In the bloodstream of primates the flagellate became a trypanosome, *Trypanosoma cruzi*. Sick children were found to habour the organism. In later years acute and chronic phases were defined, and in the latter Chagas observed heart disease and dilatation of the gut. Subsequently many Brazilian reports of patients with megacolon or megaoesophagus have appeared. These include two good reviews of the subject in English (Köberle, 1963; Ferreira-Santos and Carrill, 1964).

Megacolon, megarectum and megaoesophagus are very common in rural areas of central Brazil. Over an eight-year period 100 patients underwent operation for megacolon at Ribeirao Preto School of Medicine. During the same period 69 megacolons were found in 556 consecutive autopsies (Ferreira-Santos and Carrill, 1964). In this region two areas, each with a population of less than 50 000 inhabitants, yielded 1514 (Mineiro, 1958) and 2000 (Freitas, 1950) cases of megaoesophagus. The regional prevalence of dilatation of the oesophagus and colon corresponds with the area of endemicity of *T. cruzi* infection. Ninety-five per cent of patients with such lesions have positive complement-fixation tests to this organism, strengthening the link between the two conditions.

T. cruzi is transmitted to man by bloodsucking insects of the subfamily Triatominae. The insects often bite the face, particularly around the mouth (hence the nickname 'kissing bugs'). Trypanosomes from an animal reservoir (usually wild mammals such as monkeys and armadillos) infect the vector and multiply in its intestine. They are present in its faeces, and when the human bite is rubbed, the trypanosomes enter through the skin. The parasites multiply locally and then enter the bloodstream. After a few days they invade smooth and skeletal muscle and myocardium, where they settle as Leishmania. These divide further, making small colonies which destroy the surrounding tissue with an acute inflammatory response, producing the picture—in voluntary muscle—of focal polymyositis, and the formation of pseudocysts. These eventually rupture liberating further showers of trypanosomes. Reinfection of the blood occurs. Several such cycles may be completed within the first few weeks of infection.

The patients show the clinical features of an acute generalised infection—fever, lymphadenopathy and hepatosplenomegaly. In severe cases there may be meningitic or encephalitic signs. Mortality is high in this acute phase, being 10 per cent overall and even more in the very young or very old. Diagnosis may be possible at this stage, either by scrutiny of blood smears for the presence of parasites or by looking for trypanosomes in the faeces of a laboratory-bred Triatome that has bitten the patient.

Survivors from the acute phase harbour very few organisms. After a variable time interval they pass into a chronic phase, the manifestations of which are due to neuronal damage. Making an analogy with syphilis is irresistible, if naïve. In this phase there is heart block, with cardiac enlargement and sometimes intractable chronic or acute heart failure. Seventy per cent of a group of patients with megacolon (Ferreira-Santos and Carrill, 1964) had ECG evidence of right bundle branch block, indicating that myocardial involvement occurs frequently. However, cardiac symptoms are overshadowed by alimentary ones, especially chronic constipation, abdominal distension and dysphagia, at times so severe as to produce cachexia. These symptoms are due to intestinal dilatation. Megacolon and megaoesophagus, as already noted, are common in Chagas' disease, but gross dilatation of stomach, duodenum and jejunum may also occur although they are rare. Other hollow viscera are occasionally affected (Köberle, 1963). Megaureters and enlarged bladders are sometimes encountered, while 5 per cent of patients with Chagas' disease show bronchiectasis, which may or may not be a related lesion. Acute abdominal complications occasionally supervene. These include volvulus and perforation of the sigmoid colon.

The underlying lesion is neuropathological, namely death of the intrinsic neurones of the alimentary canal, occurring as a delayed consequence of smooth muscle colonisation by *T. cruzi*. Quantitative studies of ganglion cells in large bowel, oesophagus and myocardium (Köberle, 1963) indicate their virtual absence in those cases with a clinically obvious lesion. Significantly, cases of Chagas' disease without megaoesophagus or megacolon show marked reduction in numbers of intrinsic neurones. Barbara Smith (1972) has examined three cases of megacolon. Thick, silver-impregnated preparations showed the myenteric plexus to consist in places of extrinsic fibres only, the neurones and intrinsic axons having been destroyed. Some inflammatory cells and neuronal remnants were found, as well as thick, single aberrant fibres in the muscle coats, away from the plexus.

Achalasia of the cardia

As in Chagas' disease, loss of oesophageal myenteric neurones is responsible for this condition, which is, however, familiar to physicians and surgeons in many parts of the world. Achalasia is a disease of adults, and although it has been claimed that it is occasionally due to an exogenous agent none has been firmly incriminated. Perhaps the condition is best thought of as a localised neuronal 'abiotrophy'.

When appropriately examined, the oesophagus shows replacement of the myenteric plexus by a tangle of Schwann cells, fibrous tissue and a little argyrophilic débris. No neurones are seen. Vagal fibres appear normal. There is no inflammatory reaction. These findings (Smith, 1972) support the idea of a primary neuronal degeneration being responsible. At various times it has been suggested that an inflammatory (possibly 'autoimmune') process might be the cause of neuronal loss. Some workers (Hurst and Rake, 1930) have found small round cells in the oesophageal myenteric plexuses, but Lendrum (1937) pointed out that these were just as likely to be neuronal satellite cells as lymphocytes. Others (Cassella et al, 1964) have reported pathological changes in the preganglionic (vagal) nerve fibres, but changes at this level and in brainstem vagal nuclei are hard to accept on the strength of published information.

The functional effect on the oesophagus of denervation of the cardia is to destroy the reflex pathway through which the gastro-oesophageal segment relaxes in response to a bolus of food (Smith, 1972). Denervation is followed by local thickening. Dilatation above the thickened zone is a secondary effect. These changes produce the familiar clinical picture of dysphagia, retrosternal pain, regurgitation, and variable weight loss, which in some patients may proceed rapidly to advanced cachexia. A progression of symptoms from an early severe phase, through a 'compensated' asymptomatic phase (in which marked oesophageal dilatation is occurring), to a late, severe, complicated 'decompensated' phase has been well described by Ellis (Adams et al, 1961). Radiological diagnosis may not be possible in the first of these three stages.

Infantile pyloric stenosis

The circular muscle forming the pyloric sphincter is hypertrophied in this relatively common condition. Boys are mainly affected and symptoms of pyloric obstruction develop after the age of three weeks. Infantile hypertrophic pyloric stenosis is the result of denervation: there are many observations that the neurones of the pyloric canal are abnormal in both structure and function.

Friesen, Boley and Miller (1956) found that the pyloric myenteric ganglia contained many small 'immature', 'undifferentiated' neurones. The final maturation of neuroblasts into functional neurones, which normally occurs two to four weeks after birth at this site, was apparently delayed. Friesen and Pearse (1963) later published histochemical findings in support of this view: cholinesterase was present in large amounts in the abnormal ganglion cells, indicating some kind of function, yet the small cells contained no oxidative enzymes, showing that they were still dependent on glycolysis, the respiratory pathway shared by many fetal cells.

A number of other authors (Belding and Kernohan, 1953; Alarotu, 1956; Nielsen, 1956) have published reports claiming the presence of a variety of 'degenerative' changes in pyloric neurones. These minor variations in cell morphology do not stand up to critical scrutiny. The recognition of 'exhausted' neurones in routinely stained paraffin sections (Belding and Kernohan, 1953), or of multiple grades of 'degeneration' on the basis of nuclear staining with gallocyanin (Alarotu, 1956) is purely subjective, and pertains to the realm of psycho-histology.

Current opinion of the pathogenesis of this disorder (Rintoul and Kirkman, 1961) is that the pyloric mesenteric plexus is defective. The defect is probably one of neuronal maturation, and there is little evidence that degeneration of mature ganglion cells has occurred.

Hirschsprung's disease (congenital megacolon)

Hirschsprung's disease produces constipation in childhood. It may present as intestinal obstruction in the neonate, although milder cases may not become apparent until later in life. The gross defect is a narrow, contracted, non-motile rectal segment, proximal to which the large bowel is dilated. These two zones are joined by a funnel-shaped transitional zone. Dilatation is the result of constriction, the pathological basis of which is well established.

Absence of ganglion cells in the constricted segment was clearly demonstrated in an autopsied case by Robertson and Kernohan (1938). In 1948 Whitehouse and Kernohan reported on 11 cases: in the majority neuronal loss extended into the transitional zone and into the sigmoid colon. In all cases the affected regions of rectum contained nerve bundles in the myenteric plexus which were not present in controls. Bodian, Stephens and Ward (1949) confirmed these findings.

Little has been added to knowledge of the subject over the past 25 years. Formalin-induced fluorescence has been used to study adrenergic nerves in surgical specimens (Bennett, Garrett and Howard, 1968). The abnormal nerves discovered by Whitehouse and Kernohan are in part adrenergic and presumably come from overgrowth of sympathetic fibres in this denervated area. Barbara Smith's techniques show characteristic changes in surgical specimens, with replacement of the plexus in the contracted segment by unmyelinated fibre networks and anatomical abnormalities of the plexus in the dilated segment right up to the margin of the resection (Smith, 1972).

Ganglioneuromatous involvement of the intestines

McMahon and Davies (1945) reported the case of a 16-year-old girl who had had diarrhoea and episodic abdominal pain and vomiting since early childhood. During painful episodes an epigastric mass was often palpable. At operation, an abnormal segment of terminal ileum, 33 inches long, was removed. Its walls were diffusely thickened, and contained many bundles of nerves and fibrous tissue, interspersed with large numbers of ganglion cells. This was a diffuse ganglioneuroma, a benign tumour of intrinsic nerve elements, and was plainly responsible for many of her symptoms.

Until the mid-1960s gastrointestinal ganglioneuromas were nothing but a pathological curiosity. Dahl, Waugh and Dahlin (1957) were able to collect only 12 cases from published accounts. Five of these were restricted to the appendix. Several of the 12 were polypoid, circumscribed masses, but a number produced diffuse thickening of the muscle coats. Abdominal symptoms were variable, and diarrhoea was not a regular feature. Despite the well-recognised association of adrenal and thoracic ganglioneuromas with von Recklinghausen's disease, as well as the occurrence in this disease of plexiform neuromas (which these alimentary lesions resemble) none of the 12 cases showed evidence of neurofibromatosis, though a family history was obtained in one (Oberndorfer, 1921).

In the 1960s, Williams provoked much interest in medullary carcinoma of the thyroid with his accounts of the tumour, his ideas of its origin from parafollicular (C) cells, and his description of its clinical syndromes and pathological associations. One of these associations (Williams and Pollock, 1966) included intestinal ganglioneuromas. This pointed to a relationship between medullary carcinoma of the thyroid, neurofibromatosis, and phaeochromocytomas, all tumours now believed to be derived from neuroectoderm (see p. 199).

The syndrome reported by Williams and Pollock (1966) comprised multiple neuromas of eyelids, lips and tongue, multiple phaeochromocytomas, and medullary carcinoma of the thyroid. Additional lesions were present in one of the two patients described. This was a girl aged 19 with severe watery diarrhoea, for which no cause was apparent after hospital investigation. At laparotomy a diffusely thickened colon was found, and partial colectomy carried out. She died postoperatively, and was shown at autopsy to have other intestinal lesions, including diffuse thickening of the small intestine and multiple submucous nodules in the oesophagus. Under the microscope the lesions in small and large bowel were shown to be diffuse ganglioneuromatosis, characterised by small and large irregular conglomerations of nerve fibres and ganglion cells replacing Auerbach's and Meissner's plexus.

Other patients with this syndrome and similar intestinal lesions have since been described (Ruppert, Buerger and Chang, 1966; Schimke et al, 1968). It should be pointed out that intestinal ganglioneuromatosis may well not be the cause of the diarrhoea in these cases. Diarrhoea is a prominent symptom of medullary carcinoma in the absence of alimentary lesions, and is present in a third of all cases (Williams, 1966; Bernier et al, 1969). A hormone produced by the thyroid tumour is believed to cause this symptom. It is not known whether calcitonin, serotonin, a prostaglandin, or one of the substances mentioned in relation to 'pancreatic cholera' (p. 200) is the agent responsible.

References

Smooth muscle involvement in diseases of voluntary muscles

Berblinger, W. & Dukens, J. (1929). Der kardio-intestinale Symptomenkomplex bei der progressiven Muskeldystrophie; 1. Klinische und pathologisch-anatomische Beobachtungen. *Zeitschrift für Kinderheilkunde*, **47**, 1–26.

Bevans, M. (1945). Changes in the musculature of the gastrointestinal tract and in the myocardium in progressive muscular dystrophy. *Archives of Pathology*, **40**, 225–238.

Bunting, C. H. (1908). Chronic fibrous myocarditis in progressive muscular dystrophy. *American Journal of the Medical Sciences*, **135**, 244–251.

Crowe, G. G. (1961). Acute dilatation of stomach as a complication of muscular dystrophy. *British Medical Journal*, **1**, 1371.

Huvos, A. G. & Pruzanski, W. (1967). Smooth muscle involvement in primary muscle disease. II. Progressive muscular atrophy. *Archives of Pathology*, **83**, 234–240.

Patterson, M., Ong, H. & Drake, A. (1964). Intestinal absorption in muscular dystrophy patients. *Archives of Internal Medicine*, **114**, 67–70.

Patterson, M. & Rios, G. (1959). Disturbed gastrointestinal motility: an unusual manifestation of systemic muscular disorder; polymyositis or progressive muscular dystrophy. *Gastroenterology*, **36**, 261–268.

Robin, G. C. & Falewski, G. de L. (1963). Acute gastric dilatation in progressive muscular dystrophy. *Lancet*, **2**, 171–172.

Smooth muscle involvement in extrinsic nervous disease

Appenzeller, O. (1969). The vegetative nervous system. In *Handbook of Clinical Neurology. Volume* 1, *Disturbances of Nervous Function*, ed. Vinken, P. J. & Bruyn, G. W., pp. 427–535. Amsterdam: North-Holland.

Bariety, M., Coury, C., Paillas, J., Thibault, P. & Leymarios, J. (1961). A propos d'un cas de dilatation gastrique au cours d'une sclérose latérale amyotrophique. *Presse médicale*, **69**, 1673–1674.

Berge, K. G., Sprague, R. G. & Bennett, W. A. (1956). The intestinal tract in diabetic diarrhea. *Diabetes*, **5**, 289–294.

Bosma, J. F. & Brodie, D. R. (1969). Disabilities of the pharynx in amyotrophic lateral sclerosis as demonstrated by cineradiography. *Radiology*, **92**, 97–103.

Boudin, G., Barbizet, J., Hillemand, B. & Lote, J. (1954). Atonie et dilatation gastro-oesophagienne au cours de la sclérose latérale amyotrophique. *Bulletins et Mémoires de la Société médicale des Hôpitaux de Paris*, **70**, 641–648.

Connell, A. M., Frankel, H. & Guttmann, L. (1963). The motility of the pelvic colon following complete lesions of the spinal cord. *Paraplegia*, **1**, 98–115.

Eadie, M. J. (1963). The pathology of certain medullary nuclei in Parkinsonism. *Brain*, **86**, 781–792.

Eadie, M. J. & Tyrer, J. H. (1965). Radiological abnormalities of the upper part of the alimentary tract in Parkinsonism. *Australasian Annals of Medicine*, **14**, 23–27.

Fischer, R. A., Ellison, G. W., Thayer, W. R., Spiro, H. M. & Glaser, G. H. (1965). Esophageal motility in neuromuscular disorders. *Annals of Internal Medicine*, **63**, 229–248.

Grossiord, A., Chérigié, E., Bourdon, R. & Held, J. P. (1956). Contribution à l'étude radio-cinématographique des troubles de la déglutition en neurologie et particulièrement dans la maladie de Parkinson (présentation d'un film). *Bulletins et Mémoires de la Société médicale des Hôpitaux de Paris*, **72**, 82–86.

Hensley, G. T. & Soergel, K. H. (1968). Neuropathologic findings in diabetic diarrhea. *Archives of Pathology*, **85**, 587–597.

Hillemand, B. (1955). *Manifestations digestives au cours des atteintes du système nerveux central.* Thesis. Paris: Foulon.

Hodges, F. J., Rundles, R. W. & Hanelin, J. (1947). Roentgenologic study of the small intestine. II. Dysfunction associated with neurologic disease. *Radiology*, **49**, 659–673.

Lawyer, T. Jr & Netsky, M. G. (1953). Amyotrophic lateral sclerosis. A clinicoanatomic study of fifty-three cases. *Archives of Neurology and Psychiatry*, **69**, 171–192

Léri, A. (1902). Atrophie généralisée de la musculature de tous les viscères dans une amyotrophie progressive type Aran-Duchenne. *Revue neurologique*, **10**, 394–401.

Malins, J. M. & French, J. M. (1957). Diabetic diarrhoea. *Quarterly Journal of Medicine*, **26**, 467–480.

Pallis, C. A. (1971). Parkinsonism: natural history and clinical features. *British Medical Journal*, **3**, 683–690.

Rundles, R. W. (1945). Diabetic neuropathy. *Medicine (Baltimore)*, **24**, 111–160.

Sheridan, E. P. & Bailey, C. C. (1946). Diabetic nocturnal diarrhea. *Journal of the American Medical Association*, **130**, 632–634.
Smith, A. W. M., Mulder, D. W. & Code, C. F. (1957). Esophageal motility in amyotrophic lateral sclerosis. *Proceedings of the Staff Meetings of the Mayo Clinic*, **32**, 438–441.
Walters, W. & Belding, H. (1951). Clinical studies on 130 patients one to four years after vagotomy. *Proceedings of the Staff Meetings of the Mayo Clinic*, **26**, 199–208.
Wruble, L. D. & Kalser, M. H. (1964). Diabetic steatorrhea: a distinct entity. *American Journal of Medicine*, **37**, 118–129.

Gastrointestinal disease due to lesions of intrinsic bowel innervation

Adams, C. W. M., Brain, R. H. F., Ellis, F. E., Kauntze, R. & Trounce, J. R. (1961). Achalasia of the cardia. *Guy's Hospital Reports*, **110**, 191–236.
Alarotu, H. (1956). The histopathological changes in the myenteric plexus of the pylorus in hypertrophic pyloric stenosis of infants (pylorospasm). *Acta paediatrica* (*Uppsala*), **45**, Supplementum 107, 1–131.
Belding, H. H., III & Kernohan, J. W. (1953). A morphological study of the myenteric plexus and musculature of the pylorus with special reference to the changes in hypertrophic pyloric stenosis. *Surgery, Gynecology and Obstetrics*, **97**, 322–334.
Bennett, A., Garrett, J. R. & Howard, E. R. (1968). Adrenergic myenteric nerves in Hirschsprung's disease. *British Medical Journal*, **1**, 487–489.
Bernier, J. J., Rambaud, J. C., Cattan, D. & Prost, A. (1969). Diarrhoea associated with medullary carcinoma of the thyroid. *Gut*, **10**, 980–985.
Bodian, M., Stephens, F. D. & Ward, B. C. H. (1949). Hirschsprung's disease and idiopathic megacolon. *Lancet*, **1**, 6–11.
Cassella, R. R., Brown, A. L. Jr, Sayre, G. P. & Ellis, F. H. Jr (1964). Achalasia of the esophagus: pathologic and etiologic considerations. *Annals of Surgery*, **160**, 474–487.
Castro, F. de (1932). Sympathetic ganglia. Normal and pathological. In *Cytology and Cellular Pathology of the Nervous system*, ed. W. Penfield. Vol. 1, pp. 317–379. New York: Hoeber.
Chagas, C. (1909). Nova tripanozomiaze humana. Estudos sobre a morfologia e o ciclo evolutivo do *Schizotrypanum cruzi n. gen., n. sp.*, ajente etiologico de nova entidade mortida do homem. *Memorias do Instituto Oswaldo Cruz*, **1**, 159–218.
Dahl, E. V., Waugh, J. M. & Dahlin, D. C. (1957). Gastrointestinal ganglioneuromas: brief review with report of a duodenal ganglioneuroma. *American Journal of Pathology*, **33**, 953–965.
Ferreira-Santos, R. & Carrill, C. F. (1964). Acquired megacolon in Chagas' disease. *Diseases of the Colon and Rectum*, **7**, 353–364.
Freitas, S. V. Jr (1950). Megacolo e magaesofago no Brasil central. *Resenha clinico cientifica*, **19**, 411–423.
Friesen, S. R., Boley, J. O. & Miller, D. R. (1956). The myenteric plexus in the pylorus: its early normal development and its changes in hypertrophic pyloric stenosis. *Surgery*, **39**, 21–29.
Friesen, S. R. & Pearse, A. G. E. (1963). Pathogenesis of congenital pyloric stenosis: histochemical analyses of pyloric ganglion cells. *Surgery*, **53**, 604–608.
Hurst, A. F. & Rake, G. W. (1930). Achalasia of the cardia (so-called cardiospasm). *Quarterly Journal of Medicine*, **23**, 491–508.
Köberle, F. (1963). Enteromegaly and cardiomegaly in Chagas' disease. *Gut*, **4**, 399–405.
Lendrum, F. C. (1937). Anatomic features of the cardiac orifice of the stomach with special reference to cardiospasm. *Archives of Internal Medicine*, **59**, 474–511.
McMahon, J. S. & Davies, G. F. S. (1945). Plexiform ganglioneuroma of the small intestine. *Australian and New Zealand Journal of Surgery*, **15**, 50–53.
Mineiro, V. (1958). Contribuicão a etiologia do megaesofago. *Revista goiana de Medicina*, **4**, 29–34.
Nielsen, O. S. (1956). Histological changes of the pyloric myenteric plexus in infantile pyloric stenosis. Studies on surgical biopsy specimens. *Acta paediatrica* (*Uppsala*), **45**, 636–647.
Oberndorfer (1921). Partieller, primärer Riesenwuchs des Wurmfortsatzes, kombiniert mit Ganglioneuromatose. (Ein Beitrag zur Entstehung der Ganglienzellen.) *Zeitschrift für die gesamte Neurologie und Psychiatrie*, **72**, 105–118.

Rintoul, J. R. & Kirkman, N. F. (1961). The myenteric plexus in infantile hypertrophic pyloric stenosis. *Archives of Disease in Childhood*, **36,** 474–480.
Robertson, H. E. & Kernohan, J. W. (1938). The myenteric plexus in congenital megacolon. *Proceedings of the Staff Meetings of the Mayo Clinic*, **13,** 123–125.
Ruppert, R. D., Buerger, L. F. & Chang, W. W. (1966). Pheochromocytoma, neurofibromatosis and thyroid carcinoma. *Metabolism*, **15,** 537–541.
Schimke, R. N., Hartmann, W. H., Prout, T. E. & Rimoin, D. L. (1968). Syndrome of bilateral pheochromocytoma, medullary thyroid carcinoma and multiple neuromas. *New England Journal of Medicine*, **279,** 1–7.
Smith, B. (1972). *The Neuropathology of the Alimentary Tract*. London: Arnold.
Whitehouse, F. R. & Kernohan, J. W. (1948). Myenteric plexus in congenital megacolon. Study of eleven cases. *Archives of Internal Medicine*, **82,** 75–111.
Williams, E. D. (1966). Diarrhoea and thyroid carcinoma. *Proceedings of the Royal Society of Medicine*, **59,** 602–603.
Williams, E. D. & Pollock, D. J. (1966). Multiple mucosal neuromata with endocrine tumours: a syndrome allied to von Recklinghausen's disease. *Journal of Pathology and Bacteriology*, **91,** 71–80.
World Health Organisation Study Group (1960). Chagas' disease. Report of a study group. *World Health Organisation Technical Report Series*, **202,** 1–21.

Index